AF621752

THE UNDERLYING MOLECULAR, CELLULAR, AND IMMUNOLOGICAL FACTORS IN CANCER AND AGING

ADVANCES IN EXPERIMENTAL MEDICINE AND BIOLOGY

Editorial Board:

NATHAN BACK, *State University of New York at Buffalo*

IRUN R. COHEN, *The Weizmann Institute of Science*

DAVID KRITCHEVSKY, *Wistar Institute*

ABEL LAJTHA, *N. S. Kline Institute for Psychiatric Research*

RODOLFO PAOLETTI, *University of Milan*

Recent Volumes in this Series

Volume 323
MECHANISMS OF LYMPHOCYTE ACTIVATION AND IMMUNE REGULATION IV: Cellular Communications
Edited by Sudhir Gupta and Thomas A. Waldmann

Volume 324
PROSTATE CANCER AND BONE METASTASIS
Edited by James P. Karr and Hidetoshi Yamanaka

Volume 325
RECOVERY FROM BRAIN DAMAGE: Reflections and Directions
Edited by F. D. Rose and D. A. Johnson

Volume 326
THE USE OF RESEALED ERYTHROCYTES AS CARRIERS AND BIOREACTORS
Edited by Mauro Magnani and John R. DeLoach

Volume 327
GENETICALLY ENGINEERED VACCINES
Edited by Joseph E. Ciardi, Jerry R. McGhee, and Jerry M. Keith

Volume 328
ENZYMOLOGY AND MOLECULAR BIOLOGY OF CARBONYL METABOLISM 4
Edited by Henry Weiner, David W. Crabb, and T. Geoffrey Flynn

Volume 329
DENDRITIC CELLS IN FUNDAMENTAL AND CLINICAL IMMUNOLOGY
Edited by Eduard W. A. Kamperdijk, Paul Nieuwenhuis, and Elisabeth C. M. Hoefsmit

Volume 330
THE UNDERLYING MOLECULAR, CELLULAR, AND IMMUNOLOGICAL FACTORS IN CANCER AND AGING
Edited by Stringner Sue Yang and Huber R. Warner

Volume 331
FRONTIERS IN CEREBRAL VASCULAR BIOLOGY: Transport and Its Regulation
Edited by Lester R. Drewes and A. Lorris Betz

A Continuation Order Plan is available for this series. A continuation order will bring delivery of each new volume immediately upon publication. Volumes are billed only upon actual shipment. For further information please contact the publisher.

THE UNDERLYING MOLECULAR, CELLULAR, AND IMMUNOLOGICAL FACTORS IN CANCER AND AGING

Edited by

Stringner Sue Yang

National Cancer Institute
Bethesda, Maryland

and

Huber R. Warner

National Institute on Aging
Bethesda, Maryland

SPRINGER SCIENCE+BUSINESS MEDIA, LLC

Library of Congress Cataloging in Publication Data

The underlying molecular, cellular, and immunological factors in cancer and aging / edited by Stringner Sue Yang and Huber R. Warner.

p. cm.—(Advances in experimental medicine and biology; v. 330)

"Proceedings of a Workshop on the Underlying Molecular, Cellular, and Immunological Factors in Age-Related Cancers, held June 4–6, 1990, in Annapolis, Maryland"—T.p. verso.

Includes bibliographical references and index.

ISBN 978-0-306-44411-1 ISBN 978-1-4615-2926-2 (eBook)

DOI 10.1007/978-1-4615-2926-2

1. Cancer—Immunological aspects—Congresses. 2. Cancer—Age factors—Congresses. I. Yang, Stringner, Sue. II. Warner, Huber R. III. Workshop on the Underlying Molecular, Cellular, and Immunological Factors in Age-Related Cancers (1990: Annapolis, Md.) IV. Series.

[DNLM: 1. Neoplasms—genetics—congresses. 2. Neoplasms—immunology—congresses. 3. Aging—genetics—congresses. W1 AD559 v.330 1993 / QZ 200 U512 1990]

RC268.3.U53 1993

618.97'6994079—dc20

DNLM/DLC 93-1447

for Library of Congress CIP

Proceedings of a workshop on The Underlying Molecular, Cellular, and Immunological Factors in Age-Related Cancers, held June 4–6, 1990, in Annapolis, Maryland

ISBN 978-0-306-44411-1

©1993 Springer Science+Business Media New York

Originally published by Plenum Press, New York in 1993

All rights reserved

No part of this book may be reproduced, stored in retrieval system, or transmitted in any format or by any means, electronic, mechanical, photocopying, microfilming, recording, or otherwise, without written permission from the Publisher

PREFACE

Background

Cancer is a variety of malignancies generally associated with aging. As the overall health technology and health care delivery improved with the advances made in medicine and science in the United States, the life expectancy of the population also increased. The average life expectancy in the U.S.A. has increased from 49 years at the end of 1900 to 75 years today in 1990 [(1-3)]. The population of 65 years and older that constituted 25.5 million or 11.3% of the total U. S. population in 1980[(4)] has now increased to 31.1 million or 12.5% of the population according to the 1990[(5)] census. As cancer diagnosis and treatment have improved, cancer mortality among patients under 55 has been significantly reduced within recent years[*1]; however, cancer incidence under 55 is still increasing at about 0.4% per year (as compared to 1.0% for all ages or 0.6% for <65) according to the 1990 review of the 15 year trends in the *Cancer Statistics Review 1973-1987*, published by the Surveillance, Epidemiology, and End Results (SEER) Program of the National Cancer Institute (NCI). In contrast, both cancer incidence and mortality have been increasing among the population 65 and over[*2] at a rate of 1.4% and 1.0% respectively per year between 1973-1987[(6)]. Whereas persons 65 years of age and over constitute approximately 12% of the total population, statistics showed that over 50% of all cancers occur in this age group. In specific cases like breast cancer, approximate 80% of cases occur in women over the age of 50[(6)], suggesting that cancer tends to target elderly persons. Confronting the increasing cancer incidence among the aged, the National Cancer Institute implements special measures aiming at reducing cancer mortality among the underserved population of age 65 years and over.

[*1]For age group of 45-55 in the years of 1973, 1977, 1982 and 1987, the respective cancer mortality rates per 100,000 are 179.0, 179.2, 172.1 and 170.7 respectively age-adjusted, all sites combined.[(6)]

[*2]For 1973, 1977, 1982 and 1987 the mortality rates of populations 65+ are 929.6, 962.3, 1023, and 1057 per 100,000 respectively.[(6)]

Rationale, Opportunity and Strategy for the Future

A panel of experts including William Ershler, Michael Gottesman, Arnold Levine, James O'Leary and Bert Vogelstein, was convened to discuss with program staff the merits and impacts of such statistical findings and to explore the scientific research opportunities, state-of-the-art technology, and the relative readiness for a multidisciplinary approach to achieve a better understanding of why cancer incidence increases with the aged and how to reduce cancer mortality among the underserved population over 65. Areas that need to be examined in detail are:

- o Are there age-related differences in the phenotypic and genotypic properties of tumor cells derived from the same organ?

- o What factors might contribute to altered tumor behavior? Is a tumor in an older patient (age 65 and over) more aggressive than the same tumor in a young patient (under 65) in terms of growth rate and metastatic potential or *vice versa*?

- o Within an identical environment, does a tumor from an old patient grow at the same or equivalent rate as the same tumor from a young patient? Why do some tumors grow more slowly in elderly patients? Does the elderly host present a "*hostile milieu*" to the tumor cell as compared with a young host?

- o Is the increase in mortality among patients over 65 years of age a true reflection of cancer deaths? If so, what accounts for the slow growth observed with some tumors in old patients? Does growth rate have any relationship to the malignancy of a tumor?

- o To what extent does genetic instability play a role in tumor heterogeneity in elderly patients as compared with the same in young patients? Does genetic dominance exist in certain tumor cells and are these dominant tumor cells derived primarily from older patients' tumors? Can such a hypothesis be tested *in vitro* and/or *in vivo*?

- o What is the nature of the negative genetic control of tumorigenesis as expressed by suppressor genes, e.g. RB-1 and p53, and their gene products. What interplay exists at the genetic level with respect to aging and cancers? What results may be expected from transfer of suppressor genes in transgenic animal studies with respect to age-related cancers?

- o To what extent do the physiological and metabolic changes of the host during aging affect the tumor cell response to anti-cancer drugs and thus the overall tumor behavior?

After a day of discussion, the panel concluded that, notwithstanding certain shortcomings in the available statistical information, the trend of the cancer statistics (1972-1986) with respect to increasing incidence and mortality rates among the aged, and the poor survival of the elderly within this fifteen-year period, demands special research emphasis in aging and cancer. There is a scarcity of information in many of the issues addressed above. Nevertheless, there are rational, testable, experimental hypotheses that can be proposed in a number of areas discussed in age-related cancer. A database desperately needs to be established specifically for age-related cancer patients' response to anti-cancer drugs, drug transport, drug metabolism and drug-resistance.

It was the expressed opinion of the advisory panel that a forum whereby the state-of-the-art presentations, followed by open and frank exchanges, would provide opportunities to (1) identify areas of critical concern in cancers among the underserved population over 65, and (2) stimulate research collaboration among scientists of diverse disciplines.

As an initial effort to stimulate the awareness of the scientific community, a workshop on *The Underlying Molecular, Cellular and Immunological Factors in Age-related Cancers* was convened on June 3-6, 1990 in Annapolis, Maryland. The purpose of the workshop was to bring together scientists from diverse disciplines in cancer biology, epidemiology, molecular biology, genetics, immunology, gerontology and drug resistance to discuss the possible underlying factors that may account for the increase in cancer incidence and mortality among the elderly. The National Cancer Institute considers it a high priority to identify the intrinsic (genetic, molecular, and cellular) and extrinsic (epigenetic, immunological, drug-induced, chemical and viral) factors that may play a critical role and account for increases in certain cancer incidence and mortality among the aged.

The workshop was co-sponsored by the Division of Cancer Biology, Diagnosis, and Centers of the NCI and the Biomedical Research and Clinical Medicine Program of the Institute on Aging. Its goal was to identify such factors in cancers of the elderly and compare with those in the younger patients, to assess the state-of-the-art in Cancer and Aging, and to stimulate the awareness of scientists and clinicians to face the challenge in reducing the cancer mortality of the underserved population of age 65 and over.

This book, developed from the proceedings of this workshop, is dedicated to Samuel Broder, Director of the National Cancer Institute, and to Brian W. Kimes[*3], Associate Director, Centers, Training and Resources Program, Division of Cancer Biology, Diagnosis and Centers, NCI, for their very keen insights in identifying cancer problems and their leadership in providing opportunities for innovative and creative approaches in areas of molecular biology, clinical medicine and technology tranfer.

Stringner Sue Yang

October 1, 1990

REFERENCES

1. Health United States: 1986, publication (PHS) 87-1232. Washington, D.C., U.S. DHHS (1987).

2. Fries, J.F. Aging, natural death, and the compression of morbidity. *N. England J. Med.* 303:130-135 (1980).

3. Kennedy, B.J.: Aging and Cancer. *J. Clinical Oncology* 6:1903-1911 (1988).

4. U.S. Bureau of the Census: Estimates of the population of the United States by age, sex, and race: 1980-1986. Washington, D.C. Current population reports, Series P-25, No. 1000, February (1987).

5. U.S. Bureau of the Census: 1990 Census data file (1990 STF-S3 MARS for Counties, April 1, 1990 counts).

6. Ries, L.A.G., Hankey, B.F. and Edwards, B.K. Cancer Statistics Review, 1973-1987. NIH Publication No. 90-2789. U.S. DHHS, National Cancer Institute, Bethesda, MD (1990).

[*3] Formerly Associate Director of the Extramural Research Program

ACKNOWLEDGMENTS

We would like to thank the members of the Program Committee, Brian W. Kimes, Colette S. Freeman, Stringner S. Yang of The National Cancer Institute and Huber R. Warner and Anna McCormick of The Institute on Aging for their effort in putting together this multifaceted program. We would also like to acknowledge the contribution of Richard Wundruff and Evan C. Hadley during the very initial planning phase and of Franklin T. Williams, Director, of The Institute on Aging, for his support of this Workshop. We thank the speakers, chairpersons and the authors for their participation and important contribution to the overall success of this Workshop. Lastly we like to extend special thanks to Marilyn Goldberg, Regina Berthold and Donna Gillis for retyping the manuscripts.

CONTENTS

BACKGROUND

GENETICS AND EPIGENETICS

INFLUENCE OF PHYSIOLOGICAL CHANGES IN THE IMMUNE CONSTITUTIONS IN AGING AND CANCER

MOLECULAR BIOLOGY OF AGE-RELATED CHANGES IN SOME TYPES OF CANCER

I. BREAST CANCER

II. PROSTATE CANCER

MOLECULAR EPIDEMIOLOGY AND TREATMENT MODALITY IN PATIENTS OF DIFFERENT AGES WITH LEUKEMIAS

DRUG RESISTANCE

SUMMATION AND SYNTHESIS

AGING, COMORBIDITY, AND BREAST CANCER SURVIVAL : AN EPIDEMIOLOGIC VIEW*

William A. Satariano

School of Public Health
University of California at Berkeley
Berkeley, CA 94720

ABSTRACT

This is a review of epidemiologic studies, which suggest that comorbidity (e.g., diabetes and heart disease) has an adverse effect on survival among women with incident, invasive breast cancer, adjusting for chronological age and stage of breast cancer at diagnosis. As part of this review, recent results are presented from a series of 463 breast cancer cases, identified through the Metropolitan Detroit Cancer Surveillance System. Women with two or more concurrent health conditions were 2.2 times more likely than breast cancer cases without comorbidity to die from their breast cancer over a four-year period (95% CI: 1.13, 4.18). Limiting heart disease was especially problematic. Recommendations are made for future research in this area.

INTRODUCTION

Breast cancer is the leading form of cancer in women. The age-adjusted incidence rate for the disease among women in the United States between 1986 and 1987 was 108.9 per 100,000[1]. This is over two times greater than the age-adjusted incidence

---

*Support for this project was provided through NIA Grant RO1-AG-04969, NCI Contract N01-CN-55423, and by the United Foundation of Detroit.

rate for cancer of the colon, the second leading form of cancer in women. It is well known that the risk of breast cancer increases with age[1]. The incidence rate for the disease among women under the age of 50 is only 34.4 per 100,000, compared to 351.1 for women aged 50 and over.

Although the risk of developing breast cancer increases dramatically with age, differences in five-year relative survival rates by age are far less pronounced. Recent data from the National Cancer Institute indicate that for white women the poorest survival rates are found both for those under the age of 35 and those over the age of 75 at the time of diagnosis (Table 1).[1] On the other hand, for black women, those with the poorest survival are aged 55 to 64. The reasons for these age (and race) differences in survival are still unclear.

TABLE 1. The Five-Year Relative Survival Rates for Black And White Women with Incident, Invasive Breast Cancer by Age at Diagnosis

Surveillance, Epidemiology, and End Results Program
National Cancer Institute, 1974-1986

Age at Diagnosis	Black Women %	White Women %
< 35	63.5	69.3
35 - 44	63.5	77.2
45 - 54	66.1	77.6
55 - 64	62.8	75.1
65 - 74	64.6	77.3
75 +	63.0	74.4

Source: Ries, L.A.C.; Hankey, B.F.; Edwards, B.K. (ed.) Cancer Statistics Review, 1973-87. Bethesda, MD: National Cancer Institute (NIH Publication No. 90-2789).

Tumor and host characteristics have been implicated in breast cancer prognosis. Most research has focused on tumor characteristics, such as the number of affected axillary lymph nodes, estrogen receptor status, the degree of vascularization, and the size and grade of the tumor[2-7]. With regard to host characteristics, a number of studies have pointed to obesity as a risk factor[8,9]. Obese women are less likely than women with normal body mass to survive following breast cancer. In addition, there is a growing body of research, which suggests that the prevalence of concurrent health conditions, such as heart disease and diabetes, elevate the risk of death[10,11]. Given that the prevalence of concurrent health conditions in the general population increases with age, research in this area may be particularly fruitful for understanding breast cancer prognosis in older women[12].

COMORBIDITY AND BREAST CANCER SURVIVAL

The purpose of this chapter is to review recent epidemiologic research on the association between comorbidity and breast cancer survival. In addition, areas of needed research will be identified to understand more clearly the underlying mechanisms affecting prognosis following the diagnosis of breast cancer.

Attempts have been made to develop a comorbidity index to assess the risk of dying from specific concurrent conditions among women diagnosed with breast cancer. It is reported that an index of this kind would aid in designing clinical trials to better assess therapeutic interventions; people with serious comorbid conditions could be randomized separately from patients with fewer or less serious comorbid conditions. Along these lines, an index was developed by Charlson and colleagues[10] from a review of a sample of 607 patients admitted to the medical service at New York Hospital-Cornell Medical Center during a one-month period in 1984. The number and severity of comorbid diseases were recorded at the time of admission. Survival was measured in months from the date of admission to either the date of death or one year following the admission. A prognostic weight was assigned to each health condition. The weight was derived from the relative risk of death associated with the specific diagnosis. The final score was based on the sum of the weights of each condition exhibited by the patient at the time of admission.

The index was then used to evaluate the prognostic significance of comorbidity for a second cohort of women diagnosed with breast cancer. This cohort consisted of 685 women with histologically-confirmed primary carcinoma of the breast, who received their first treatment at Yale New Haven Hospital. In addition to clinical characteristics of the cancer itself, e.g., stage at diagnosis, the number and severity of comorbid diseases also were recorded. Survival was assessed over a 10-year period, with deaths being restricted to those due to a comorbid disease. Deaths due to breast cancer were censored, i.e., "withdrawn" from the analysis. Moreover, patients with metastases at death, but whose death was caused by a comorbid condition (e.g., myocardial infarction) were categorized as cancer deaths and thus censored.

The number and severity of comorbidity were associated with poorer survival.

Specifically, the relative risk of comorbid death for each increasing level of the index was 2.3 (95% CI: 1.9, 2.8). This is similar to risk associated with each decade of age (2.4; 95% CI: 2.0, 2.9). Charlson and colleagues conclude that the risk of dying from comorbid disease posed by an additional decade of age was equivalent to an increase of "1" in the comorbidity index.

In another study, comorbidity was found to be associated with the risk of death from all causes[11]. The study was based on 463 breast cancer cases aged 55 to 84 identified through the Metropolitan Detroit Cancer Surveillance System, a population-based cancer registry. Information about comorbidity was obtained from an interview with the cases conducted three months after diagnosis. The interview included questions concerning the number and types of diagnosed chronic conditions, as well as the resulting functional limitations. A chart of 20 different conditions was adapted from that used by the Human Population Laboratory (HPL) in Alameda County[13]. The HPL self-reported health assessment has been demonstrated to be both reliable and valid in several evaluation studies[14-16]. In another study on health surveys in older populations, Bush *et al.*[17] reports "good to excellent" agreement between the medical record and the reports of respondents aged 65 and over, especially for common conditions, such as stroke, diabetes, myocardial infarction, and hypertension. Reading through the list of conditions, respondents in the Detroit study were asked whether they had ever been diagnosed with the condition by a physician and if so, in what year they were first diagnosed[11]. Those reporting a diagnosis were then asked whether the condition currently limits any of their daily activities.

Of the 463 women with breast cancer interviewed three months after diagnosis, 63 or 13.6% died during a 2-year period. Comorbidity was associated with the risk of death. Sixty-two percent of the 63 women who died within the first two years reported one or more comorbid conditions three months after diagnosis. In contrast, only 38% of the 400 women who survived at least two years reported comorbid conditions at the first interview (three months after diagnosis).

The number of limiting conditions increased the risk of death from all causes, independently of age and stage of disease. Stage of disease was classified as either "local" (invasive cancer confined to the breast), "regional" (spread to adjacent organs by direct extension or to regional lymph nodes), or "remote" (extension or metastases to distant organs or distant lymph nodes). Women reporting one comorbid condition were 2.5 times more likely to die than those women without any comorbid conditions. Among women with two or more conditions, the risk was 3.4 compared to women without any conditions. The number of non-limiting conditions was not associated with the risk of death. Advanced age, obesity, past cigarette smoking, and current alcohol consumption were all associated with an elevated risk of comorbidity.

More recently, analyses have been conducted in this population to determine whether comorbidity also elevates the risk of death from breast cancer. This was done to determine whether comorbidity aggravates the course of the disease itself. After approximately 4 years, 101 (21.8%) of the 463 interviewed cases had died. Breast cancer was listed on the death certificate as the underlying cause for 61 of the decedents. The analysis was restricted to these decedents. As in our past work[11], analysis of duration of survival was based on Cox proportional hazards models. The

TABLE 2. Number of Comorbid Conditions and Risk of Death from Breast Cancer among Women Aged 55 to 84 with Invasive Breast Cancer of The Detroit Metropolitan Area

	Relative Hazard	95% Confidence Interval
Race		
Black vs. White	1.28	0.70, 2.34
Age		
65-74 vs. 55-64	0.60	0.32, 1.12
75-84 vs. 55-64	0.79	0.41, 1.54
Stage of Disease		
Regional vs. Local	4.35	2.05, 9.23
Remote vs. Local	28.83	12.77, 65.10
Number of Comorbid Conditions		
1 vs. 0	1.45	0.75, 2.81
2+ vs. 0	2.17	1.13, 4.18
Limiting Breast Cancer		
Yes vs. No	0.80	0.46, 1.39

Cox model provides an estimate of the relative hazards associated with each independent variable. The risk estimate is the average of estimated relative risks for various small intervals over the survival period, in this case, approximately 4 years. The Cox analysis also allows adjustment for a variety of covariates, providing an estimate of the independent effect of each factor associated with survival.

Table 2 compares the risk estimates for age, race, stage of disease, and the number of limiting comorbid conditions. In addition, we included the patient's report of whether the breast cancer itself currently limits her daily activities. Although there was no elevated risk for women with only one limiting condition, those with two or more concurrent conditions were 2.2 times more likely than women without comorbid conditions to die from breast cancer, adjusting for other factors (95% CI: 1.13, 4.18).

The prognostic significance of individual conditions also was assessed. Limiting heart disease, hypertension, arthritis were the three most common conditions reported by the breast cancer cases[11]. Individual risk estimates were obtained for each of these conditions, adjusting for race, age, stage of disease at diagnosis, as well as the number of remaining limiting conditions.

Women with limiting heart disease were 2.4 times more likely than women without limiting heart disease to die from breast cancer, adjusting for other factors (95% CI: 1.07, 5.52) (Table 3). Limiting arthritis and hypertension were not associated with an elevated risk of death. Women with two or more other limiting conditions (i.e., not arthritis, hypertension, or heart disease) continued to have an elevated risk of death.

These preliminary studies suggest that comorbidity has an adverse effect on survival, independently of age and how advanced the breast cancer is at the time of diagnosis. In spite of these promising findings, additional research is needed to clarify this association, especially as a way of understanding more clearly the underlying mechanisms associated with survival.

RESEARCH ISSUES AND FUTURE DIRECTIONS

Cause of Death

Determining the cause of death is of utmost importance in conducting survival studies. In most survival studies in epidemiology, deaths are restricted to those in which the index condition, in this case, breast cancer, is listed as the underlying cause of death. Deaths from other causes, such as heart disease, are "censored" and treated similarly to those cases who have been lost to follow-up. Restricting the analysis to deaths due to breast cancer may prevent, however, a comprehensive view of the risks associated with comorbidity. Indeed, Charlson and colleagues[10] were specifically interested in determining whether comorbidity elevates the risk of death from causes other than breast cancer. Innovative procedures may be required to obtain a more

TABLE 3. Selected Comorbid Conditions and Risk of Death from Breast Cancer among Women Aged 55 to 84 with Invasive Breast Cancer of The Detroit Metropolitan Area

	Relative Hazard	95% Confidence Interval
Race		
Black vs. White	1.43	0.76, 2.67
Age		
66-74 vs. 55-64	0.61	0.33, 1.13
75-84 vs. 55-64	0.72	0.36, 1.44
Stage of Disease		
Regional vs. Local	4.73	2.22, 10.07
Remote vs. Local	32.93	14.14, 76.73
Limiting Heart Disease		
Yes vs. No	2.43	1.07, 5.52
Limiting Arthritis		
Yes vs. No	1.03	0.52, 2.07
Limiting Hypertension		
Yes vs. No	0.46	0.14, 1.59
Limiting Breast Cancer		
Yes vs. No	0.82	0.47, 1.44
Remaining Limiting Comorbidity		
1 vs. 0	1.03	0.50, 2.11
2+ vs. 0	2.83	1.18, 6.77

complete picture of survival using both underlying and contributory causes of death. It is also important to keep in mind that in some instances it is difficult to determine the cause of death. In the presence of other health problems, how does one establish whether a death was due to breast cancer or to some other cause? To what extent is the decision affected by the number and severity of health problems facing the person? Moreover, do differences in the time interval between diagnosis and death determine why one condition is listed as the underlying cause of death rather than some other condition? In light of these difficulties, it is advisable to examine the risk of breast cancer recurrence associated with comorbidity. Indeed, recurrence may be a more precise measure of whether comorbidity affects the course of the cancer itself.

Measurement of Comorbidity

Research in this area depends on clear criteria for defining and measuring comorbidity. As a first step, it is necessary to determine whether comorbid conditions are antecedent, concurrent, or subsequent to the diagnosis of the breast cancer. Determining the timing of the condition is important for establishing both the etiology of the concurrent health condition and its effect on survival. There may be instances when the comorbid condition itself increases the risk of the breast cancer. Diabetes and hypertension, for example, elevate the risk of endometrial cancer[18]. On the other hand, some forms of cancer treatment may lead to the development of health problems. Certain chemotherapeutic agents, such as doxorubicin (Adriamycin), are known in some cases to have cardiotoxic side effects[19].

The severity of comorbid conditions also needs to be established. It should be emphasized that the level of severity does not depend simply on the number of concurrent health conditions. Instead, the potential seriousness or impact of each condition must be considered. As noted previously, researchers have scored health conditions in terms of either the risk of death or disability associated with each condition[10]. Others have asked respondents through health surveys to assess the extent to which a prevalent condition limits their daily activities[11]. It would be worthwhile to determine whether data from medical records and health surveys could be used together to develop a more comprehensive comorbidity index. Scores could be based on both the risk of death as well as expected functional limitations associated with each concurrent health condition.

Research to date has focused on either the prognostic significance of individual conditions or the total number and severity of conditions exhibited by the cancer patient. Research is needed to address the prognostic significance of specific combinations of conditions. It is also important to establish more precise measures of severity. Most summary measures are additive. The Charlson index, for example, is based on the assumption that the overall degree of severity of comorbidity equals the sum of the weights of each individual condition. It may be, however, that the severity of particular combinations of conditions is not additive. Together, some conditions may be especially lethal, reflecting a multiplicative or synergistic relationship. In other instances, the presence of an additional condition may not elevate the overall risk of death beyond the level of risk associated with the most serious concurrent condition.

Comorbidity and Tumor Characteristics

It is again well known that the risk of death following breast cancer depends on the size and grade of the tumor as well the number of affected axillary lymph nodes. It is unknown, however, whether particular combinations of comorbid conditions are associated with these tumor characteristics. In addition to a physiologic relationship, comorbidity may affect the stage of disease at diagnosis by affecting the likelihood of screening. Are women with particular comorbid conditions more likely than others not to be screened, thus elevating the risks of being diagnosed with advanced disease? Are there other instances, however, in which the presence of particular conditions, for example, those being monitored by a physician, actually improve the chances that an incident breast cancer will be identified? In addition, the prognostic significance of comorbidity itself may be affected by the stage of the breast cancer at diagnosis. The risk of death associated with comorbidity may be greater for women with local and regional disease than it is for women with remote disease, those for whom the risk of death is already high. The prognostic significance of comorbidity must be determined in conjunction with detailed assessments of tumor characteristics, e.g., tumor size and grade. With the exception of ongoing research from the Breast Cancer Prognostic Study at the Michigan Cancer Foundation, the effects of comorbidity on survival have not been assessed in conjunction with detailed specifications of tumor characteristics.

Comorbidity and Host Characteristics

Comorbidity either may determine or simply serve as an indicator of the host's immunological status. The risk of death associated with comorbidity also may depend on the host's chronological age. Is the prognostic significance of comorbidity greater for older women than it is younger women? This question has yet to be addressed. Comorbidity also may help to clarify the reasons for the elevated risk associated with other host characteristics, such as body mass. It is hypothesized that obesity has an adverse effect on survival through hormonal mechanisms involving changes in prolactin, gonadotropins, or estrogen levels. Serum albumin, commonly used as an indicator of nutritional status and more specifically, amino acid intake, also has been associated with breast cancer prognosis[20]. Women with low serum albumin have poor immune function, which may impede recovery following disease. Obesity and serum albumin level also may affect survival through unknown mechanisms. For example, it may be hypothesized that obesity and level of serum albumin elevate the risk for other, concurrent health conditions, such as heart disease and diabetes, which, in turn, may have an adverse effect on the course of the breast cancer following diagnosis. Obesity and other nutritional factors, therefore, may adversely affect survival both directly (e.g., through hormonal mechanisms) and indirectly (through the development and/or aggravation of other, concurrent health conditions).

CONCLUSION

Preliminary evidence suggests that comorbidity has an independent effect on prognosis following the diagnosis of breast cancer. Data on the number, type, and severity of concurrent health conditions may provide prognostic information about the host beyond what is available from data on chronological age and body mass. More important, the study of comorbidity may provide an excellent opportunity for collaboration between epidemiology and molecular biology to understand more clearly the mechanisms affecting survival for women with breast cancer.

REFERENCES

1. Ries, L.A.G.; Hankey, B.F.; Edwards, B.K. (ed.) Cancer Statistics Review, 1973-87. Bethesda, MD: National Cancer Institute (NIH Publication No. 90-2789) (1990).

2. Kelsey, J.L. A review of the epidemiology of human breast cancer. *Epid. Rev.* 1:74 (1980).

3. Miller, A.B.; Bulbrook, R.D. The epidemiology and etiology of breast cancer. *New England J. Med.* 303:1246 (1980).

4. Pitelka, D.R.; Unemori, E.N.; Field, M.F. Cell-cell and cell stroma interactions in metastasis. In: Rich, M.A., Hager, J.C., Furmanski, P. (eds.) Understanding Breast Cancer: Clinical and Laboratory Aspects. Dekker, New York. 99 (1984).

5. Bertuzzi, A.; Daidone, M.O.; DiFronzo, G.; Silverstrini, R. Relationship among estrogen receptors, proliferative activity and menopausal status in breast cancer. *Breast Cancer Res. Treat.* 1:253 (1981).

6. Boyle, P.; Leake, R. Progress in understanding breast cancer: epidemiological and biological interactions. *Breast Cancer Res. Treat.* 11:91 (1988).

7. Russo, J.; Frederick, J.; Ownby, H.E.; Fine, G.; Hussain, M.; Krickstein, H.I.; Robbins, T.O.; Rosenberg, B. Predictors of recurrence and survival of patients with breast cancer. *Amer. J. of Clin. Path.* 88:123 (1987).

8. Donegan, W.L.; Hartz, A.J.; Rimm, A.A. The association of body weight with recurrent cancer of the breast. *Cancer* 41:1590 (1978).

9. Mohle-Boetani, J.; Grosser, S.; Whittemore, A.S.; Malec, M.; Kampert, J.B.; Paffenbarger, R.S. Body size, reproductive factors, and breast cancer survival. *Prev. Med.* 17:634 (1988).

10. Charlson, M.E.; Pompei, P.; Ales, K.L.; MacKenzie, C.R. A new method of classifying prognostic comorbidity in longitudinal studies: Development and validation. *J Chron. Dis.* 40:373 (1987).

11. Satariano, W.A.; Ragheb, N.E.; Dupuis, M.A. Comorbidity in older women with breast cancer: an epidemiologic approach. In: Yancik, R.; Yates, J. (eds.) Cancer in the Elderly: Approaches to Early Detection and Treatment. Springer, New York. 71 (1989).

12. Verbrugge, L.M.; Lepkowski, J.M.; Imanaka, Y. Comorbidity and its impact on disability. *Milbank Q.* 67:450 (1989).

13. Berkman, L.F.; Breslow, L. Health and Ways of Living: The Alameda County Study. Oxford University, New York (1983).

14. Kaplan, G.A.; Camacho, T. Perceived health and mortality: A 9-year follow-up of the Human Population Laboratory cohort. *Amer. J. Epid.* 117:293 (1983).

15. Kaplan, G.A.; Kotler, P.L. Self-reports predictive of mortality from ischemic heart disease: A nine-year follow-up of the Human Population Laboratory cohort. *J. Chron. Dis.* 38:196 (1985).

16. Wiley, J.A.; Camacho, T.c. Life-style and future health: evidence from the Alameda County Study. *Prev. Med.* 9:1 (1980).

17. Bush, T.L.; Miller, S.R.; Golden, A.L.; Hale, W.E. Self-report and medical record agreement of selected medical conditions in the elderly. *Amer. J. Publ. Health* 79:1554 (1989).

18. Centers for Disease Control Cancer and Steroid Study. Oral contraceptice use and the risk of endometrial cancer. *J. Amer. Med. Assn.* 49:1600 (1983).

19. Von Hoff, D.D.; Layard, M.W.; Basa, P.; Davis, H.L.; Von Hoff, A.L.; Rozencweig, M.; Muggia, F.M. Risk factors for doxorubicin-induced congestive heart failure. *Ann. Intern. Med.* 91:710 (1979).

20. Goates, R.J.; Clark, W.S.; Eley, J.W.; Greenberg, R.S.; Huguley, C.M.; Brown, R.L. Race, nutritional status, and survival from breast cancer. *J. Nat. Cancer Inst.* 82:1684 (1990).

SQUAMOUS CELL CANCER OF THE CERVIX, IMMUNE SENESCENCE AND HPV: IS CERVICAL CANCER AN AGE-RELATED NEOPLASM ?

Jeanne Mandelblatt

Memorial Sloan-Kettering Cancer Center
Division of Cancer Control
New York, New York 10021

ABSTRACT

Relationships between cancer and aging will assume greater scientific importance over the coming decades as the number and proportion of elderly increase. Contrary to popular belief, cervical cancer remains an important disease into old age. This paper will briefly review what is known about immune senescence, cervical cancer and immune function, and the relationship between human papilloma virus and immunity, to support the hypothesis that these factors may contribute to the continued occurrence of invasive cervical cancer in the elderly.

INTRODUCTION

Relationships between cancer and aging will assume greater scientific importance over the coming decades as the number and proportion of elderly increase (Butler, Gastel, 1979). Contrary to popular belief, cervical cancer remains an important disease into old age. While cervical carcinoma in-situ (CIS) incidence peaks prior to menopause and then rapidly declines, invasive cervical cancer (ICC) incidence continues to rise with advancing age (Figure 1). These contrasting incidence patterns may be due to several factors, including: the natural history of the disease with its long, but detectable, pre-invasive phase, under-representation of post-menopausal and elderly women in population screening programs, and/or biological and physiologic changes associated with aging, such as lower hormonal production or declining immune competence, which may facilitate carcinogenesis in the elderly. Cervical neoplasia is considered to develop along a continuum, with neoplastic cells occupying progressively larger portion of the squamous epithelium (Figure 2). Invasive cancer occurs when these cells invade through the basement membrane and extend into the stroma. This process is estimated to take between three and ten years.

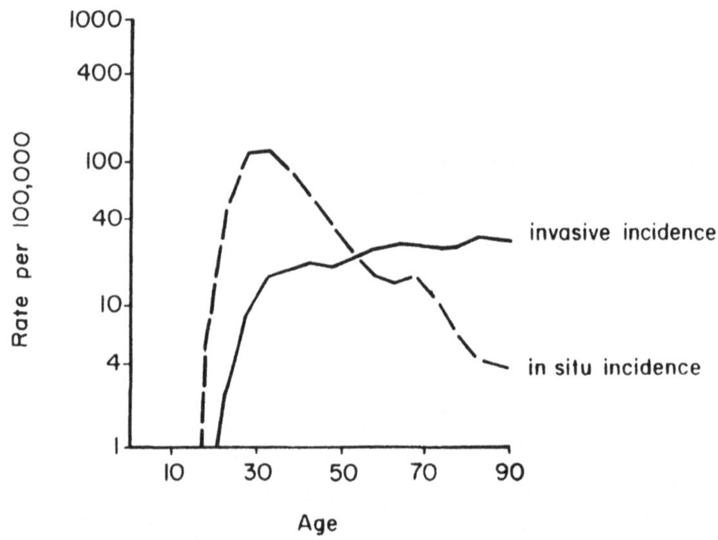

Figure 1. *Age-Specific Cervical Cancer Rates*

Thus, the observation of increased incidence of invasive cervical cancer in the aged may be an artifact of the progressive nature of cervical neoplasia and when disease is detected in this course. For example, if a woman is receiving regular Pap tests, as many younger women are likely to, her disease can be detected prior to invasion. If no screening is occurring, as is more often the case for elderly women, the same disease will be detected at an invasive state, when it is more likely to produce abnormal symptoms, such as bleeding. Thus, older women, by virtue of their non-use of screening, may be diagnosed at the end of a given state of cervical neoplasia and thus appear to have higher rates of ICC than younger women.

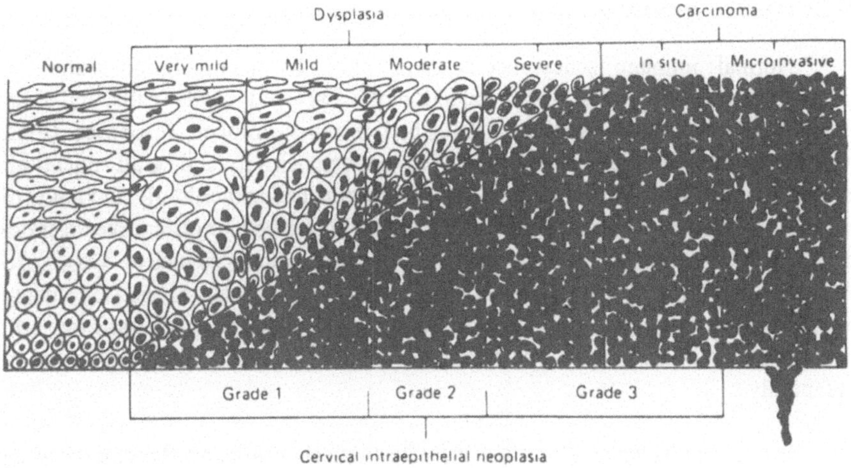

Source: Frenczy A, in Blaustein: Pathology of the Female Genital Tract, 1977

Figure 2. *The Progression of Squamous Cell Cancer of The Cervix*

If no screening occurred and all CIS cases presented with symptomatic invasive cancer, say, 10 years later, we would expect the two incidence curves to overlap. However, if we adjust the incidence curves under this assumption, the curves do not overlap and the incidence of invasive disease in the older age groups still exceeds that expected solely from the progression of CIS.

Therefore, the incidence of invasive disease in the older age groups depends on factors beyond screening patterns. One possibility is to postulate either a proportion of slow growing CIS cases which finally invade after, say, twenty to thirty years, or a substantial portion of CIS cases arising postmenopausally which rapidly progress to invasive disease. A recent review of the natural history of cervical cancer in the elderly concluded that the data regarding disease progression are inconclusive, but suggestive of the latter scenario (Muller, *et al.*, 1990).

What, then, is the mechanism whereby cervical neoplasia may arise in older women and, once it has developed, progress to invasive cancer? This paper will briefly review what is known about immune senescence, cervical cancer and immune function and the relationship between human papilloma virus and immunity to support the hypothesis that these factors may contribute to the continued occurrence of invasive cervical cancer in the elderly.

IMMUNE SENESCENCE

Normal immune senescence is characterized by an involution of the thymus gland, a decrease in T cells, with a reduction of CD4+ and CD8+ cells, and reduction in the helper/suppressor ratio and diminished *in vitro* mitogen responses (Fletcher, 1986; Weksler, 1982; Kay, 1978). Delayed hypersensitivity and graft rejection, two manifestations of cell-mediated immunity, are diminished in the elderly, including muted reactions to Candida, Mumps and PPD and a diminished proliferative response to mitogens. When lymphocytes of the elderly are exposed to antigens such as *Mycobacterium tuberculosis* or *varicella-zoster* virus they do not proliferate to the same degree as do lymphocytes of younger individuals. Not only do there seem to be fewer mitogen responsive cells in the elderly, but these cells are also impaired in their ability to divide sequentially.

It has been suggested that the increased susceptibility of the elderly to cancer may be a consequence, in part, of these immune deficits associated with senescence (Weksler, 1982). In animal models the evidence for a role of the aging immune system in carcinogenesis is more direct. Basically, animal models show a loss of tumor-specific immunity with increasing age (Flood *et al.*, 1981); and the ability of mice to reject tumors diminishes with increasing age as a result of defects in cellular responsiveness (Urban, Schreiber, 1984).

CERVICAL CANCER AND IMMUNITY

Is immune status, then, in turn, related to cervical neoplasia? The primary immune response of the cervical squamous cell epithelium is of the cell-mediated variety. Cell-mediated immunity has also been noted as the primary immune response in cervical cancer patients (Goldstein, *et al.*, 1971; Chen, *et al.*, 1975; Chiang, *et al.*, 1976). Interestingly, the alterations in immune function noted among cervical cancer patients are remarkably similar to those seen with normal aging. Patients with histologically proven invasive squamous cell carcinoma of the cervix have been noted to have immune deficits characterized by a decrease in T cell counts, a decrease in CD4+ helper cells, a decreased CD4+/CD8+ ratio, a decreased lymphocytic response to mitogens, and impaired function of Langerhans's cells, compared to healthy controls (Levy, *et al.*, 1978; Ishiguro, *et al.*, 1980; Castello, *et al.*, 1986; Park, Kim 1989).

In one study, T-cell counts were evaluated in women with dysplasia, CIS, and early (stage 1 and 2) and late (stage 3 and 4) invasive cervical cancer. The authors noted a general decline in T-cell counts with advancing stage of disease, although there was an initial increase early in the invasive process. They concluded that this overall depression of cell-mediated immunity was responsible for the initiation of cervical cancer and that the temporary increase in T-cells may represent a reaction against invasion of the malignant cells through the basement membrane (Ishiguro, *et al.*, 1980). Other groups, based on similar findings, have also concluded that cervical cancer progression is related to immune suppression (Castello, *et al.*, 1986).

In addition, the Langerhans's cells, which exist throughout the cervical squamous epithelium, have also been proposed as part of the immune response (Morris, *et al.*, 1983) and surveillance (Streilein, Berggstresser, 1980) system of the cervix. Patients with papilloma virus infection have been noted to have reductions or absence of Langerhans's cells and a depletion of T-lymphocytes (Morris, *et al.* 1983). The Langerhans's cells which were present in viral infected cervices showed poor differentiation of cytoplasmic processes and a loss of dendritic arborizations (Morris, *et al.* 1983), indicating a loss of normal functioning. Other studies have also shown either a decrease in the number of Langerhans's cells with CIN lesions (Tay, *et al.*, 1987) or the presence of morphological abnormalities (Morris, *et al.*, 1983). These findings suggest an interaction of immune response and cervical neoplasia which may be further promoted by viral agents.

Studies in other settings have also noted a strong association between cervical cancer and immune function. For example, women with iatrogenic immunosuppression have been observed to have higher than expected rates of cervical neoplasia (Porreco, 1975, Schneider, *et al.*, 1983, Fraumeni, Hoover, 1977) and this increase may be as high as ten to fourteen-fold, compared to healthy women (Sillman, *et al.*, 1984, Porreco, Penn, Droegemueller *et al.*, 1975); and women with HIV (HTLV III) infection and disease have been observed to have high rates of cervical neoplasia, correcting for other confounders (Koss, 1987). However, since all of these relationships between cervical cancer and immune deficits are from either case-control or cross-sectional studies, the temporal sequence of events cannot, by design, be determined.

HPV AND IMMUNITY

Recent epidemiological and biologic evidence suggest that human papilloma virus (HPV) may either be an initiating or promoting agent in cervical carcinogenesis (zur Hausen, 1982; Meisels, Fortin, 1976; Purola, Savia, 1977; Koss, 1987). The overall prevalence of HPV in normal Pap smears has been noted to range from a low of 1.3% (Reid, *et al.*, 1980) and 3% (Meisels, Morin, 1981; Grubb, 1986), to a high of 10% (Devilliers, *et al.*, 1987); in women with cervical neoplasia, HPV is contained in 50% to 95% of lesions (Nelson, Averette, Richart, 1988). From these, and other data, it has been estimated that HPV may increase the risk of cervical neoplasia by as much as between 10 to 30-fold (Reeves, 1989).

It also appears that HPV typing may be useful to predict the course of cervical disease (Syrjanen, *et al.*, 1985). Several viral types (16, 18) have been observed in as many as 95% of cases with invasive cervical cancer, whereas other types (6, 11) are only rarely observed in malignant lesions (Nelson, *et al.*, 1988; Schneider, *et al.*, 1987; Campoin, *et al.*, 1986). Table 1 summarizes the types of HPV typed to date and their disease associations.

Next, is there evidence for a relationship between altered immunity and the development of HPV infections? In the normal cervix the CD4+ helper and CD8+ suppressor cells are present in the same proportions to that found in the peripheral circulation. However, women with either multiple genital papillomas and intraepithelial neoplasia or contemporaneous HPV infection and CIN have been noted to have a decreased CD4+/CD8+ ratio (generally as a result of decreased CD4+ cells) and diminished responses of lymphocytes to mitogens, compared to control populations (Carson, Twiggs, Fukushima *et al.*, 1986; Tay, Jenkins, Maddox *et al.*, 1987). Also, a near complete depletion of Langerhans's cells in women with cervical neoplasia and HPV suggests a local immunodeficiency state (Tay, Jenkins, Maddox *et al.*, 1987, McArdle, Muller, 1986).

There are also several lines of indirect evidence linking HPV and impaired immune function:

1) women who have been both iatrogenically immunosuppressed and have HPV infection have been observed to rapidly develop ICC (Shokri–Tabibzadeh, *et al.*, 1981; Schneider, Kay, Lee, 1983; Porreco, *et al.*, 1975; Sillman, *et al.*, 1984);

2) pregnant women, who experience a non–pathological state of immunosuppression, have been noted to have a higher rate of all types of HPV and specifically a higher HPV 16 replication rate, compared to controls (Schneider, *et al.*, 1985, 1986, 1987);

3) women with HIV and HPV have markedly increased incidence of cervical cancer; women with concurrent HPV and HIV infection are 42 times more likely to have CIN than women without either virus (Feingold, Vermund, Burk, 1990).

Unfortunately, from the present evidence it is not possible to determine whether immunosuppression promotes the activation of oncogenic viruses or whether HPV infection suppresses the natural immune system. However, HPV is not reported to be a lymphotropic virus that selectively infects and destroys the CD4+ subset of T cells, supporting the idea that HPV infection may be facilitated by a pre–existing decrease in immune competence.

Is there, then, an association between HPV and age? In Germany, one group examined more than 9,000 women for HPV types 16/18 and 6/11; 10% of the study

Table 1. Anogenital Human Papillomaviruses[1]

HPV TYPE	DISEASE ASSOCIATION	ONCOGENIC ASSOCIATION
6	Condylomata acuminata Low-grade dysplasias	Rarely malignant
11	Condylomata acuminata Low-grade dysplasias	Rarely malignant
16	CIN 1-3, Bowenoid papulosis; Bowen's disease Cervical, vulvar, and anal ulcers	Malignant
18	CIN 3; rarely CIN 1-2 Cervical cancers	Highly malignant
31	CIN 1-3, cancers	Malignant
33	CIN 1-3, cancers	Malignant
35	Cervical intraepithelial neoplasias	Malignant
39	Bowenoid papulosis	Rarely malignant
41	Condylomata	Benign
42	Flat condylomata Bowenoid papulosis	Benign
43	Low-grade dysplasias	Benign
44	Condylomata acuminata Low-grade dysplasias	Benign
45	Condylomata	Rarely malignant
51	Low-grade CIN ?	Benign
52, 56	Condylomata CIN 1-2, cancers	Malignant
53-56	Genital HPV	?

[1]Source: Adapted from Nelson, Averette, Richart, 1989.
HPV types with insufficient data to determine association with neoplasia have been designated with a question mark.

sample were aged 60, and older (DeVilliers, *et al.*, 1987). They found that the association between HPV and CIN and HPV and normal smears generally decreased with age, although there is some suggestion that the age-specific distribution of HPV in CIN lesions is bimodal, with the second peak at about age 75. In contrast, they also noted that HPV was present more often in elderly women with ICC, compared to younger women with ICC (DeVilliers, *et al.*, 1987) (Fig.3).

Also, in a recent report of HPV in Latin America, Reeves *et al.*, noted that HPV types 16 and 18 were associated with cervical cancer and that this association increased with increasing age of the woman (Table 2). Meanwell also noted that the chance of a woman's being HPV 16 positive has been noted to increase with age, whether she had cervical cancer, or not (Meanwell, 1987). These observations support the hypothesis that age-related changes may interact with HPV and the neoplastic process.

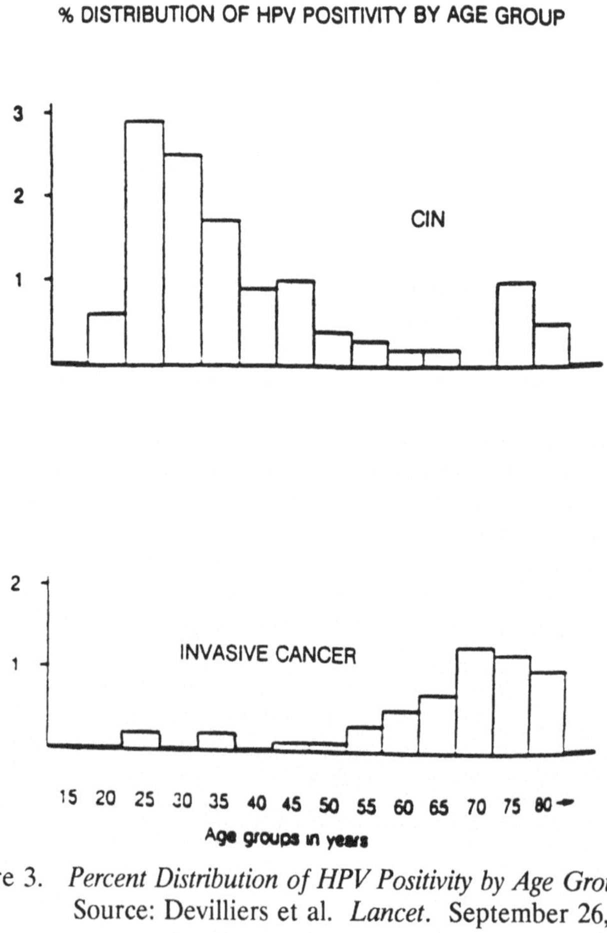

Figure 3. *Percent Distribution of HPV Positivity by Age Group*
Source: Devilliers et al. *Lancet*. September 26, 1987.

Table 2. Risks of Cervical Cancer Associated with HPV

RISKS	NEGATIVE for HPV	POSITIVE for HPV 16/18
Age	**Adjusted Relative Risk***	
<40	1.00	4.08
40-49	0.98	4.51
50-59	0.78	4.72
≥60	0.75	5.63
Cigarettes		
None	1.00	4.66
<10	1.03	5.91
≥10	1.02	8.00
No. of Sexual Partners		
1	1.00	4.72
2 or 3	1.56	8.00
≥4	1.35	8.69
Age at First Intercourse		
≥18	1.00	4.56
16 or 17	1.35	5.53
<16	1.42	10.38
Oral Contraceptives		
Never Used	1.00	5.31
Used	1.35	6.34

*Adjusted for age, number of partners, age of first intercourse, number of births, interval since Pap, and education.

From: Reeves *et al.*, *New England Journal of Medicine* 320:1437 (1989).

Table 3. Results of PAP Smear Screening for Elderly Women

AGE	RACE	PAP	HISTOLOTY
83	black	+ ca	vaginal squamous ca
88	white	+ ca	invasive squamous ca
65	black	+ ca	invasive squamous ca
65	black	CIN 1	CIN 1
67	white	CIN II	CIN II
67	white	koilocytes	CIN 1
77	white	CIS	CIS
73	hispanic	koilocytes	CIN 1
77	oriental	+ ca	invasive squamous ca
73	black	suspicious ca	CIN 3/CIS
74	white	suspicious ca	CIS

There have been no studies in the United State of HPV infection in elderly women. In our previous work, we screened over 1,500 elderly women attending a public hospital medical clinic. In that program the average age of the patients was 74 years, 25% of the women had never been screened before and only 25% reported regular past screening. We found 11 abnormal Pap smears among 816 women who agreed to be screened, for a rate of 13.5 per 1,000. Interestingly, two patients, or 18% of the abnormal smears were reported as having koilocytosis (Table 3) (Mandelblatt et al., 1986).

We are currently conducting a case-control study of the relationship between HPV infection and cervical neoplasia in a group of high-risk elderly women. Briefly, we are studying the association between HPV types 16/18, 6/11, 31/33/35 and abnormal Pap smears (as defined as CIN, or worse) among a group of 1,000 black women aged 65 to 99 living in Harlem, NYC. Preliminary results suggest that women who are HPV DNA positive are significantly more likely to have an abnormal Pap smear than those who are HPV negative.

CONCLUSION

It appears that when the immune system is compromised, either iatrogenically or by changes in physiologic functioning, such as aging, conditions favorable to both neoplasia and the maturation of the HPV may be created (Koss, 1987; Meisels, Morin, 1981;). It seems plausible to postulate, given the epidemiologic and molecular biologic evidence, that there may be an interaction between HPV infection, immune status, or other factors in elderly women which promote the expression of cervical neoplasia, making cervical cancer an age-related cancer.

Other factors which may also contribute to the relationship between aging and cervical cancer include hormonal status, genetic factors, as well as yet un-delineated factors. The paradox of CIS incidence dramatically declining after a peak at age 30 in contrast to the increase, or plateau, in invasive cancer rates with increasing age cannot be explained by screening utilization patterns alone. The elucidation of the factors which interact with age in promoting invasive cervical cancer could contribute to our understanding of age-related carcinogenesis.

REFERENCES

Butler, R.N., Gastel, B. Aging and cancer management, part ii: Research perspectives. *Ca - A Ca. J. Clinicians* 29:6 (1979).

Campoin, M.J., McCance, D.J., Cuzjic, J. Progressive potential of mild cervical atypia: Prospective cytological, colposcopic, and virological study. *Lancet* 1:237-240 (1986).

Castello, G., Esposito, G., Stellato, G., Mora, L.D., Abate, G., Germano, A. Immunological abnormalities in patients with cervical carcinoma. *Gynecol. Oncol.* 25:61-64 (1986).

Chen, S.S., Koffler, D., Cohen, C.J. Cellular hypersensitivity in patients with squamous cell carcinoma of the cervix. *Am. J. Obstet. Gynecol.* 121:91-95 (1975).

Chiang, W.T., Wei, P.Y., Alexander, E.R. Circulatory and cellular immune responses to squamous cell carcinoma of the cervix. *Am. J. Obstet. Gynecol.* 126:116-121 (1976).

deVilliers, E.M., Wagner, D., Schneider, A., Wesch, H., Kiklaw, H. Wahrendorf, J., Papendick, U., Zur Hausen, H. Human papillomavirus infections in women with and without abnormal cervical cytology. *Lancet* 2:703-705 (1987).

Fraumeni, J.F. Jr, Hoover, R. Immuno-surveillance and cancer: epidemiologic observations. *Natl. Cancer Inst. Monogr.* 47:121-126 (1977).

Goldstein, M.S., Shore, B., Gusberg, S.B. Cellular immunity as a host response to squamous carcinoma of the cervix. *Am. J. Obstet. Gynecol.* 111:751-755 (1971).

Grubb, G.S. Human papillomavirus and cervical neoplasia: Epidemiological considerations. *International Journal of Epidemiology* 15:1-7 (1986).

Ishiguro, T., Sugitachi, I., Katoh, K. T and B lymphocytes in patients with squamous cell carcinoma of the uterine cervix. *Gynecol. Oncol.* 9:80-85 (1980).

Kay, M.M.B. The effects of aging on immune function. In Waters, H. ed., The Handbook of Cancer Immunology. Garland STPM Press, New York, Volume I, pp. 63-93 (1978).

Koss, L.G., Durfee, G.R. Unusual patterns of squamous epithelium of the uterine cervix: Cytologic and pathologic study of koilocytotic atypia. *Ann. N.Y. Acad. Sci.* 63:1245-1261 (1956).

Koss, L.G. Cytologic and histologic manifestations of human papillomavirus infection of the female genital tract and their clinical significance. *Cancer* 60:1942-1950 (1987).

Levy, S., Kopersztych, S., Musatti, C.C., Souen, J.S., Salvatore, C.A., Mendes, N.F. Cellular immunity in squamous cell carcinoma of the uterine cervix. *Am. J. Obstet. Gynecol.* 130:160-164 (1978).

Mandelblatt, J.S., Gopaul, I., Wistreich, M. Gynecological care of elderly women in a primary care setting: Another look at Papanicolaou smear testing. *J. Amer. Medical Assoc.* 256:367-371 (1986).

Meanwell, C., Cox, M., Blackledge, G., Maitland, N. HPV 16 DNA in normal and malignant cervical epithelium: implications for the aetioogy and behaviour of cervical neoplasia. *Lancet*: 1:703-707 (1987).

Meisels, A., Fortin, R. Condylomatous lesions of the cervix and vagina: Cytologic patterns. *Acta Cytol.* (Baltimore) 20:505-509 (1976).

Morris, H.H.B., Gatter, K.C., Sykes, G., Casemore, V. Langerhans's cells in human cervical epithelium: Effects of wart virus infection and intraepthelial neoplasia. *British J. of Obstet. and Gynec.* 90:412-420 (1983).

Muller, C.M., Mandelblatt, J., Schecther, C. The Costs Effectiveness of Screening for Cervical Cancer in Elderly Women. In the OTA's Series on Preventive Services Under Medicare. Health Program, Office of Technology Assessment, U.S. Congress, Washington, DC, February, 1990.

Porreco, R., Penn, I., Droegemueller, W., Greer, B., Makowski, E. Gynecologic malignancies in immunosuppressed organ homograft recipients. *Obstet. Gynecol.* 45:359-364 (1975).

Purola, E., Savia, E. Cytology of gynecologic condyloma acuminatum. *Acta Cytol.* (Baltimore) 21: 26-31 (1977).

Reeves, W.C., Brinton, L.A., Garcia, M., Brenes, M.M., Herrero, R., Gaitan, E., Tenorio, F., de Britton, R.C., Rawls, W.E. Human papillomavirus infection and cervical cancer in Latin America. *New Engl. J. Med.* 320:1437-1441 (1989).

Reid, R., Laverty, C.R., Coppleson, M., Isarangkul, W., Hills, E. Noncondylomatous cervical wart virus infection. *Obstet. Gynecol.* 55:476-483 (1980).

Schneider, A., Kraus, H., Schuhmann, R., Gissmann, L. Papillomavirus infection of the lower genital tract. *Int. J. Cancer* 35:443-446 (1985).

Schneider, A., Hotz, M., Gissmann, L. Prevalence of genital HPV infections in pregnant women. In Cold Spring Harbor Symposium on Papillomaviruses (1986).

Schneider, A., Sawada, E., Gissman, L., Shah, K. Human papillomaviruses in women with a history of abnormal Papanicolaou smears and in their male partners. *Obstet. and Gynecol.* 69:554-562 (1987).

Schneider, A., Kay, S., Lee, H.M. Immunosuppression: High risk factor for the development of condyloma acuminata and squamous neoplasia of the cervix. *Acta Cytol.* (Baltimore) 27:220-224 (1983).

Shokri-Tabibzadeh, S., Koss, L., Molnar, J., Romney, S. Association of human papillomavirus with neoplastic processes in genital tract of four women with impaired immunity. *Gynecol. Oncol.* 12:S129-S140 (1981).

Sillman, F., Stanek, A., Sedlis, A., Rosenthal, J., Lanks, K.W., Buchhagen, D., Nicastri, A., Boyce, J. The relationship between human papillomavirus and lower genital intraepithelial neoplasia in immunosuppressed women. *American Journal of Obstetrics and Gynecology* 150:300-308 (1984),

Streilein, J.W., Bergstresser, P.R. Ia antigens and epidermal Langerhans cells. *Transplantation* 30:319-323 (1980).

Syrjanen, K., Parkinen, S., Mantyjarni, R., Vayrynen, M., Syrjanen, S., Holopainen, H., Saarikoski, S., Castren, O. Human papillomavirus (HPV) type as an important determinant of the natural history of HPV infections in uterine cervix. *Eur. J. Epidemiol.* 1:180-187 (1985).

Tay, S.K., Jenkins, D., Maddox, P., Campoin, M., Singer, A. Subpopulations of Langerhan's cells in cervical neoplasia. *British J. of Obstet. and Gynecol.* 94:10-15 (1987).

Urban, J.L., Schreiber, H. Rescue of the tumor-specific immune response of aged mice *in vitro*. *J. of Immunology* 133: 527-534 (1984).

Weksler, M.E. Age-associated changes in the immune response. *J. Amer. Geriatrics Soc.* 30:718-723 (1982).

zur Hausen, H. Human papillomavirus and their possible role in squamous cell carcinomas. *Curr. Topics Microbiol. Immunol.* 78:1-30 (1977).

zur Hausen, H. Human Genital Cancer: Synergism between two virus infections or synergism between a virus infection and initiating events? *Lancet* 2:1370-1372 (1982).

GENETIC AND MOLECULAR BASIS FOR CELLULAR SENESCENCE

J. Carl Barrett, Lois A. Annab, and P. Andrew Futreal

Laboratory of Molecular Carcinogenesis
National Institute of Environmental Health Sciences
Research Triangle Park, North Carolina 27709

ABSTRACT

Normal human and rodent cells in culture exhibit a finite life span at the end of which they exhibit morphological changes and cease proliferating, a process termed cellular senescence or cellular aging. Many cancer cells differ from normal cells in that they do not senesce and have an indefinite life span in culture, suggesting that alterations relating to cellular senescence are involved in the neoplastic evolution of tumor cells. Recent experimental results strongly support a genetic basis for cellular senescence. Defects in the senescence program in transformed cells can be corrected by introduction of a specific chromosome from normal cells into the abnormal cells. Using this approach, possible senescence genes have been mapped to specific chromosomes. Cell cycle control genes that regulate entry into the DNA synthetic phase of the cell cycle must be altered in senescent cells. Recent findings suggest that phosphorylation of the retinoblastoma gene is altered in senescent cells. It is possible, but not yet proven, that aging at the cellular level contributes to the aging of the individual. Therefore, an understanding of cellular senescence at the genetic and molecular levels may provide new insights into both the cancer and aging processes.

INTRODUCTION

Nearly thirty years ago, Hayflick and Moorhead reported that normal human embryo fibroblasts are able to undergo a limited, fixed number of cell divisions after which they cease proliferation[1]. Human embryonic fibroblasts can be grown for 50-60 population doublings before senescence. The failure of the cells to grow beyond this

The Underlying Molecular, Cellular, and Immunological Factors in Cancer and Aging, Edited by S.S. Yang and H.R.Warner, Plenum Press, New York, 1993

limit is an inherent property of the cells that cannot be explained simply by inadequate media components[1]. The key determinant in the life span of cells in culture is the number of cell doublings, not the length of time in culture[1]. Normal cells transplanted serially in vivo also exhibit a finite life span, suggesting that cellular senescence is not a cell culture artifact[2].

Three lines of evidence suggest that the aging of cells in culture may be related to the aging of the organism[1,3]:

(1) The doubling potential of cells in culture is inversely proportional to the age of the donor. Cells from embryonic tissue exhibit the longest life span 50-60 cell doublings). Cells from adult tissue can be grown for only 14 to 29 doublings, and there is a general decrease in the life span of cells in culture with increasing age of the donor tissue.

(2) Cells derived from individuals who exhibit premature aging have a decreased life span in culture. Patients with progeria (Hutchinson-Gilford syndrome) manifest signs of aging at the end of their first decade of life that are typical of normal individuals in the seventh decade of life. Werner syndrome individuals also have accelerated aging but in later years--the mean age of death is 47. The main causes of death in these individuals are cancer and cardiovascular disease, similar to normal individuals. Fibroblasts derived from individuals with the premature aging characteristics senesce prematurely in culture, after only 2 to 10 population doublings.

(3) The life span of cells in culture is correlated in general with the maximum life span of the species, although the variability in this experimental data isgreat. Cells from humans (maximum life span = 100-120 years) can be grown for 50-60 population doublings, whereas cells from rodents (3-5 year life span) can be grown for only 20-40 population doublings. Cells from the Galapagos tortoise, which has a life span of 175-200 years, undergo a greater number of population doublings (90-125) in culture than human cells.

These lines of evidence, although not conclusive, provide provocative support for the hypothesis that aging of cells is related to the aging process of the organism. Escape from cellular senescence is an important step in neoplastic progression of human and rodent cancers[4]. Many, but not all, tumor cells can be grown indefinitely in culture and therefore have escaped senescence and are termed immortal. It is not clear whether the failure of some tumor cells to grow in culture is a technical artifact or an indication that escape from senescence is not required for these cancers. Many of these tumors cannot be maintained in vivo in nude mice, suggesting that only a small growth fraction of cells exists in the tumor. Improvements in cell culture techniques have led to the establishment of many cell lines from most tumor types, suggesting that it is possible to obtain immortal cell lines if the culture conditions are optimal. Since no property of cancer cells is universal, it is not necessary to demonstrate that escape from senescence has occurred in every cancer. However, in those cancers where this change is evident, it is probably a critical change based on the following additional lines of evidence[4].

The observation that treatment of normal cells with diverse carcinogenic agents, including chemical carcinogens, viruses, and oncogenes, allows cells to escape senescence indicates that this change is important in cancer induction. While immortality is not sufficient for neoplastic transformation, most immortal cells have an increased propensity for spontaneous, carcinogen-induced or oncogene-induced neoplastic progression[4]. Therefore, escape from senescence is a preneoplastic change that predisposes a cell to neoplastic conversion. It is clear that immortal cells are further along the multistep pathway to neoplasia than normal cells[4].

Cellular senescence may be one of the mechanisms by which tumor suppression occurs[4, 5]. Tumor suppression is controlled by a family of normal cellular genes that must be inactivated, lost, or mutated in cancer cells. Since cellular senescence limits the growth of cells, it is reasonable that senescence might be one mechanism by which tumor suppressor genes operate.

Two major theories of cellular senescence have been proposed for many years[1,3]. One is the error catastrophe or damage model, which proposes that random accumulation of damage or mutations in DNA, RNA, or protein leads to the loss of proliferative capacity. The experimental evidence support the error accumulation hypothesis has been criticized[3]. A second hypothesis is that senescence is a genetically programmed process, and support for a genetic basis for senescence was provided by the recent experiments of Pereira-Smith and Smith[6] and of Sugawara et al.[7] It is possible to fuse cells of different origins and then to select for the hybrid cells using biochemical markers for drug sensitivity or resistance that differ in the parental cells. When cells with a finite life span are fused to immortal cells with an indefinite life span, the majority of these hybrids senesce, indicating that senescence is dominant over immortality[6, 8]. Even hybridization of two different immortal human cell lines with each other can result in senescence, indicating that different complementation groups exist for the senescence function lost in these hybrid cells. Four complementation groups have been established, suggesting that loss or inactivation of one of multiple genes might allow escape from senescence[6]. If this hypothesis is correct, it should be possible to map the genes involved in cellular senescence. Recent findings with hamster and human interspecies hybrids have mapped putative senescence genes to specific human chromosomes[7, 9].

MATERIALS AND METHODS

All the materials and methods have been previously described[7-10].

RESULTS

Mapping Genes for Cellular Senescence

When normal human cells with a finite life span are fused to immortal hamster cells, the hybrids that form exhibit a finite life span characteristic of the normal human cells. At the end of this life span, the cells display signs of cellular senescence characteristic of the parental human cells at the end of their life span. Criteria for senescence include cellular enlargement and flattening, and cessation of proliferation as measured by the failure to increase cell number in two weeks, failure to subculture, failure to form colonies at clonal density, and lack of significant incorporation of 3H-thymidine as measured by labeled nuclei (<2%) following autoradiograph[7].

When MRC-5 cells, which are normal human lung fibroblasts with a life span of 60 population doublings, were used at a population doubling level of 40, the human-hamster hybrids grew for approximately 20 population doublings, i.e., the remaining life span of the parental human cells. Since the cell hybrids grew extensively before dying, the cessation of growth was not due to a toxic effect of the fusion protocol or some other trivial reason. Furthermore, when earlier passage MRC-5 cells were used (population doubling level 30), the hybrids grew longer, for up to 30 population doublings, again achieving the life span of the parental cells. Therefore, the senescence of the hybrids is an active process dictated by the senescence program of the normal human cells. The limited life span of the hybrids indicates that cellular senescence is dominant in these hamster-human hybrids. A similar conclusion was drawn from studies of intraspecies, i.e., human-human and hamster-hamster hybrids[6, 8].

Although the majority of the hamster-human hybrids senesced, some of the hybrids ultimately escaped senescence (Fig. 1). Senescent cells appeared in all of the hybrid clones after two to three passages. In some of the clones a few nonsenescent cells persisted and continued to proliferate, achieved >100 population doublings, and had high labelling indexes and colony forming efficiencies[7]. These results indicated that these hybrid clones had escaped senescence. Since it is known that human chromosomes are usually lost in interspecies hybrids, the possibility that escape from senescence is due to loss of an essential chromosome or chromosomes was examined by karyotypic examination of the hybrids after escape from senescence (approximately 40 population doublings). Since it is possible to distinguish human and hamster chromosomes, the simple question was asked whether escape from senescence involved the loss of any specific human chromosome. Without exception, all of the human-hamster hybrid clones that escaped senescence had lost both copies of human chromosome 1. All other human chromosomes were present in one or two copies in at least one of the immortal hybrids[7].

In order to determine whether the loss of chromosome 1 in non-senescent hybrids was the fortuitous consequence of human chromosome loss in the hybrid or an indication that a gene on this chromosome influenced the senescence process, two additional approaches were undertaken. The hamster cells used in these experiments lacked HPRT gene activity[7]. Hamster-human hybrid clones were selected in HAT medium, which requires the cells to retain the HPRT gene located on the long arm of human chromosome. Karyotypic analysis confirmed that all immortal hybrids retained a human chromosome X. Normal human fibroblasts with a translocation between the human chromosome X and either chromosome 1 or chromosome 11 were obtained. The translocated portion of the chromosome contained the HPRT gene located on the long arm of the X chromosome. Both cell strains had a finite life span and hybrids between the human cells and hamster cells senesced. The percentage of senescent

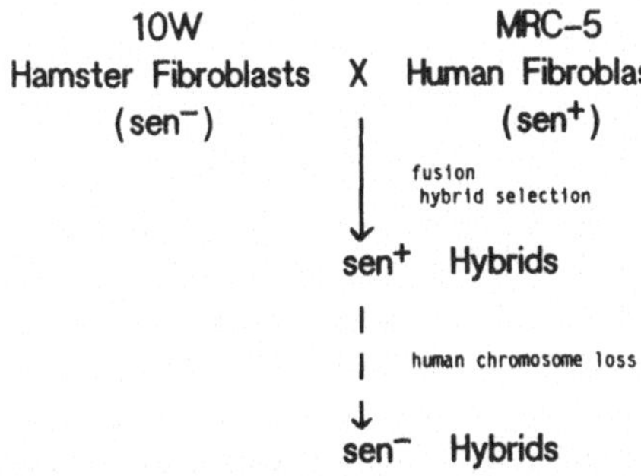

Fig. 1. *Hybrids between immortal (sen-) hamster cells and normal human cells senescence (sen+). Rare variants escape senescence (sen-) after losing human chromosomes.*

hybrids was 40% in the case of fusions between hamster cells and human cells with a t(X;11) chromosome, similar to the percentage with normal diploid human MRC-5 and hamster cells. In contrast, nearly 90% of the cell hybrids between the hamster cells and human cells with a t(X;1) chromosome senesced. This increased frequency of senescent hybrids is consistent with the hypothesis that chromosome 1 contains a gene(s) involved in the senescence process. The gene(s) must be on the long arm of the chromosome 1 since only this portion of chromosome 1 is present on the translocated chromosome. The few hybrids that escaped senescence were examined karyotypically and no intact t(X;1) chromosome was observed. We interpret these results to indicate that a deletion of the critical portion of chromosome 1 occurred, which allowed these hybrids to escape senescence. Since the cells still grow in HAT media, the HPRT gene on chromosome X must be retained in these cells.

To further confirm the role of human chromosome 1 in the senescence of hamster cells, transfer of a single copy of chromosome 1 into immortal hamster cells by the microcell transfer technique was attempted[7]. Mouse A9 cells containing a single human chromosome 1 or 11 tagged with a dominant selectable marker (neomycin) were isolated by techniques previously described[10]. Chromosome 1 or chromosome 11 was transferred by microcell fusions to immortal Syrian hamster cell lines and mouse A9 cells. Numerous colonies were observed following transfer of chromosome 11 into the hamster cells, and no colonies senesced. The frequency of colonies following transfer of chromosome 1 into the mouse A9 cells was similar to that observed with chromosome 11, but only one large colony was observed in 10 experiments with the hamster cell line (the frequency was reduced by at least two orders of magnitude). This clone, however, senesced after 4 weeks and failed to grow to more than 1000 cells. Several small, senescent colonies (8 to 20 cells) were observed following transfer of chromosome 1 into the hamster cells, but these colonies ceased proliferating and sometimes detached from the dish.

The data presented above suggest that a gene or genes on human chromosome 1 are involved in the senescence of hamster-human hybrids. This conclusion is based on three experimental approaches: interspecies cell hybrids with diploid human cells, interspecies cell hybrids with human cells carrying X;autosomal chromosome translocations, and microcell hybrids with individual human chromosomes. Each experimental approach alone is inconclusive, but taken together the results strongly implicate human chromosome 1 in cellular senescence.

Recently, in collaboration with Dr. Max Costa and coworkers, we have mapped another senescence gene to chromosome X[9]. In addition, Ning, Pereira-Smith and Smith (personal communication) have mapped a senescence gene for HeLa cells to chromosome 4. Thus, three senescence genes have now been mapped (Table 1).

POSSIBLE ROLE OF PHOSPHORYLATION OF RETINOBLASTOMAMA GENE IN CELLULAR SENESENCE

The Rb susceptibility gene encodes a nuclear phosphoprotein of 110 kilodaltons[11,12]. Inactivation of both alleles of this gene leads to the development of retinoblastoma and has been implicated in several other malignancies including osteosarcoma, soft tissue sarcomas, lung carcinoma and breast carcinoma[13-18]. Recent work has shown that the Rb protein is differentially phosphorylated during the cell cycle[19-23]. It was found that the Rb protein is unphosphorylated in the G_1/G_o compartment of the cell cycle and is phosphorylated as cells enter into S phase. The protein is increasingly phosphorylated as the cells progress through G_2 and M and is again primarily in the unphosphorylated form as cells re-enter G_1[19-23]. Also, the RB protein was found to be unphosphorylated in cells induced to differentiate[20, 23]. These data suggest that the unphosphorylated form of the protein is growth inhibitory and that the tumor suppressor function of the RB protein may be linked to cell cycle control and differentiation. Therefore, we examined whether the product of the retinoblastoma tumor suppressor gene may be a key regulator of cellular senescence[24].

Examination of RB protein expression levels in senescent SHE cells was accomplished by PAGE separation of cellular lysates followed by the Western blotting procedure and immunochemical detection using monoclonal antibodies to the human retinoblastoma protein[24]. This antibody detected bands of approximately 110 to 116 kD by Western blot in the hamster cells, which is similar to the reported sizes of both human and mouse RB proteins[12,25,26]. Senescent SHE cell cultures expressed comparable levels of RB protein to young cells; however, only the unphosphorylated form of RB was observed.

Table 1. Mapping of Putative Senescence Genes

Chromosome Localization of Sen+ Gene	Cell Line(s)	Reference
Chromosome 1	Syrian hamster 10W Syrian hamster BHK Human endometrial	Sugawara et al., 1990 Annab & Barrett, unpublished Yamada et al., 1990
Chromosome 4	Cervical carcinoma (HeLa)	Ning, Smith & Pereira-Smith, unpublished
Chromosome X	Chinese hamster (Ni-2)	Klein et al., 1991

We examined whether the senescent cells could be stimulated to phosphorylate the RB protein in response to growth stimulatory signals[24]. When cultures of young or senescent cells were maintained for 48 hours in media containing 0.5% serum, both young and senescent cells exhibited only the unphosphorylated form of the RB protein as determined by Western blot analysis. When the cells were stimulated with media containing 10% serum, the phosphorylated form of the RB protein was observed in the young cells by 10 hours after serum stimulation, peaking at 20 hours, which corresponds to the time course for stimulation of DNA synthesis under similar conditions. In the senescent cells, the Rb protein remained unphosphorylated at all time points examined (up to 120 hours). This result indicates that senescent cells are blocked in their ability to phosphorylate the Rb protein in response to normal growth stimuli (Fig. 2).

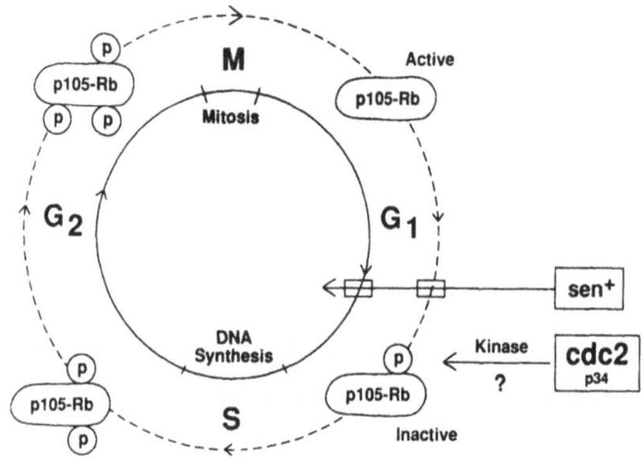

Fig. 2. *The block to DNA synthesis in senescent cells appears to be in later G_1 prior to the phosphorylation of the Rb protein.*

A recent report by Stein et al.[27] also found that the Rb protein was not phosphorylated in senescent human cells, which further substantiates the possible growth regulatory role of the unphosphorylated Rb protein in cellular senescence of cells from different species. We have shown that senescent cells no longer possess the capability to phosphorylate the Rb protein in response to growth stimulation[24]. This finding implicates upstream modifiers of Rb phosphorylation as possible crucial regulatory elements in mediating cellular senescence, with the end result being a block to proliferation caused by the presence of unphosphorylated Rb protein acting on its own or through other effector molecules. Down-regulation of a Rb kinase activity in senescent cells and/or upregulated activity of a Rb phosphatase are possible mechanisms for the alterations of Rb phosphorylation in senescent cells. Recent studies indicate that the cdc2 p34 kinase, which is a candidate Rb kinase, is downregulated in senescent hamster cells (Richter, H., Burkhart, B., Annab, L.A., Boyd, J., and Barrett, J.C., unpublished observations).

DISCUSSION

Our results indicate that it is possible to map genes involved in cellular senescence to specific chromosomes. These findings provide important support for the hypothesis that cellular senescence is a genetically programmed event. We would like to propose the following hypothesis: Cellular senescence is controlled by a set of genes that are activated or whose function becomes manifested at the end of the life span of the cell. Defects in the function of these genes can allow cells to escape the program of senescence and become immortal. Immortalization relieves one constraint on tumor cell growth, allowing malignant progression. A number of key questions relating to this hypothesis can be proposed. Most of these questions remain unanswered but a discussion of possible answers and our current understanding of these problems may help to guide future research in this area.

Question #1: What genes control the program for cell senescence?

The mapping of genes involved in cell senescence to specific chromosomes (Table 1) provides a foundation for the answer of this question. Recent findings (Futreal, P.A., Annab, L.A., and Barrett, J.C., unpublished observations) have localized the senescence gene on chromosome 1 to the region 1q23-q25 (Fig. 3). Further mapping of this region will hopefully lead to the cloning of this gene. Alterations of chromosome 1 are common in many tumor types[28-38] including gastrointestinal, breast, mesothelioma, ovarian, uterine and colon. In some cases the region 1q23 has been implicated[33-36].

Question #2: How do these genes arrest cell division?

The findings of Stein et al.[27] and Futreal and Barrett[24] that the Rb protein is unphosphorylated in senescent cells provide one possible mechanism for the arrest of cell division. However, neither our study nor the study by Stein et al.[27] can distinguish whether the lack of Rb phosphorylation in senescent cells is the cause or consequence of growth arrest. Cellular senescence is perhaps the ultimate perturbation of cell cycle progression and very few treatments are capable of extending the *in vitro* life span of normal cells in culture[4]. One of these is SV40 virus[39], and the interaction of the Rb protein with the large-T antigen of SV40 is well documented[40, 41]. It is very tempting to speculate that the mechanism of SV40-induced immortality is through its interaction with the Rb protein, which in its unphosphorylated form acts as a block to further cell cycle progression. Large T antigen binds preferentially to the unphosphorylated form of the Rb protein[41], thus targeting the growth inhibitory form for presumed inactivation. Other studies have shown that the majority of senescent cells are arrested in the G_1/G_0 compartment of the cell cycle[47], which is in agreement with such a hypothesis.

The Rb protein is a possible substrate for the cdc2 protein kinase[43]. An inability of senescent cells to express this kinase (Richter, H., unpublished observation) may result in a block to DNA replication in senescent cells. The cdc2 p34 kinase phosphorylates several possible regulatory proteins in cell cycle control[43-47]. In yeast, the gene for this kinase is called Start. It seems logical that a program which stops cell growth may operate by blocking the start point in the cell cycle.

Question #3: How do senescence genes relate to genes that control cell division in terminal differentiation and/or apoptosis (programmed cell death)?

Only after the genes involved in these processes are identified can this question be answered. However, it is highly likely that the genes involved in cellular senescence are also involved in other terminal growth arrest states.

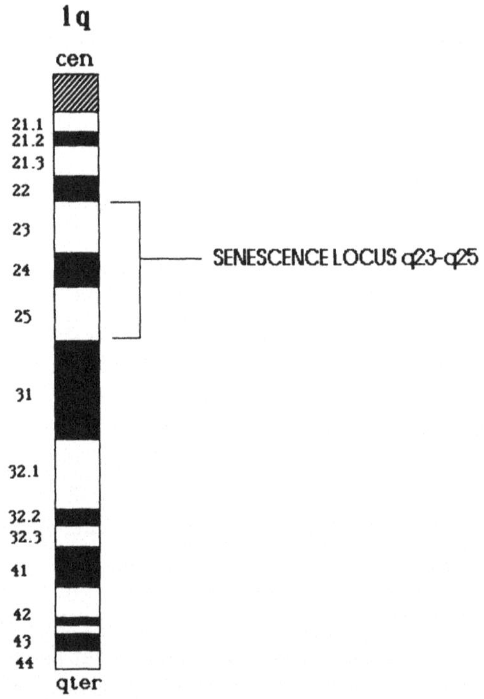

Fig. 3. *Mapping senescence gene on chromosome 1q23.*

Question #4: What is the activation switch for the senescence program?

If the cdc2 kinase is a key determinant in growth, then we have a means to explore the nature of the switch for the program that results in cell senescence. We recently observed that the activity of the senescence gene on the X chromosome appears to be regulated by DNA methylation/demethylation[9]. This may provide a mechanism for one of the switches that activates the cellular senescence program.

Question #5: What is the clock for cell senescence?

This is an intriguing biological question. Cell aging appears to be dependent on the number of cell divisions rather than time *per se*. A clock mechanism at the cellular level could be achieved by the progressive accumulation, deletion, or winding up of some cellular component at each cell division. Since normal chromosomes transferred into immortal cells can correct the defect in these cells and restore their ability to express the apparently normal senescence program, we are currently addressing whether chromosomes from young cells differ from chromosomes from old cells in their rate of induction of cellular senescence, i.e., can chromosomes tell time? Preliminary results (Annab, L.A. and Barrett, J.C., unpublished observation) are consistent with this hypothesis.

One intriguing observation is that the ends of chromosomes (telomeres) become progressively shorter in older cells[49, 50]. This could represent a clock mechanism for the chromosome and for the cell.

Question #6: What is the evolutionary advantage of cell senescence?

It seems paradoxical that a cell would have a program that is detrimental, i.e., promotes death. There must be an evolutionary advantage for cell aging. We would like to propose that the cellular senescence program is switched on in response to signals that are triggered by cellular states that are detrimental to the organism. For example, if genetic instability were to arise in a normal cell, this could lead to aberrant behavior and clonal growth of cells resulting in cancer, developmental defects, and other deleterious effects to the organism. A mechanism to eliminate such aberrant cells (e.g., senescence) would allow improved survival (and life span) for the organism.

Question #7: What is the relationship between cell senescence and aging of the organism?

This is a key unresolved question. The answer, of course, could be that there is no relationship, and the evidence supporting a relationship (as discussed in the Introduction) may only be coincidental. On the other hand, the hypothesis proposed in question #6 provides a link. Cell senescence may allow longer life span and actively delay age-related diseases in the organism. Hayflick[51] expressed this when he noted that "Why do we age?" may be the wrong question. The right question may be, "Why do we live as long as we do?"

Further studies of the genetic and molecular basis of cell aging should provide insights into both the cancer and aging processes.

Question #8: What is the role of cellular senescence in oncogenesis and/or tumor growth?

Cellular senescence may be one of the mechanisms by which tumor suppression occurs. Tumor suppression is controlled by a family of normal cellular genes that must be inactivated, lost, or mutated in cancer cells. Since cellular senescence limits the growth of cells, it is reasonable that senescence must be one mechanism by which tumor suppressor genes operate. Hayflick has shown that cells from adults can be grown in culture for 14 to 29 population doublings[1]. If all the changes necessary for tumorigenic conversion were to accumulate in an adult cell without loss or gain of life span potential, then this cell could grow to form a tumor of 16,354 cells (14 doublings or 2^{14} cells) to 5.4×10^8 cells (29 doublings or 2^{29} cells). It is estimated that a tumor formed after 30 cell doublings would be approximately 1 cm^2 in size. Interestingly, Paraskeva and coworkers have shown that colon adenomas of < 1 cm^2 in size are rarely capable of indefinite growth *in vitro* whereas cells from adenomas of >1 cm^2 are often immortal[22-24], which suggests that escape from senescence is a requirement for tumor growth beyond a certain size or cell number and is consistent with the hypothesis that cell senescence is a constraint on tumor growth.

DEDICATION

The initial phase of this work, the arduous mapping of chromosome 1 losses in human-hamster cell hybrids, was performed by Dr. Osamu Sugawara. We are sad to report that Dr. Sugawara died of amyloidosis in 1990, and we would like to dedicate this paper to the memory of this special scientist and friend.

REFERENCES

1. Hayflick, H. The cell biology of human aging. *New Engl. J. Med.* 295:1302-1308 (1976).

2. Daniel, C.W., DeOme, K.B., Young, J.T., Blair, P.B., Faulkin, L.J., Jr. The *in vivo* span of normal and preneoplastic mouse mammary glands: a serial transplantation study. *Proc. Natl. Acad. Sci. USA* 61:53-60 (1968).

3. Macieira-Coelho, A. Biology of normal proliferating cells *in vitro*. Relevance for *in vivo* aging. In: Interdisciplinary Topics in Gerontology, Volume 23, ed. by von Hang, H.P. Karger, Basel (1988).

4. Barrett, J.C. and Fletcher, W.F. Cellular and molecular mechanisms of multistep carcinogenesis in cell culture models. In: Barrett, J.C. (ed.) Mechanisms of Environmental Carcinogenesis: Multistep Models of Carcinogenesis. Volume II. CRC Press, Boca Raton, 1987.

5. Sager, R. Genetic suppression of tumor formation: a new frontier in cancer research. *Cancer Research* 46:1573-1580 (1986).

6. Pereira-Smith, O.M.; Smith, J.R. Genetic analysis of indefinite division in human cells: Identification of four complementation groups. *Proc. Natl. Acad. Sci. USA* 85:6043-6046 (1988).

7. Sugawara, O., Oshimura, M., Koi, M., Annab, L. and Barrett, J.C. Induction of cellular senescence in immortalized cells by human chromosome 1. *Science* 247:707-710 (1990).

8. Koi, M. and Barrett, J.C. Loss of tumor-suppressive function during chemically induced neoplastic progression of Syrian hamster embryo cells. *Proc. Natl. Acad. Sci. USA* 83:5992-5996 (1986).

9. Klein, C.B., Conway, K., Wang, X.W., Bhamra, R.K., Lin, X., Cohen, M.D., Annab, L., Barrett, J.C. and Costa, M. Senescence of nickel-transformed cells by a mammalian X chromosome: Possible epigenetic control. *Science* (in press, 1991).

10. Koi, M., Morita, H., Yamada, H., Satoh, H., Barrett, J.C. and Oshimura, M. Normal human chromosome 11 suppresses tumorigenicity of human cervical tumor cell line SiHa. *Molecular Carcinogenesis* 2:12-21 (1989).

11. Lee, H.-H., Shew, J.-Y., Hong, F.D., Shery, T.W., Domoso, L.A., Young, L.-J., Bookstein, R. and Lee, E. Y.-H. P. The retinoblastoma susceptibility gene encodes a nuclear phosphoprotein associated with DNA binding activity. *Nature* 329:642-645 (1987).

12. Zu, H.-J., Hu, S.-X., Hashimoto, T., Takahashi, R. and Benedict, W.F. The retinoblastoma susceptibility gene product: a characteristic pattern in normal and abnormal expression in malignant cells. *Oncogene* 4:807-812 (1989).

13. Friend, S. H., Horowitz, J.M., Gerber, M.R., Wang, X.-F., Bogenmann, E., Li, F.P. and Weinberg, R.A. Deletions of a DNA sequence in retinoblastomas

and mesenchymal tumors: organization of the sequence and its encoded protein. *Proc. Natl. Acad. Sci. USA* 84:9059-9063 (1987).

14. Weichselbaum, R. R., Beckett, M. and Diamond, A. Some retinoblastomas, osteosarcomas, and soft tissue sarcomas may share a common etiology. *Proc. Natl. Acad. Sci. USA* 85:2106-2109 (1988).

15. Lee, E.Y.-H.P., To, H., Shew, Y.-Y., Bookstein, R., Scully, P. and Lee, W.-H. Inactivation of the retinoblastoma susceptibility gene in human breast cancers. *Science* 241:218-221 (1988).

16. Harbour, J. W., Lai, S.-L., Whang-Peng, J., Gazdar, A.F., Minna, .D. and Haye, F.J. Abnormalities in structure and expression of the human etinoblastoma gene in SCLC. *Science* 241:353-357 (1988).

17. T'Ang, A., Varley, J.M., Chakraborty, S., Murphree, A.L. and Fung, Y.-K.T. Structural rearrangement of the retinoblastoma gene in human breast carcinoma. *Science* 242:263-266 (1988).

18. Stratton, M.R., Williams, S., Fisher, C., Ball, A., Westbury, G., Gusterson, B.A., Fletcher, C.D.M., Knight, J.C., Fung, Y.-K., Reeves, B.R. and Cooper, C.S. Structural alterations in the Rb1 gene in human soft tissue tumours. *Br. J. Cancer* 60:202-205 (1989).

19. DeCaprio, J. A., Ludlow, J.W., Lynch, D., Furukawa, Y., Griffin, J., Piwnica-Worms, H., Huang, C.-M. and Livingston, D.M. The product of the retinoblastoma susceptibility gene has properties of a cell cycle regulatory element. *Cell* 58:1085-1095 (1989).

20. Chen, P.-L., Scully, P., Shew, J.-Y., Wang, J.Y.J. and Lee, W.-H. Phosphorylation of the retinoblastoma gene product is modulated during the cell cycle and cellular differentiation. *Cell* 58:1193-1198 (1989).

21. Buchkovich, K., Duffy, L.A. and Harlow, E. The retinoblastoma protein is phosphorylated during specific phases of the cell cycle. *Cell* 58:1097-1105 (1989).

22. Mihara, K., Cao, X.-R., Yen, A., Chandler, S., Driscoll, B., Murphree, A.L., T'Ang, A. and Fung, Y.-K.T. Cell cycle-dependent regulation of phosphorylation of the human retinoblastoma gene product. *Science* 246:1300-1303 (1989).

23. Furukawa, Y., DeCaprio, J. A., Freedman, A., Kanakura, Y., Nakamura, M., Ernst, T. J., Livingston, D. M. and Griffin, J. D. Expression and state of phosphorylation of the retinoblastoma susceptibility gene product in cycling

phosphorylation of the retinoblastoma susceptibility gene product in cycling and noncycling human hematopoietic cells. *Proc. Natl. Acad. Sci. USA* 87: 2770-2774 (1990).

24. Futreal, P.A.; and Barrett, J.C. Failure of senescent cells to phosphorylate the Rb protein. *Oncogene* (1991, in press).

25. Shew, J.-Y., Ling, N., Yang, X., Fodstad, O. and Lee. W.-H. Antibodies detecting abnormalities of the retinoblastoma susceptibility gene product (pp110 Rb) in osteosarcomas and synovial sarcomas. *Oncogene Research* 1:205-214 (1989).

26. Bernards, R., Schackleford, G. M., Gerber, M. R., Horowitz, J. M., Friend, S. H., Schartl, M., Bogenmann, E., Rapaport, J. M., McGee, T., Dryja, T.P. and Weinberg, R.A. Structure and expvession of the murine retinoblastoma gene and characterization of its encoded protein. *Proc. Natl. Acad. Sci. USA* 86:6464-6478 (1989).

27. Stein, G. H., Beeson, M. and Gordon, L. Failure to phosphorylate the retinoblastoma gene product in senescent human fibroblasts. *Science* 249:666-669 (1990).

28. Kovacs, G. Abnormalities of chromosome No. 1 in human solid malignant tumours. *Int. J. Cancer* 21:688-694 (1978).

29. Rowley, J.D. Abnormalities of chromosome No. 1: significance in malignant transformation. *Virchows Arch.* 29:139-144 (1978).

30. Brito-Babpulle, V. and Atkin, N.B. Break points in chromosome #1 abnormalities of 218 human neoplasms. *Cancer Genet. Cytogenet.* 4:215-225 (1981).

31. Atkin, N.B. Chromosome 1 aberrations in cancer. *Cancer Genet. Cytogenet.* 1:279-285 (1986).

32. Oláh, E., Balogh, E., Kovács, I. and Kiss, A. Abnormalities of chromosome 1 in relation to human malignant diseases. *Cancer Genet. Cytogenet.* 43:179-194 (1989).

33. Fey, M.F., Hesketh, C., Wainscoat, J.S., Gendler, S. and Thein, S.L. Clonal allele loss in gastrointestinal cancers. *Br. J. Cancer* 59:750-754 (1989).

34. Chen, L.-C., Dollbaum, C. and Smith, H.S. Loss of heterozygosity in chromosome 1q in human breast cancer. *Proc. Natl. Acad. Sci. USA* 86:7204-7207 (1989).

35. Merlo, G.R., Siddiqui, J., Cropp, C.S., Liscia, D.S., Lidereau, R., Callahan, R. and Kufe, D.W. Frequent alteration of the DF3 tumor-associated antigen gene in primary human breast carcinomas. *Cancer Research* 49:6966-6971 (1989).

36. Tiainen, M., Tammilehto, L., Rautonen, J., Tuomi, T., Mattson, K. and Knuutila, S. Chromosomal abnormalities and their correlations with asbestos exposure and survival in patients with mesothelioma. *Br. J. Cancer* 60:618-626 (1989).

37. Paraskeva, C., Harvey, A., Finerty, S. and Powell, S. Possible involvement of chromosome 1 in *in vitro* immortalization: evidence from progression of a human adenoma-derived cell line *in vitro*. *Int. J. Cancer* 43:743-746 (1989).

38. Reichmann, A., Martin, P. and Levin, B. Chromosomes in human large bowel tumors. A study of chromosome #1. *Cancer Genet. Cytogenet.* 12:295-301 (1984).

39. Wright, W. E., Pereira-Smith, O.M. and Shay. J.W. Reversible cellular senescence: implications for immortalization of normal human diploid fibroblasts. *Mol. Cell. Biol.* 9:3088-3092 (1989).

40. DeCaprio, J.A., Ludlow, J.W., Figge, J., Shew, J.-Y., Huang, C.-M., Lee, W.-H., Marsilio, E., Paucha, E. and Livingston, D.M. SV40 Large tumor antigen forms a specific complex with the product of the retinoblastoma susceptibility gene. *Cell* 54:275-283 (1988).

41. Ludlow, J.W., DeCaprio, J.A., Huang, C.-M., Lee, W.-H., Paucha, E. and Livingston, D. M. SV40 Large T antigen binds preferentially to an under phosphorylated member of the retinoblastoma susceptibility gene product family. *Cell* 56:57-65 (1989).

42. Sherwood, S.W., Rush, D., Ellsworth, J.L. and Schimke, R.T. Defining cellular senescence in IMR-90 cells: a flow cytometric analysis. *Proc. Natl. Acad. Sci. USA* 85:9086-9090 (1988).

43. Draetta, G. Cell cycle control in eukaryotes: molecular mechanisms of cdc2 activation. *TIBS* 15:378-383 (1990).

44. Moreno, S. and Nurse, P. Substrates for p34cdc2: in vivo veritas? *Cell* 61:549-551 (1990).

45. D'Urso, G., Marraccino, R.L., Marshak, D.R. and Roberts, J.M. Cell cycle control of DNA replication by a homologue from human cells of the p34cdc2 protein kinase. *Science* 250:786-791 (1990).

46. Cisek, L.J. and Corden, J.L. Phosphorylation of RNA polymerase by the murine homologue of the cell-cycle control protein cdc2. *Nature* 339:679-684 (1989).

47. Sturzbecher, H.-W., Maimets, T., Chumakov, P., Brain, R., Addison, C., Simanis, V., Rudge, K. and Philip, R., Grimaldi, M., Court, W. and Jenkins, J.R. p53 Interacts with $p34^{cdc2}$ in mammalian cells: implications for cell cycle control and oncogenesis. *Oncogene* 5:795-801 (1990).

48. Lee, M. and Nurse, P. Cell cycle control genes in fission yeast and mammalian cells. *TIG* 4:287-290 (1988).

49. Harley, C.B., Futcher, A.B. and Greider, C.W. Telomeres shorten during ageing of human fibroblasts. *Nature* 345:458-460 (1990).

50. Hastie, N.D., Dempster, M., Dunlop, M.G., Thompson, A.M., Green, D.K. and Allshire, R.C. Telomere reduction in human colorectal carcinoma and with ageing. *Nature* 346:866-868 (1990).

51. Hayflick, L. Antecedents of cell aging research. *Exp. Gerontol.* 24:355-365 (1989).

52. Paraskeva,C., Finarty, S. and Powell, S. Immortalization of a human colorectal adenoma cell line by continuous *in vitro* paasage: possible involvement of chromosome 1 in tumour progression. *Int. J. Cancer* 41:908-912 (1988).

53. Paraskeva, C, Finarty, S., Mountford, R.A. and Powell, S.C. Specific cytogenetic abnormalities in two new human colorectal adenoma-derived epithelial cell lines. *Cancer Res.* 49:1282-1286 (1989).

54. Paraskeva, C., Harvey, A., Finarty, S. and Powell, S. Possible involvement of chromosome 1 in in vitro immortalization: evidence from progression of a human adenoma-derived cell line *in vitro*. *Int. J. Cancer* 43:743-746 (1989).

A SINGLE GENE CHANGE CAN EXTEND YEAST LIFE SPAN: THE ROLE OF *RAS* IN CELLULAR SENESCENCE

S. Michal Jazwinski, James B. Chen, and Jiayan Sun

Department of Biochemistry and Molecular Biology
Louisiana State University Medical Center
New Orleans, LA 70112

ABSTRACT

The budding yeast *Saccharomyces cerevisiae* has a limited life span (reproductive capacity), which is measured by the number of times an individual cell divides. There is evidence for the involvement of a senescence factor that affects cell cycle traversal in older yeast cells. Distinct alterations in the abundance of a handful of transcripts have been identified during the life span of this organism, and the genes that specify these mRNAs have been cloned. This raises the question whether the activity of one or more genes can alter the yeast life span. Indeed, the controlled expression of the transforming gene of Harvey murine sarcoma virus (v-Ha-*ras*) was found to extend the life span nearly two-fold. The normal homologs of this oncogene, *RAS*1 and *RAS*2, play a central role in the integration of cell growth and the cell cycle in yeast. Expression of v-Ha-*ras* appears to impinge on this integration. We suggest that it is the relative levels of the senescence factor and the Ras protein that determine whether a cell ceases to divide and senesces. We liken the senescence factor to the product of an anti-oncogene or tumor suppressor gene that neutralizes Ras.

INTRODUCTION

There are several points in the cell cycle at which control may be exerted. In yeast, a microbial eukaryote, there is evidence for coordination of successive cell cycles, understood as the dependence of certain events in the current cell cycle on

The Underlying Molecular, Cellular, and Immunological Factors in Cancer and Aging, Edited by S.S. Yang and H.R.Warner, Plenum Press, New York, 1993

events in previous cell cycles and not merely as a requirement for cytokinesis (Pringle and Hartwell, 1981). In a mortal cell with a finite life span (reproductive capacity), this may be the essence of the aging process. With regard to budding yeast, this statement seems paradoxical, because one can passage a yeast culture indefinitely. The resolution of this dilemma lies in the fact that yeast divide asymmetrically by budding. The yeast cell (mother) can divide many times, becoming one generation older at each division. The bud or daughter also has this capacity, but it starts from scratch. The finite nature of this process was first shown by Mortimer and Johnston (1959). Thus, the individual yeast cell is mortal, even though the culture is immortal.

Information concerning the aging and senescence of *S. cerevisiae* has been reviewed recently (Jazwinski, 1990; Jazwinski, 1990a). It is clear that yeast undergo a variety of morphological and physiological changes with increasing buddings (reproductive age). Therefore, it is appropriate to speak of an aging process in this organism. Notably, the mortality rate of yeast cells increases exponentially with age (Pohley, 1987; Jazwinski et al., 1989) similarly to what is observed in higher organisms, including humans. Studies in yeast and in other systems suggest an intimate relationship between the cell cycle and cellular life span (Jazwinski, 1990; Jazwinski, 1990a). To depict this relationship, we have proposed the Cell Spiral Model (Jazwinski et al., 1989; Jazwinski et al., 1990; Jazwinski, 1990). In this model, individual cell cycles are not isolated throughout the life span, but rather they are connected in a downward spiral that reflects the aging process. The successive cell cycles are coordinated up and down this spiral, indicating the operation of a "molecular memory". As in other systems, the senescent phenotype is a dominant feature in yeast (Egilmez and Jazwinski, 1989). Evidence has been accumulated for a senescence factor that arrests normal mammalian cells at the G_1/S boundary of the cell cycle at the limits of their population doubling capacity in culture (Smith, 1990). A similar senescence factor appears to be operative in yeast cells (Egilmez and Jazwinski, 1989), and the importance of the G_1/S boundary for determining the life span in this organism has been demonstrated (Jazwinski et al., 1989; Jazwinski et al., 1990). Using a differential hybridization approach, we have cloned six genes that are differentially expressed during the yeast life span (Egilmez et al., 1989). Five of these are young cell-specific and one is old cell-specific, and our results indicate that aging in yeast does not involve random alterations in gene expression. Among these genes, perhaps, we will find the senescence factor gene.

CONTROLLED EXPRESSION OF *RAS* IN YEAST EXTENDS LIFE SPAN

The demonstration of alterations in gene activity during the life span of yeast raises the question whether the converse is true; namely, can a change in the activity of one or more genes alter the yeast life span. To examine this question, we have chosen to express the transforming gene of Harvey murine sarcoma virus, v-Ha-*ras*, in yeast cells (Chen et al., 1990). This gene was chosen because yeast possess two normal homologs of *ras*, called *RAS*1 and *RAS*2 (Gibbs and Marshall, 1989). The v-Ha-*ras* oncogene was placed under the control of the galactose-inducible yeast promoter *GAL*10 by subcloning portions of the Harvey murine sarcoma virus genome spanning *ras* (Fig. 1) from the plasmid HB11 (Ellis et al., 1981) into the yeast shuttle vector pBM150 (Johnston and Davis, 1984). This construction enables the stable

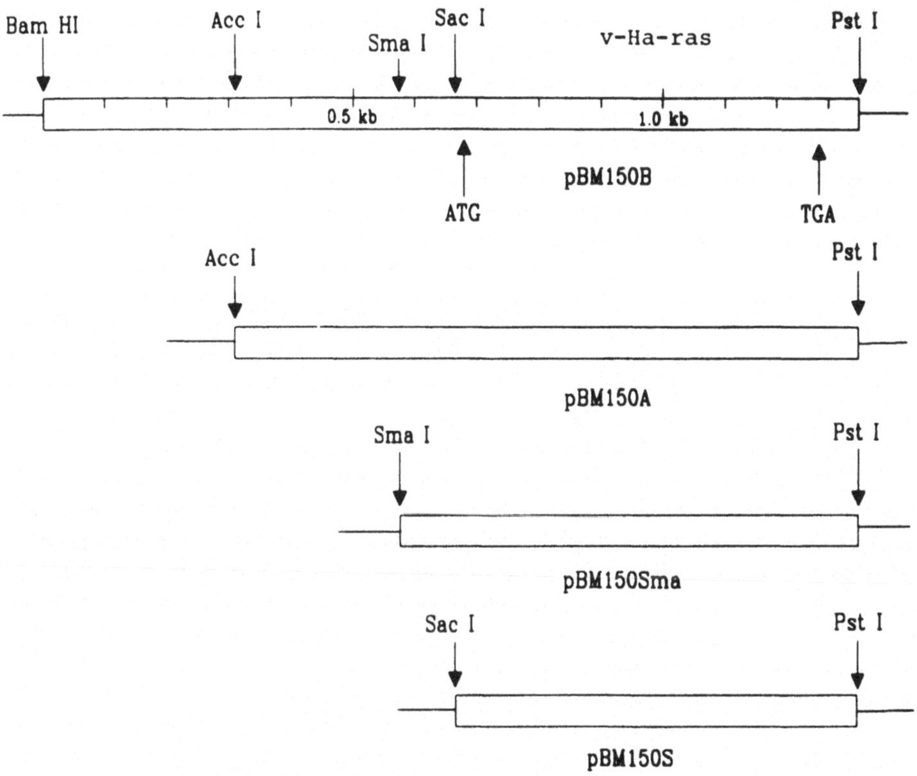

Fig. 1. *Construction of* v-Ha-*ras expression plasmids.*
Various restriction fragments derived from Harvey murine sarcoma virus DNA that span the transforming gene v-Ha-*ras* were inserted into the yeast shuttle vector pBM150 behind the *GAL*10 transcription start site using standard recombinant DNA techniques (Ausubel et al., 1989). All of these fragments shared a common *Pst*I site downstream of the TGA translational stop codon of *ras*. The fragments differed in the length of viral DNA upstream of the ATG start codon of *ras*, and they were obtained by digestion with different restriction enzymes: *Bam*HI, *Acc*I, *Sma*I and *Sac*I in the case of pBM150B, pBM150A, pBM150Sma and pBM150S, respectively. The restriction fragments were filled in by the Klenow fragment of *Escherichia coli* DNA polymerase I, *Eco*RI linkers were added with T4 DNA ligase, and then they were ligated into the *EcoR*I site of pBM150.

maintenance of v-Ha-*ras* in the yeast cell in single copy and its induction by the addition of galactose to the growth medium. As indicated in Fig. 1, several constructs were made that differed in the length of Harvey murine sarcoma virus DNA upstream of *ras*.

The induced levels of v-Ha-*ras* mRNA were determined by Northern blot analysis after transformation of yeast cells with the various constructs, as well as with pBM150 plasmid DNA as a control (data not shown). Significant levels of v-Ha-*ras* mRNA were detected upon induction of cells transformed with pBM150S. Interestingly, in cells transformed by pBM150A, these mRNA levels were approximately 5-fold lower. The v-Ha-*ras* mRNA levels expressed in cells transformed by pBM150Sma and pBM150B were similar to those detected in pBM150S- and pBM150A-transformed cells, respectively. The difference in v-Ha-*ras* mRNA levels found in cells transformed by pBM150A and pBM150S was reflected by the v-*ras* protein levels, as determined in immunoblot experiments (data not shown). It is not clear at present how the excess Harvey murine sarcoma virus DNA upstream of v-Ha-*ras* in pBM150A and pBM150B leads to a reduction in v-Ha-*ras* mRNA.

The effect of induced expression of v-Ha-*ras* on yeast life span was determined in cells transformed by the various plasmids (Fig. 2). The expression of v-Ha-*ras* from both pBM150A and pBM150B resulted in a substantial extension of yeast longevity. For pBM150A, an approximately 70% extension of both mean and maximum life span of individual yeast cells was observed as compared to control cells transformed by pBM150 alone. Interestingly, the 5-fold higher levels of expression in cells transformed by pBM150S abrogated this prolongation of yeast life span. Similarly, cells expressing v-Ha-*ras* from pBM150Sma showed no extension of life span (data not shown). The effects of v-Ha-*ras* expression on yeast life span presented in Fig. 2 were observed in several separate experiments with individually transformed sets of cells. Thus, appropriately controlled expression of v-Ha-*ras* leads to a near doubling of not only the life expectancy but also the yeast life span. It should be noted that the yeast cell is at the same time the intact yeast organism.

ROLE OF *RAS* IN YEAST LONGEVITY

The lack of life span extension in cells expressing higher levels of v-Ha-*ras* (Fig. 2) was surprising. One possibility was that the higher levels of v-Ha-*ras* in pBM150S and pBM150Sma transformants decreased cell viability. However, exponentially growing cells in which v-Ha-*ras* expression was induced by the addition of galactose to the growth medium displayed virtually identical viability throughout the logarithmic and stationary phases of growth regardless of the level of oncogene expression (data not shown).

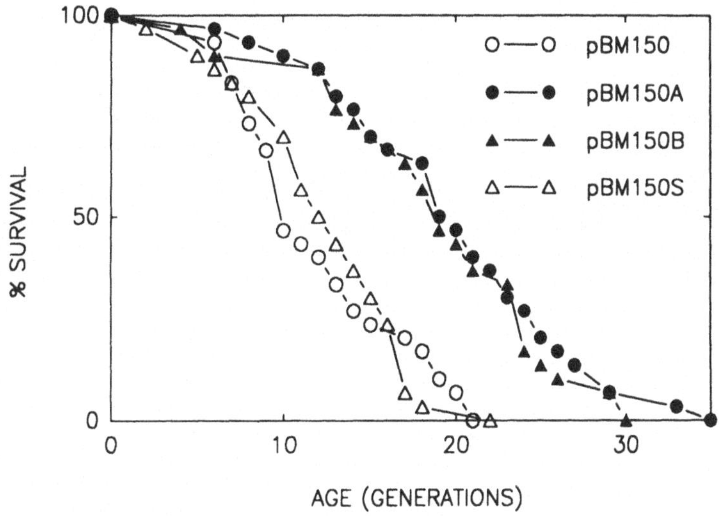

Fig. 2. *Extension of life span by* v-Ha-*ras*.
S. cerevisiae SP1 (*MAT*a, *leu*2, *ura*3, *trp*1, *ade*8, *can*1, *his*3, *gal*2) was transformed separately by the various plasmids indicated by the procedure of Ito et al. (1983). Transformants were selected by their ability to grow on medium lacking uracil, which is conferred by the *URA*3 gene in pBM150. Reproductive life spans of individual cells of each of the transformants were determined on medium containing galactose, but lacking glucose which represses the *GAL*10 promoter, as described previously (Egilmez and Jazwinski, 1989). Individual cells were observed microscopically, and their buds were removed at maturity by micromanipulation. With each budding the mother cell was counted one generation older. Each life span determination was initiated with a newborn daughter cell. The differences between the mean life spans of pBM150 and pBM150S transformants were not significant. However, the differences between the mean life spans of cells transformed by pBM150A and pBM150 and between pBM150B and pBM150 were highly significant ($P << 0.0005$).

Another possibility is the existence of a homeostatic mechanism in yeast that downregulates the signal generated by increased levels of *RAS* expression leading to a secondary response of growth arrest similar to that observed in mammalian cells (Hirakawa and Ruley, 1988). The yeast *RAS* genes are highly pleiotropic and occupy a central role in the integration of cell growth and metabolism with the cell cycle (Gibbs and Marshall, 1989). *RAS*1 and *RAS*2 are part of the A complex of START, a point in the G_1 phase of the yeast cell cycle associated with commitment to cell division (Pringle and Hartwell, 1981). The *RAS*2 gene plays a particularly crucial role in the control of cell size (Baroni et al., 1989). Therefore, the effect of v-Ha-*ras* expression on cell size during the life span was examined (Fig. 3). Regardless of whether v-Ha-*ras* expression was high as in pBM150S transformants or low as in pBM150A and pBM150B transformants, there was a striking increase in cell volume early in the life span, as compared to control cells transformed with pBM150 alone. Thus, increased cell size did not always correlate with an extended life span, and the cell size-enhancement effect of *ras* could be uncoupled from its stimulatory effect on cell cycling that results in an extended life span. Inasmuch as increased size of the cell might indicate a higher cellular metabolic rate, these results suggest that the rate of metabolism or metabolic "wear-and-tear" is not likely a major factor in limiting the life span.

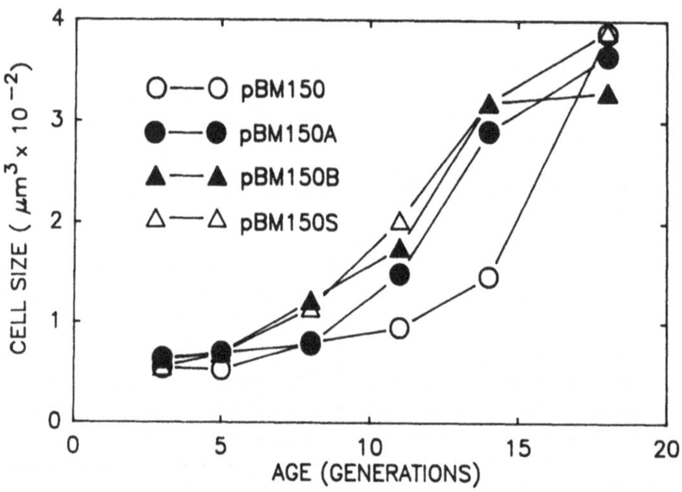

Fig. 3. *Increase in size of cells expressing v-Ha-ras.*
Cell size during the life span of transformants was determined microscopically (Egilmez et al., 1990) by measuring the major and minor axes of the cell and calculating the volume of a prolate ellipsoid. The means of measurements for 4 to 8 cells were used for each age indicated.

RAS plays a central role in cell growth and in cell division in yeast (Fig. 4). It is, in a hitherto unknown manner, involved in sensing the nutritional status of the cell (Gibbs and Marshall, 1989). *RAS* exerts its effects along at least two pathways (Gibbs and Marshall, 1989). It either stimulates adenylate cyclase and thus protein

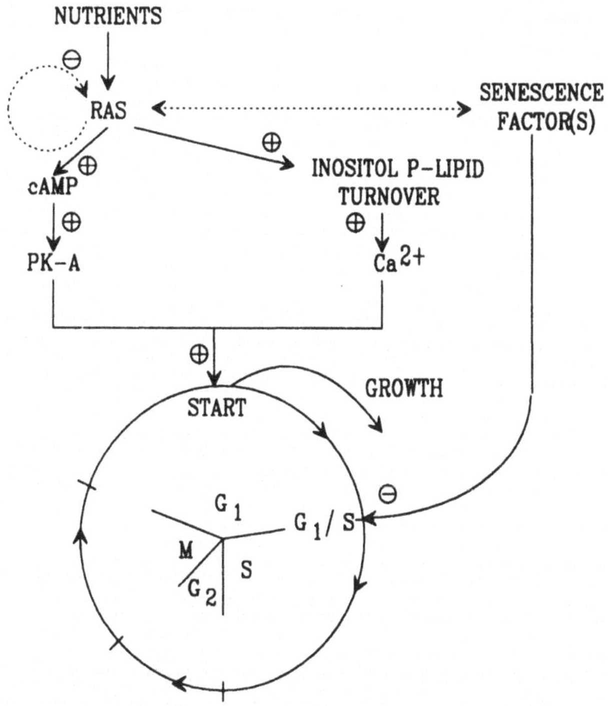

Fig. 4. *Proposed mechanism of yeast life span determination by the relative levels of* Ras *and senescence factor.*
Full description is in the text. Stimulation or activation is indicated by "+", while inhibition or downregulation by "-".

kinase A, or it stimulates inositol phospholipid turnover and calcium flux. Our observations indicate that the life span-extending effect of v-Ha-*ras* is mediated through a cAMP pathway, although some role of phospholipid turnover has not been ruled out (Sun and Jazwinski, unpublished results). In any case, the ultimate effects of *RAS* are traversal of START in the G_1 phase of the cell cycle and cell growth. Our studies indicate that these effects can be uncoupled, and we suggest that the cell cycle-stimulatory signal generated by *RAS* can be downregulated. As stated earlier, there is evidence for a senescence factor that arrests senescent cells at the G_1/S boundary of the cell cycle. We have proposed earlier that it is the relative levels of Ras and of the senescence factor that determine yeast life span (Jazwinski, 1990). The life span-extending effects of v-Ha-*ras* presented here are consistent with this hypothesis. In this case, *ras* is the oncogene and the senescence factor gene would be the anti-oncogene. Further studies will allow us to determine whether the interaction between Ras and the senescence factor is direct or indirect.

ACKNOWLEDGMENTS

This work was supported by grants from the National Institute on Aging of the National Institutes of Health and by the American Federation for Aging Research (AFAR), Inc.

REFERENCES

Ausubel, F.M., Brent, R., Kingston, R.E., Moore, D.D., Seidman, J.G., Smith, J.A., and Struhl, K., ed. Current Protocols in Molecular Biology, Volumes 1 and 2, Greene Publishing Associates and Wiley-Interscience, New York (1989).

Baroni, M.D., Martegani, E., Monti, P., and Alberghina, L. Cell size modulation by *CDC25* and *RAS2* genes in *Saccharomyces cerevisiae. Molec. Cell. Biol.* 9:2715 (1989).

Chen, J.B., Sun, J., and Jazwinski, S.M. Prolongation of the yeast life span by the v-Ha-*ras* oncogene. *Molec. Microbial.* 4:2081 (1990).

Egilmez, N.K., and Jazwinski, S.M. Evidence for the involvement of a cytoplasmic factor in the aging of the yeast *Saccharomyces cerevisiae. J. Bacteriol.* 171:37 (1989).

Egilmez, N.K., Chen, J.B., and Jazwinski, S.M. Specific alterations in transcript prevalence during the yeast life span. *J. Biol. Chem.* 264:14312 (1989).

Egilmez, N.K., Chen, J.B., and Jazwinski, S.M. Preparation and partial characterization of old yeast cells. *J. Gerontol. Biol: Sci.* 45:B9 (1990).

Ellis, R.W., DeFeo, D., Shih, T.Y., Gonda, M.A., Young, H.A., Tsuchida, N., Lowy, D.R., and Scolnick, E.M. The p21 *src* genes of Harvey and Kirsten sarcoma viruses originate from divergent members of a family of normal vertebrate genes. *Nature* 292:506 (1981).

Gibbs, J.B., and Marshall, M.S. The *ras* oncogene - an important regulatory element in lower eucaryotic organisms. *Microbiol. Rev.* 53:171 (1989).

Hirakawa, T., and Ruley, H.E. Rescue of cells from *ras* oncogene-induced growth arrest by a second, complementing, oncogene. *Proc. Natl. Acad. Sci. U.S.A.* 85:1519 (1988).

Ito, H., Fukuda, Y., Murata, K., and Kimura, A. Transformation of intact yeast cells treated with alkali cations. *J. Bacteriol.* 153:163 (1983).

Jazwinski, S.M. Aging and senescence of the budding yeast *Saccharomyces cerevisiae*. *Molec. Microbiol.* 4:337 (1990).

Jazwinski, S.M. An experimental system for the molecular analysis of the aging process: The budding yeast *Saccharomyces cerevisiae. J. Gerontol. Biol. Sci.* 45:B68 (1990a).

Jazwinski, S.M., Egilmez, N.K., and Chen, J.B. Replication control and cellular life span. *Exp. Gerontol.* 24:423 (1989).

Jazwinski, S.M., Chen, J.B., and Jeansonne, N.E. Replication control and differential gene expression in aging yeast. In: The Molecular Biology of Aging. ed. by C.E. Finch and T.E. Johnson, Wiley-Liss, New York (1990).

Johnston, M. and Davis, R.W. Sequences that regulate the divergent *GAL*1-*GAL*10 promoter in *Saccharomyces cerevisiae Molec. Cell. Biol.* 4:1440 (1984).

Mortimer, R.K. and Johnston, J.R. Life span of individual yeast cells. *Nature* 183:1751 (1959).

Pohley, H.-J. A formal mortality analysis for populations of unicellular organisms *(Saccharomyces cerevisiae). Mech. Ageing Dev.* 38:231 (1987).

Pringle, J.R., and Hartwell, L.H. The *Saccharomyces cerevisiae* cell cycle. In: The Molecular Biology of the Yeast *Saccharomyces*: Life Cycle and Inheritance. ed. by J.N. Strathern, E.W. Jones, and J.R. Broach, Cold Spring Harbor Laboratory, Cold Spring Harbor (1981).

Smith, J.R. DNA synthesis inhibitors in cellular senescence, *J. Gerontol. Biol. Sci.* 45:B32 (1990).

A COMPARISON OF THE PROPERTIES OF HUMAN P53 MUTANT ALLELES

Robin S. Quartin and Arnold J. Levine

Department of Molecular Biology
Princeton University, Princeton, NJ 08544-1014

p53 is a cellular-encoded phosphoprotein first identified in protein complexes with the large tumor (T) antigen of simian virus 40 (SV40) (Linzer and Levine, 1979; Lane and Crawford, 1979). High levels of p53 protein have been detected in both embryonal carcinoma cells and chemically induced transformed cells using antisera from animals with SV40-induced tumors or immunized with these tumorigenic lines (Linzer and Levine, 1979; DeLeo *et al.*, 1979). In addition, humans with cancer have been shown to have circulating anti-p53 antibodies (Crawford *et al.*, 1982; Caron de Fromental *et al.*, 1987). Thus, p53 was termed a tumor antigen.

While normal, non-transformed cells have been shown to express very low levels of p53 (Dippold *et al.*, 1981; Benchimol *et al.*, 1982; Thomas *et al.*, 1983; Rogel *et al.*, 1985), many transformed cells isolated from tumors or cell lines transformed by viruses or chemical treatments exhibit high metabolic levels of the protein (Linzer and Levine, 1979; Crawford *et al.*, 1981; Dippold *et al.*, 1981; Benchimol *et al.*, 1982; Rotter, 1983; Thomas et al., 1983; Koeffler *et al.*, 1986). The increased steady-state levels of p53 have been attributed to an increase in protein stability (Oren *et al.*, 1981; Reich *et al.*, 1983). The half-life of p53 in normal, non-transformed cells ranges from 6 to 20 minutes (Oren *et al.*, 1981; Reich *et al.*, 1983; Rogel *et al.*, 1985), whereas the protein is stable for many hours in transformed cells (Oren *et al.*, 1981; Reich *et al.*, 1983; Jenkins *et al.*, 1985).

A number of observations led to the original designation of p53 as an oncogene. Genomic and cDNA clones of murine p53 analyzed in transformation assays were found to cooperate with the activated (mutant) oncogene Ha-*ras* to transform cultured cells (Eliyahu *et al.*, 1984; Parada *et al.*, 1984). High levels of p53 alone resulted in cellular immortalization (Jenkins *et al.*, 1984; Rovinski and Benchimol, 1988).

The Underlying Molecular, Cellular, and Immunological Factors in Cancer and Aging, Edited by S.S. Yang and H.R.Warner, Plenum Press, New York, 1993

An oncogenic role for p53 was, however, in conflict with a series of other findings that suggested that mutation or inactivation of the p53 gene is required for transformation or tumor formation. Several Friend virus-induced murine erythroleukemic cell lines have p53 gene deletions (Mowat *et al.*, 1985; Chow *et al.*, 1987; Rovinski *et al.*, 1987; Munroe *et al.*, 1988; Ben-David *et al.*, 1988). Many leukemias of the myeloid lineage lack expression of p53 (Wolf and Rotter, 1985), and gross rearrangements in the p53 gene have been detected in humans with chronic myelogenous leukemia (Kelman *et al.*, 1989; Ahuja *et al.*, 1989). p53 allelic deletions and gene mutations have been found in human colorectal carcinomas (Baker *et al.*, 1989; Nigro *et al.*, 1989), osteogenic sarcomas (Masuda *et al.*, 1987), tumors of the lung (Takahashi *et al.*, 1989; Nigro *et al.*, 1989; Iggo *et al.*, 1990) brain and breast (Nigro *et al.*, 1989). Recently, a number of human germ-line p53 mutations have been identified that predispose family members to a variety of cancers (Malkin *et al.*, 1990).

The apparent contradictions were resolved when it was found that the p53 DNA clones that had been shown to immortalize cells and to cooperate with the *ras* oncogene to transform cells were all mutant p53 DNA clones. The wild-type p53 gene did not have these biological activities (Finlay *et al.*, 1988; Eliyahu, *et al.*, 1988; Hinds *et al.*, 1989a). Wild-type p53 has been further shown to suppress the cooperative transformation potential of ElA protein (from adenovirus) and *ras*, or of mutant p53 and *ras* (Finlay *et al.*, 1989; Eliyahu *et al.*, 1989). Transformed cell lines derived from such experiments either failed to express the p53 protein or expressed high levels of a mutant protein, suggesting that expression of wild-type p53 is antithetical to the transformation process (Finlay *et al.*, 1989). Mutations that activate the protein in these transformation assays lie within the region of amino acid residues 118-307 (Levine, *et al.*, 1989; Levine, 1990) in a protein that is 390 (murine) to 393 (human) amino acids in length.

The p53 protein may normally function to regulate cellular proliferation. Increases in p53 expression have been correlated with the cell cycle G_0- to S-phase transition (Milner and Milner, 1981; Mercer *et al.*, 1982; Reich and Levine, 1984; Lalande, 1990). Microinjection of p53-specific antibodies into cells blocked entry into S-phase (Mercer *et al.*, 1982; 1984). Expression of p53 antisense RNA has been shown to decrease cell division (Shohat *et al.*, 1987). The expression of transfected wild-type murine p53 had little or no effect upon the plating efficiency of non-transformed fibroblast cells, but inhibited foci formation of transformed cells (Finlay, *et al.*, 1989). The introduction of wild-type human p53 DNA into human tumor cell lines dramatically inhibits their growth (Baker *et al.*, 1990; Diller *et al.*, 1990; Mercer *et al.*, 1990).

Further support for the role of wild-type p53 as a tumor or growth suppressor protein is evidenced by the formation of stable complexes of p53 with various viral transformation proteins: T antigen from SV40 (Lane and Crawford, 1979; Linzer and Levine, 1979), ElB 55kd protein from adenovirus (Sarnow *et al.*, 1982), and E6 protein from human papilloma virus type 16 or 18 (Werness *et al.*, 1990). It has been proposed that complex formation with viral oncoproteins inactivates or alters the growth-suppressive function of p53 (Finlay *et al.*, 1989). Similarly, mutant p53 proteins may inhibit wild-type p53 activity through an inactivating complex. Such oligomeric complex formation has been demonstrated between mutant and wild-type p53 proteins expressed in transformed cells (Rovinski and Benchimol, 1988; Eliyahu *et al.*, 1988; Finlay *et al.*, 1989). Thus, a lack of functional p53 due to a loss of expression or inactivation through complex formation apparently confers a selective advantage for cell growth and tumorigenesis.

Analyses of the p53 genes of human colorectal carcinomas have shown that 75% of these tumors have lost one allele of the p53 gene (Baker *et al.*, 1989), and the remaining allele has suffered a missense point mutation (Nigro *et al.*, 1989). These mutations are distributed between amino acid residues 118-307, and the majority of these mutations coincide with the four most evolutionarily conserved regions of the gene defined by amino acid residues 111-136, 165-175, 230-252, 264-280 (Soussi *et al.*, 1987). Residues 175, 248, 273 and 281 represent mutational "hot spots" in p53 (Hinds, *et al.*, 1990).

A model to explain the role of mutant p53 in tumor progression proposes that initially one allele in one cell acquires a point mutation leading to the expression of an activated mutant protein that binds to and sequesters the wild-type protein (Finlay *et al.*, 1989). This cell then has a growth advantage over neighboring cells, thus increasing the probability that deletion of a wild-type allele will occur in a mutant-expressing cell. The fact that many tumors only retain a mutant allele suggests that the mutant protein may not completely dominate the wild-type protein, and that the loss of the wild-type allele confers a fully neoplastic phenotype. The predominance of missense mutants further suggests that the mutant protein has a distinct tumor-promoting function. It is apparent that a series of accumulated genetic alterations promotes normal cells to progress through a number of clinically defined stages to metastasis. Although mutation and alteration of the p53 gene is certainly not common to all types of tumors (various pathways of accumulated somatic changes may lead to a cancerous state), mutation at the p53 locus is believed to be a late event in tumorigenesis (Fearon and Vogelstein, 1990).

The tumor progression model predicts that the p53 missense proteins found in colon carcinomas should confer a growth advantage to recipient cells in culture. In co-transfection assays, human mutant p53 DNA clones were tested and compared with wild-type p53 for their ability to cooperate with an activated *ras* oncogene (which is itself unable to transform cells) to transform rat embryo fibroblasts (REF). The clones contained missense mutations at the following amino acid residues: 143

(valine to alanine), 175 (arginine to histidine), 273 (arginine to histidine) and 281 (aspartic acid to glycine). The amino acid 143 mutant clone (p53-c143A) was a cDNA, the remaining clones (p53-175H, p53-273H and p53-281G) all contained the second, third and fourth introns from the human p53 gene; all clones were under the control of the human cytomegalovirus promoter-enhancer (Hinds *et al.*, 1990).

The results of the transformation assays are detailed in Table 1. Relative transformation frequencies reflect the average number of transformed foci resulting per co-transfection experiment. The cDNA (p53-cWT) and the intron-containing (p53-WT) wild-type p53 clones did not cooperate with *ras* to produce foci above the level of *ras*-only transfections. Furthermore, no permanent cell lines could be cloned from the few foci obtained from transfections with p53-WT plus *ras*.

TABLE 1. Human p53 DNA Clones Tested in Transformation Assay with *ras*

Mutant residue	Relative transformation frequency	Cloning efficiency (%)	1/2 life protein	hsc70 bound
cWT[a]	0	5	20 min.	--
143A	1.6	22	1.5-2 hrs.	+
WT[b]	0	0	ND[c]	ND
175H	11.5	58	3.6-6.4 hrs.	+
273H	4.7	30	7 hrs.	--
281G	1.9	20	1.4 hrs.	--

[a]Wild-type sequence as defined by three independent studies (Zakut-Houri *et al.*, 1985; Matlashewski *et al.*, 1984; Lamb *et al.*, 1986).
[b]The DNA clones in the bottom of the table contained the second, third and fourth introns from the p53 gene.
[c]ND - not determined.

All four human missense mutant clones cooperated with activated *ras* to transform REF. The relatively low transformation frequency for p53-c143A plus *ras* transfections may be due to the lack of introns in this clone. Focus formation efficiency and cell line establishment were previously found to be higher for murine mutant p53 constructs containing introns than for their cDNA counterparts (Hinds *et al.*, 1989).

p53-175H was the most efficient transforming DNA clone, 6-fold more efficient than p53-281G and about 2.5-fold more effective than p53-273H. These differences in relative efficiencies of transformation were reproducible and significant.

The proteins expressed in the cloned, transformed lines were examined to further investigate the role of the mutant clones in the transformation process. The cell lines derived from p53-c143A plus *ras* and from p53-175H plus *ras* transfections expressed high levels of human p53 that formed tight complexes with both the endogenous wild-type rat p53 and the constitutively expressed heat shock protein hsc70, as had been shown for many activated murine p53 mutant proteins (Hinds *et al.*, 1987; Pinhasi-Kimhi *et al.*, 1986; Sturzbecher *et al.*, 1987).

The cell lines derived from p53-273H plus *ras* and from p53-281G plus *ras* transfections also expressed high levels of human p53 that complexed with the endogenous rat protein, but no interactions between either mutant p53 protein and the hsc70 protein were detected. These results indicate that interaction with the rat hsc70 is dependent upon the type of mutation, and that hsc70 binding is not a strict requirement for p53 activation. Additionally, half-life analyses indicated that all four mutant proteins had extended metabolic stabilities. The single line derived from a *ras* plus p53-cWT focus expressed a protein with characteristics of endogenous wild-type p53 in that the protein was found at low levels, possessed a short half-life, and did not associate with hsc70. Some other secondary event may have occurred to complement mutant *ras* in this cell line.

These results demonstrate that several of the human p53 mutants identified in colorectal carcinomas can cooperate with the ras oncoprotein to transform primary rat embryo fibroblasts in cell culture. Three of the mutants examined (175H, 273H and 281G) contain "hot spot" mutations. The cell lines transformed by the mutant clones expressed elevated levels of the mutant p53 proteins with extended metabolic stabilities. This is consistent with the high levels of p53 detected by immunohistochemical staining of various tumor tissues (Iggo *et al.*, 1990). The wild-type human p53 does not exhibit these characteristics. These data further support the growth-promoting role of p53 missense mutants in the process of tumorigenesis.

A murine p53 mutant with an amino acid substitution at residue 270 (analogous to 273 in the human protein) has been described that has characteristics similar to those of the 273H and 281G human mutants. Although it possessed an extended metabolic stability and complexed with the wild-type protein, it exhibited decreased transforming activity in the co-transfection assay and did not interact with the hsc70 protein (Halevy *et al.*, 1990).

Missense mutant p53 proteins may affect cell growth through 1) the gain of a new function and 2) the dominant loss of the wild-type, growth suppressor function. The expression of an exogenous mutant p53 protein in a cell line lacking endogenous p53 expression resulted in enhanced tumorigenicity (Wolf *et al.*, 1984). This new growth potential is indicative of a gain of function due to the presence of the mutation. The inactivation of wild-type function through complexes formed between exogenous mutant p53 proteins and endogenous wild-type p53, which often includes the hsc70 protein (Finlay *et al.*, 1989), results in the dominant loss of the normal wild-type function in the cell. The possible association of different mutant alleles with one or more of these functional changes is also suggested by the results of transactivation analyses. In such analyses two murine mutations, that highly activate p53 in the transformation assay, abolished the transactivating potential of the wild-type p53 protein (Raycroft *et al.*, 1990). while the 273H mutant was equivalent to the wild-type in promoting transcription (Fields and Jang, 1990).

There are immunologically defined conformational differences between the various tumor-associated human missense mutants. The epitope of the mutant-specific monoclonal antibody PAb240 is hidden in the properly folded (native) p53 protein, and is only made fully accessible in mutant proteins by certain mutations (Bartek *et al.*, 1990). These conformational differences may correlate with the different biological characteristics exhibited by the mutant p53 proteins. Analyses of murine p53 proteins have shown that the activated mutants that complex with hsc70 lack a conformational epitope recognized by a wild-type, murine-specific antibody (Finlay *et al.*, 1988).

Thus, two classes of p53 missense mutant proteins may be distinguished: mutants, including 175H, that efficiently cooperate with a mutant ras oncoprotein to transform primary cells and that form tight complexes with hsc70; and mutants, including 273H and 281G, that exhibit decreased transforming activities, and do not interact with hsc70.

It will be particularly important to determine the biological significance of these phenotypic differences in vivo, given the various possible backgrounds of activated oncogenes and inactivated suppressor genes in which missense p53 mutant proteins are expressed in tumor cells.

REFERENCES

Ahuja, H., Bar-Eli, M., Advani, S.H., Benchimol, S. and Cline, M.J. Alterations in the p53 gene and the clonal evolution of the blast crisis of chronic myelocytic leukemia. *Proc. Natl. Acad. Sci. U.S.A.* 86:6783, 1989.

Baker, S.J., Fearon, E.R., Nigro, J.M., Hamilton, S.R., Preisinger, A.C., Jessup, J.M., van Tuinen, P., Ledbetter, D.H., Barker, D.F., Nakamura, Y., White, R. and Vogelstein, B. Chromosome 17 deletions and p53 gene mutations in colorectal carcinomas. *Science* 244:217, 1989.

Baker, S.J., Markowitz, S., Fearon, E.R., Wilson, J.K.U., and Vogelstein, B. Suppression of human colorectal carcinoma cell growth by wild-type p53. *Science* 249:912, 1990.

Bartek, J., Iggo, R., Gannon, J., and Lane, D. Genetic and immunological analysis of mutant p53 in human breast cancer cell lines. *Oncogene* 5:893, 1990.

Ben-David, Y., Prideaux, V.R., Chow, V., Benchimol, S. and Bernstein, A. Inactivation of the p53 oncogene by internal deletion or retroviral integration in erythroleukemia cell lines induced by Friend leukemia virus. *Oncogene* 3:179, 1988.

Benchimol, S., Pim, D. and Crawford, L. Radioimmunoassay of the cellular protein p53 in mouse and human cell lines. *EMBO J.* 1:1055, 1982.

Caron de Fromental, C., May-Levin, F., Mouriesse, H., Lemerle, J., Chandrasekaran, K. and May, P. Presence of circulating antibodies against cellular protein p53 in a notable proportion of children with B-cell lymphoma. *Int. J. Cancer* 39:185, 1987.

Chow, V., Ben-David, Y., Bernstein, A., Benchimol, S. and Mowat, M. Multistage Friend erythroleukemia: Independent origin of tumor clones with normal or rearranged p53 cellular oncogene. *J. Virol.* 61:2777, 1987.

Crawford, L.V., Pim, D.C., and Bulbrook, R.D. Detection of antibodies against the cellular protein p53 in sera from patients with breast cancer. *Int. J. Cancer* 30:403, 1982.

DeLeo, A.B., Jay, G., Appella, E., Dubois, G.C., Law, L.W. and Old, L.J. Detection of a transformation related antigen in chemically induced sarcomas and other transformed cells of the mouse. *Proc. Natl. Acad. Sci. USA.* 76:2420, 1979.

Diller, L., Kassel, J., Nelson, C.E., Gryka, M.A., Litwak, G., Gebhardt, M., Bressac, B., Ozturk, M., Baker, S.J., Vogelstein, B., and Friend, S.H. p53 Suppresses the growth of osteosarcoma cells and blocks cell cycle progression. *Mol. Cell. Biol.* 10:5772, 1990.

Dippold, W.G., Jay, G., DeLeo, A.B., Khoury, G. and Old, L.J. p53 transformation-related protein: Detection by monoclonal antibody in mouse and human cells. *Proc. Natl. Acad. Sci. USA* 78:1695, 1981.

Eliyahu, D., Raz, A., Gruss, P., Givol, D. and Oren, M. Participation of p53 cellular tumour antigen in transformation of normal embryonic cells. *Nature* 312:646, 1984.

Eliyahu, D., Goldfinger, N., Pinhasi-Kimhi, 0., Shaulsky, G., Skurnik, Y., Arai, N., Rotter, V. and Oren, M. Meth A fibrosarcoma cells express two transforming mutant p53 species. *Oncogene* 3:313, 1988.

Eliyahu, D., Michalovitz, D., Eliyahu, S., Pinhasi-Kimhi, 0. and Oren, M. Wild-type p53 can inhibit oncogene-mediated focus formation. *Proc. Natl. Acad. Sci. USA* 86:8763, 1989.

Fearon, E.R. and Vogelstein, B. A genetic model for colorectal tumorigenesis. *Cell* 61:759, 1990.

Fields, S. Presence of a potent transcription activating sequence in the p53 protein. *Science* 249:1046, 1990.

Finlay, C.A., Hinds, P.W., Tan, T.-H., Eliyahu, D., Oren, M. and Levine, A.J. Activating mutations for transformation by p53 produce a gene product that forms an hsc70-p53 complex with an altered half-life. *Mol. Cell. Biol.* 8:531, 1988.

Finlay, C.A., Hinds, P.W. and Levine, A.J. The p53 proto-oncogene can act as a suppressor of transformation. *Cell* 57:1083, 1989.

Halevy, 0., Michalovitz, D. and Oren, M. Different tumor-derived p53 mutants exhibit distinct biological activities. *Science* 250:113, 1990.

Hinds, P., Finlay, C., Frey, A. and Levine, A.J. Immunological evidence for the association of p53 with a heat shock protein, hsc70, in p53 plus ras transformed cell lines. *Mol. Cell. Biol.* 7:2863, 1987.

Hinds, P., Finlay, C. and Levine, A.J. Mutation is required to activate the p53 gene for cooperation with the ras oncogene and transformation. *J. Virol.* 63:739, 1989.

Hinds, P.W., Finlay, C.A., Quartin, R.S., Baker, S.J., Fearon, E.R., Vogelstein, B. and Levine, A.J. Mutant p53 DNAs from human colorectal carcinomas can cooperate with *ras* in transforming primary rat cells: A comparison of the "hot spot" mutant phenotypes. *Cell Growth Differ.* 1:571, 1990.

Iggo, R., Gatter, K., Bartek, J., Lane, D. and Harris, A.L. Increased expression of mutant forms of p53 oncogene in primary lung cancer. *The Lancet* 335:675, 1990.

Jenkins, J.R., Rudge, K. and Currie, G.A. Cellular immortalization by a cDNA clone encoding the transformation-associated phosphoprotein p53. *Nature* 312:651, 1984.

Jenkins, J.R., Rudge, K., Chumakov, P. and Currie, G.A. The cellular oncogene p53 can be activated by mutagenesis. *Nature* 317:816, 1985.

Kelman, Z., Prokocimer, M., Peller, S., Kahn, Y., Rechavi, G., Manor, Y., Cohen, A. and Rotter, V. Rearrangements in the p53 gene in Philadelphia chromosome positive chronic myelogenous leukemia, *Blood* 74:2318, 1989.

Koeffler, H.P., Miller, C., Nicolson, M.A., Ranyard, J. and Bosselman, R.A. Increased expression of p53 protein in human leukemia cells. *Proc. Natl. Acad. Sci. USA* 83:4035, 1986.

Lalande, M. A reversible arrest point in the late Gl phase of the mammalian cell cycle. *Expt. Cell Res.*, 186:332, 1990.

Lane, D.P. and Crawford, L.V. T antigen is bound to a host protein in SV40-transformed cells. *Nature* 278:261, 1979.

Levine, A.J., Finlay, C.A. and Hinds, P.W. The p53 proto-oncogene and its product, in: "Common Mechanisms of Transformation by Small DNA Tumor Viruses," edited by L.P. Villarreal. American Society for Microbiology, Washington, DC, 1989.

Levine, A.J. The p53 protein and its interactions with the oncogene products of the small DNA tumor viruses. *Virology* 177:419, 1990.

Linzer, D.I.H. and Levine, A.J. Characterization of a 54,000 MW cellular SV40 tumor antigen present in SV40-transformed cells and uninfected embryonal carcinoma cells. *Cell* 17:43, 1979.

Malkin, D., Li, F.P., Strong, L.C., Fraumeni, J.F., Nelson, C.E., Kim, D.H., Kassel, J., Gryka, M.A., Bischoff, F.Z., Tainsky, M.A. and Friend, S.H. Germ line p53 mutations in a familial syndrome of breast cancer, sarcomas, and other neoplasms. *Science* 250:1233, 1990.

Masuda, H., Miller, C., Keoffler, H.P., Battifora, H. and Cline, M.J. Rearrangement of the p53 gene in human osteogenic sarcomas. *Proc. Natl. Acad. Sci. USA*. 84:7716, 1987.

Mercer, W.E., Nelson, D., DeLeo, A.B., Old, L.J. and Baserga, R. Microinjection of monoclonal antibody to protein p53 inhibits serum-induced DNA synthesis in 3T3 cells. *Proc. Natl. Acad. Sci. USA*. 79:6309, 1982.

Mercer, W.E., Avignolo, C. and Baserga, R. Role of the p53 protein in cell proliferation as studied by microinjection of monoclonal antibodies. *Mol. Cell. Biol.* 4:276, 1984.

Mercer, W.F., Shields, M.T., Amin, M., Suave, G.J., Appella, E., Ullrich, S.J., and Romano, J.W. Antiproliferative effects of wild-type human p53. *J. Cell. Biochem.* 14C:285, 1990.

Milner, J. and Milner, S. SV40-53K antigen: A possible role for p53 in normal cells. *Virology* 112:785, 1981.

Mowat, M., Cheng, A., Kimura, N., Bernstein, A. and Benchimol, S. Rearrangements of the cellular p53 gene in erythroleukaemia cells transformed by Friend virus. *Nature* 314:633, 1985.

Munroe, D.G., Rovinski, B., Bernstein, A. and Benchimol, S. Loss of a highly conserved domain on p53 as a result of gene deletion during Friend virus-induced erythroleukemia. *Oncogene* 2:621, 1988.

Nigro, J.M., Baker, S.J., Preisinger, A.C., Jessup, J.M., Hostetter, R., Cleary, K., Bigner, S.H., Davidson, N., Baylin, S., Devilee, P., Glover, T., Collins, F.S., Weston, A., Modali, R., Harris, C.C. and Vogelstein, B. Mutations in the p53 gene occur in diverse human tumour types. *Nature* 342:705, 1989.

Oren, M., Maltzman, W. and Levine, A.J. Post-translational regulation of the 54K cellular tumor antigen in normal and transformed cells. *Mol. Cell. Biol.* 1:101, 1981.

Parada, L.F., Land, H., Weinberg, R.A., Wolf, D. and Rotter, V. Cooperation between gene encoding p53 tumour antigen and ras in cellular transformation. *Nature* 312:649, 1984.

Pinhasi-Kimhi, 0., Michalovitz, D., Ben-Zeev, A. and Oren, M. Specific interaction between the p53 cellular tumor antigen and major heat shock proteins. *Nature* 320:182, 1986.

Raycroft, L., Wu, H., and Lozano, G. Transcriptional activation by wild-type but not transforming mutants of the p53 anti-oncogene. *Science* 249:1049, 1990.

Reich, N.C., Oren, M. and Levine, A.J. Two distinct mechanisms regulate the levels of a cellular tumor antigen, p53. *Mol. Cell. Biol.* 3:2143, 1983.

Rogel, A., Popliker, M., Webb, C.G. and Oren, M. p53 cellular tumor antigen: Analysis of mRNA levels in normal adult tissues, embryos and tumors. *Mol. Cell. Biol.* 5:2851, 1985.

Rovinski, B., Munroe, D., Peacock, J., Mowat, M., Bernstein, A. and Benchimol, S. Deletion of 5'-coding sequences of the cellular p53 gene in mouse erythroleukemia: A novel mechanism of oncogene regulation. *Mol. Cell. Biol.* 7:847, 1987.

Rovinski, B. and Benchimol, S. Immortalization of rat embryo fibroblasts by the cellular p53 oncogene. *Oncogene* 2:445, 1988.

Sarnow, P., Ho, Y.S., Williams, J. and Levine, A.J. Adenovirus Elb-58kd tumor antigen and SV40 large tumor antigen are physically associated with the same 54kd cellular protein in transformed cells. *Cell* 28:387, 1982.

Shohat, 0., Greenberg, M., Reisman, D., Oren, M. and Rotter, V. Inhibition of cell growth mediated by plasmids encoding p53 anti-sense. *Oncogene* 1:277, 1987.

Soussi, T., deFromental, C.C., Mechali, M., May, P. and Kress, M. Cloning and characterization of a cDNA from Xenopus laevis coding for a protein homologous to human and murine p53. *Oncogene* 1:71, 1987.

Sturzbecher, H.-W., Chumakov, P., Welch, W.J. and Jenkins, J.R. Mutant p53 proteins bind hsp72/73 cellular heat shock-related proteins in SV40-transformed monkey cells. *Oncogene* 1:201, 1987.

Takahashi, T., Nau, M.M., Chiba, I., Birrer, M.J., Rosenberg, R.K., Vinocour, M., Levitt, M., Pass, H., Gazdar, A.D. and Minna, J.D. p53: A frequent target for genetic abnormalities in lung cancer. *Science* 246:491, 1989.

Thomas, R., Kaplan, L., Reich, N., Lane, D.P. and Levine, A.J. Characterization of human p53 antigens employing primate specific monoclonal antibodies. *Virology* 131:502, 1983.

Werness, B.A., Levine, A.J. and Howley, P.M. The E6 proteins encoded by human papillomavirus types 16 and 18 can complex p53 *in vitro*. *Science* 248:76, 1990.

Wolf, D., Harris, N. and Rotter, V. Reconstitution of p53 expression in a nonproducer Ab-MuLV-transformed cell line by transfection of a functional p53 gene. *Cell* 38:119, 1984.

Wolf, D. and Rotter, V. Major deletions in the gene encoding the p53 tumor antigen cause lack of p53 expression in HL-60 cells. *Proc. Natl. Acad. Sci. U.S.A.* 82:790, 1985.

GENE STRUCTURE AND EXPRESSION IN COLORECTAL CANCER

James M. Pipas[1], Kay Pogue-Geile[1], Gene G. Finley[2], Christine A. Cartwright[3], and Arnold I. Meiesler[2]

[1]Department of Biological Sciences
University of Pittsburgh
Pittsburgh, PA 15260

[2]Department of Medicine And VA Medical Center
University of Pittsburgh School of Medicine
Pittsburgh, PA 15240

[3]Division of Gastroenterology
Department of Medicine, S 069
Stanford University, Stanford, CA 94305

ABSTRACT

Colorectal cancer provides a unique model for the study of molecular changes that are associated with tumorigenesis. The cancer evolves as an apparent ordered sequence from a benign to a malignant lesion in histopathological recognizable stages. Since it is relatively easy to isolate tissue representing each of these stages, studies of molecular events associated with tumor progression are feasible. Such studies have shown that multiple changes in gene structure, expression and activity occur during tumorigenesis.

INTRODUCTION

One of the hallmarks of many and perhaps all cancers are their apparent ability to evolve through a series of stages with each successive stage having a higher invasive or metastatic potential than the previous. Epidemiology data indicate that

The Underlying Molecular, Cellular, and Immunological Factors in Cancer and Aging, Edited by S.S. Yang and H.R.Warner, Plenum Press, New York, 1993

multiple events are required for the initiation of cancer coupled with an array of data demonstrating that genetic mutations from an integral part of this process has led to the hypothesis that cancer cells acquire their malignant phenotype through the acquisition of mutations. These alter the structure, expression or activity of proteins involved in regulating cell proliferation and survival. That is the acquisition of mutations in specific loci contribute to the development and behavior of the tumor. Thus, one of the goals of cancer biology is to identify molecular events responsible for different stages of tumorigenesis and to identify those that directly effect tumor behavior.

Colorectal cancer provides a model system for the study of molecular events that occur during the genesis and progression of tumors. Invasive adenocarcinomas are thought to arise from benign neoplasms called adenomatous polyps (Muto *et al.*, 1975). Both tumors and polyps occur as different classes distinguishable by histological criteria. Furthermore, therapy dictates that tumors and polyps, and the surrounding normal colon be surgically removed from an affected individual then they are identified. Thus, colorectal cancer provides an opportunity to obtain normal, premalignant and malignant tissue in quantities suitable for molecular analysis, from the same patient. The existence of genetic syndromes such as familial polyposis coli, that predispose of the development of colorectal cancer provide additional material for study.

Molecular genetic hypotheses for the genesis of colorectal cancer predict that mutation affecting a specific set of genes leads to the formation of an adenomatous polyp from normally regulated colonic epithelium and that mutations in an additional collection of genes leads to the invasive phenotype characteristic of adenocarcinoma. Similarly mutations at specific loci should contribute to the metastatic potential of the tumor. The identification of the loci affected at each stage of tumorigenesis is an important task since such changes might provide hallmarks that are predictive of tumor behavior and thus be of therapeutic significance. A number of laboratories have begun cataloging changes that occurring gene structure, expression and activity at different stages of colorectal cancer. In this manuscript we discuss our efforts and those of others and the problems inherent with this strategy.

Expression of the *Myc* Gene Family in Colorectal Cancer

The *myc* gene family consists of three members, c-*myc*, N-*myc* and L-*myc* each of which encodes a nuclear phosphoprotein those precise roles in cellular metabolism are not understood (Cole, 1986; Bishop, 1987). Evidence from a variety of sources suggests that these proteins may play a role in controlling cell proliferation or both. All three are oncogenes in that they are capable of inducing neoplastic transformation and/or immortalization in cell culture systems and in the case of c-*myc*, of inducing tumors in transgenic animals. In addition, expression of c-*myc* is elevated when quiescent cells are stimulated with serum or purified growth factors. Changes in structure and expression of all three members of the gene family have been observed in human tumors.

Several laboratories have reported that the c-*myc* gene is over expressed in a majority of adenocarcinomas of the colon (Erisman *et al.*, 1985; Stewart *et al., 1986; Erisman et al.*, 1988; Calabretta *et al.*, 1989; Finley *et al.*, 1989). Our studies indicated that the L-myc and N-*myc* genes also frequently show increased levels of expression in colorectal cancer (Finley *et al.*, 1989). These changes in expression usually occur without gross structural alterations in the gene, although occasionally the c-*myc* gene is amplified 2.3 fold in tumors relative to normal mucosa. These studies indicated that two-thirds of adenocarcinomas of the colon show increased levels of the c-*myc* transcript as detected by Northern hybridization and normalization to the signal obtained from histologically normal colon adjacent to the tumor. There was no obvious correlation between the levels of *myc* RNA and the pathology, stage of clinical outcome of the disease.

We extended previous studies by examining expression of the *myc* family in adenomatous polyps, presumed precursor to carcinoma (Finley *et al.*, 1989). Approximately two-thirds of these neoplasms showed increased levels of *myc*-related transcripts relative to normal mucosa. Again no clear correlation was evident between the histology of the polyp and the level of *myc* expression. The fact that over expression of *myc* genes is detected in adenomatous polyps indicate that deregulation of this gene family is a relatively early event in the course of tumorigenesis and that this deregulation persists through the transition from the benign to the malignant state.

Northern hybridization analysis is not ideal for these studies. The fact that tumor tissue is necessarily a collection of neoplastic epithelium mixed with other tissue, i.e., muscle, vessels, and nerves that are present and not easily separable from pure tumor cells could lead to: (1) an underestimation of the amount of *myc* transcripts present in the tumor if these genes are not expressed at high levels in extraneous tissue and if contamination of tumor cells with non-tumor tissue is significant; or (2) an overestimation of transcript levels if expression in the tumor cells is normal, but transcript levels are increased in the extraneous tissue. Our preliminary experiments using immunohistochemistry to detect *myc* protein levels in individual cells indicate that the former is the case. That is all adenocarcinomas and adenomatous polyps show increased levels of *myc* proteins (Melham *et at.*, manuscript in preparation). Moreover, it appears that not all tumor cells within a tumor express the *myc* protein nor are all cells expressing the protein proliferating as determined by simultaneous measurement of the proliferation associated antigen, Ki-67.

Activation of pp60$^{c\text{-}src}$ in Colon Carcinomas and Adenomas

The Rous sarcoma virus transforming gene v-*src*, and its cellular homologue c-*src*, encode 60-kilodalton, membrane associated protein-tyrosine kinases. Transformation by the viral protein (pp60$^{v\text{-}src}$) or by mutants of the cellular protein (pp60$^{c\text{-}src}$) is closely correlated to elevated specific activity of the enzyme. All transforming mutants of pp60$^{c\text{-}src}$ tested have higher specific activity than normal pp60$^{c\text{-}src}$.

Bolen and coworkers reported that pp60$^{c\text{-}src}$ from human neuroblastoma (Bolen *et at.*, 1985) breast adenocarcinoma (Rosen *et at.*, 1986) or co1on carcinoma (Bolen *et at.*, 1987) had higher in *vitro* protein tyrosine kinase activity than pp60$^{c\text{-}src}$ from normal mucosa adjacent to the tumor. The most consistent and striking elevation in pp60$^{c\text{-}src}$ activity was observed in colon cancer.

We also measured the *in vitro* protein kinase activity pp60$^{c\text{-}src}$ from human colon carcinoma cell lines and tumors (Cartwright *et at.*, 1989). The activity of pp60$^{c\text{-}src}$ from 6 to 9 carcinoma cell lines was higher (on average, 5-fold as measured by enolase phosphorylation, or 8-fold as as measured by autophosphorylation) than that of pp60$^{c\text{-}src}$ from colonic mucosal cells, or human or rodent fibroblasts. Similarly, the activity of pp60$^{c\text{-}src}$ from 13 of 21 primary colon carcinomas was 5 or 7 fold higher than that of pp60$^{c\text{-}src}$ from normal colonic mucosa adjacent to the tumor. Overall, we observed elevated pp60$^{c\text{-}src}$ protein kinase activity in two thirds of colon carcinoma cell lines and tumor tested. The increased pp60$^{c\text{-}src}$ activity did not result solely from and increase in the level of pp60$^{c\text{-}src}$ protein, suggesting that the specific activity of the pp60$^{c\text{-}src}$ kinase is elevated in the tumor cells.

Using immunoblotting with antibodies to phosphotyrosine we identified substrates of protein-tyrosine kinases in colonic cells (Cartwright *et at.*, 1989). Three phosphotyrosine containing proteins of approximately 145, 125 and 57 kDa were detected at significantly higher levels in most colon carcinoma cell lines than in normal colonic mucosal cells, normal human mammary cells, or normal human or rat fibroblast cell lines. The data indicate that active protein tyrosine kinases, inactive protein-tyrosine phosphatases, or both, are present in colon carcinoma cells. The observation that all colon carcinoma cell lines with elevated pp60$^{c\text{-}src}$, activity as measured *in vitro*, show increased phosphorylation of proteins on tyrosine *in vivo*, suggests that pp60$^{c\text{-}src}$ is activated in the cells and is possibly one of the kinases phosphorylating these proteins.

To determine whether pp60$^{c\text{-}src}$ is activated in colonic tissue at risk for carcinoma, we measured the *in vitro* protein kinase activity of pp60$^{c\text{-}src}$ from 22 colonic polyps and adjacent normal mucosa, from 18 patients (Cartwright *et at.*, 1990). The polyps varied in size (0.5 - 8.0 cm). Histology (tubular, tubulovillous and villous architecture) and degree of dysplasia (mild, moderate and severe). $pp60^{c\text{-}src}$ activity in $\leq$ 2 cm benign polyps was not significantly different from activity in normal mucosa adjacent to the polyp. In contrast, $pp60^{c\text{-}src}$ activity in > 2 cm benign polyps was significantly higher than activity in smaller polyps or in normal mucosa. A close correlation existed between increased $pp60^{c\text{-}src}$ activity and increased cancer risk as predicted by polyp size, histology, and degree of dysplasia and/or cancer. Thus $pp60^{c\text{-}src}$ activation occurs in benign polyps that are at greatest risk for developing cancer. The data suggest that activation of $pp60^{c\text{-}src}$ is an early event, although not the genesis of human colon carcinoma.

Changes in mRNA Levels between Normal Mucosa and Tumors

Most work directed towards finding genes important for tumorigenesis has centered on genes known to play a role in controlling proliferation or inducing transformation in cell culture systems. Thus most of these studies have utilized previously characterized oncogenes. More recently several groups have turned the differential screening of cDNA libraries prepared from normal and malignant tissue to identify genes whose level of expression is altered (Bartsch *et al.*, 1986; Augenlicht *et al.*, 1987). Again, colorectal cancer offers a unique opportunity for such studies since both tumor and adjacent normal mucosa are removed upon surgical resection in quantities suitable for library preparation.

Our initial experiments as well as those of others indicate that a large number of genes show changes in expression levels when adenocarcinoma is compared to normal colonic epithelium. Many of these genes have been identified by comparing their nucleotide sequence to a sequence data base. In colorectal cancer these include a laminin binding protein, cytochrome c oxidase, type I and type II keratin genes and the gene for ribosomal protein L31 (Yow *et al.*, 1988; Chester *et al.*, 1989; Heerdte *et al.*, 1990; Schwinfest *et al.*, 1990). In addition, several genes of unknown function whose sequence has not been previously reported have been identified by this procedure. In these cases the problem will be to identify those whose change in expression contributes in some way to the transformed phenotype from those whose change is a result of transformation and therefore irrelevant to the molecular mechanism(s) involved in tumorigenesis.

We have recently cloned and identified a cDNA encoding the human S3 ribosomal protein from such a differential cDNA library screen (Pogue-Geile *et al.*, in preparation). The transcript for this gene is over-expressed in both adenocarcinomas and adenomatous polyps indicating that the increased expression is a relatively early event in tumorigenesis. We also examined the levels of transcripts for several other ribosomal protein genes and found that these too were over-expressed in both malignant and premalignant tissue. We hypothesize that this indicates that increased expression of the genes for ribosomal proteins and thus presumably increased number of ribosomes is an event that occurs coordinately with or soon after the initial onset of neoplasia in this tissue.

DISCUSSION

Colorectal cancer provides a unique opportunity to study the molecular changes in gene structure and expression associated with the early stages and progression of tumorigenesis. A number of laboratories have set out to catalogue these changes in premalignant and invasive tumors. These studies have demonstrated a large number of such alterations. Thus, mutational activation of K-*ras* oncogene (Bos et al.; 1987; Forrester *et al.*, 1987), loss of heterozygosity and mutation of the p53 locus (Baker *et al.*, 1989; Nigro *et al.*, 1989), over-expression of the *myc* gene family (Erisman *et al.*, 1985; Stewart *et al.*, 1986; Calabretta *et al.*, 1989; Finley et al. 1989), over-expression of the c-*erb*B-2 gene product (D'Emilia *et al.*, 1989), activation of *src* tyrosine kinase activity (Bolen *et al.*, 1987, Cartwright , 1989; Cartwright *et al.*, 1990) and mutation of the DCC locus (Fearon *et al.*, 1990) have all been observed as frequent events in colorectal cancer. In addition alterations on chromosome 5 have been associated with familial polyposis and/or sporadic cancer suggesting that a gene on this chromosome may play an early role in neoplasia of the colon (Bodmer *et al.*, 1987; Leppert *et al.*, 1987; Solomon *et al.*, 1987: Okamoto *et al.*, 1988; Vogelstein *et al.*, 1988).

The significance of any of these events in relation to tumor behavior is unclear. The problem is that it is difficult to distinguish a gene product whose function is to restrict (negatively regulate) or stimulate cell proliferation from one whose expression or activity is deleterious or advantageous to the growth and survival of a cell in an abnormal environment for reasons unrelated to neoplasia *per se*. Thus it will be necessary to couple the observations made in primary human tumors with systematic animal studies where the changes can be introduced one at a time or in combination to study their effects on cell behavior.

ACKNOWLEDGEMENTS

This work was supported by grants CA46547 (J.M.P.) from the NIH, VA Merit Review S21 (A.I.M), D-400 from the American Cancer Society (C.A.C.) and by funds from BRSG 2S07RR07084-23 and the Pittsburgh Cancer Institute.

REFERENCES

Augenlicht, L. H., Wahrman, M.Z., Anderson, L., Taylor, J. and Lipkin, M. Expression of Cloned Sequences in Biopsies of Human Colonic Tissue and in Colonic Carcinoma Cells Induced to Differentiate *in vitro*. *Cancer Research* 47:6017, 1987.

Baker, S.J., Fearon, E. Nigro, J. Hamilton, S. Preisinger, A. C., Jessup, J. M., VanTuinen, P., Ledbetter, D. H., Barker, D.F., Nakamura, Y., White, R., and Vogelstein, B. Chromosome 17 deletions and p53 gene mutations in colorectal carcinomas. *Science* 244:217, 1989.

Bartsch, R. A., Joannou, C., Talbot, I. C. and Bailey, D.S. Cloning of mRNA sequences from the human colon: Preliminary characterization of defined mRNAs in normal and neoplastic tissues. *Brit. J. Cancer* 54:791, 1986.

Bishop, J.M. The molecular genetics of cancer. *Science* 235:305, 1987.

Bodmer, W. F., Bailey, C. J., Bodmer, J., Bussey, H.J.R., Ellis, A., Gorman, P., Luciobello, F. C., Murday, V. A., Rider, S. H., Scambler, Sheer, Solomon, E. and Spurr, N. K. Localization of the gene for familial adenomatous polylposis on chromosome 5. *Nature* 328:614, 1987.

Bolen, J. B., Rosen, N. and lsrael, M.A. Increased $pp60^{c\text{-}src}$ tyrosine kinase activity in human neuroblastomas is associated with amino-terminal tyrosine phosphorylation of the *src* gene product. *Proc. Natl. Acad. Sci. USA* 82:7275, 1985.

Bolen, J.B., Veillette, A., Schwartz, A.M., DeSeau, V. and Rosen, N. Activation of $pp60^{c\text{-}src}$ protein kinase activity in human tumor cell lines. *Proc. Natl. Acad. Sci. USA.* 84: 2251, 1987.

Bos, J.L., Fearon, E.R., Hamilton, S.R., Verlaan-deVries, M., van Boom, J. H., van der Eb, A. J. and Vogelstein, B. Prevalence of *ras* gene mutations in human colorectal cancers. *Nature (London)* 327:293, 1987.

Calabretta, B., Kaczmarek, L., L. Ming, P. M. L., Au, F., and Ming, S.-C. Expression of c-*myc* and other cell cycle-dependent genes in human colon neoplasia. *Cancer Research* 45:6000, 1985.

Cartwright, C. A., Kamps, M. P., Meisler, A.I., Pipas, J. M., and Eckhart, W. $pp60^{c\text{-}src}$ activation in human colon carcinoma. *J. Clin. Invest.* 83: 2025, 1989.

Cartwright, C. A., Meisler, A.I., and Eckhart, W. Activation of the $pp60^{c\text{-}src}$ protein kinase is an early event in colonic carcinogenesis. *Proc. Natl. Acad. Sci. USA* 87:558, 1990.

Chester, K. A., Robson, L., Begent, R. H.J., Talbot, I. Pringle, J. H., Primrose, L., Macpherson, A. J. S., Boxer, G., Southall, P. and Malcolm, A. D. B. Identification of a human ribosomal protein mRNA with increased expression in colorectal tumors. *Biochimica et Bioohvsica Acta* 1009:297, 1989.

Cole, M.D. The *myc* oncogene: Its role in transformation and differentiation. *Ann. Rev. Genet.* 20:361, 1986.

Finley, G. G., Schulz, N. T., Hill, S. A., Geiser, J. R., Pipas, J. M., and Meisler, A. I. Expression of the *myc* gene family in different stages of human colorectal cancer. *Oncogene* 4:963, 1989.

Forrester, K., Almoguera, C., Han, K., Grizzle, W. E., and Perucho, M. Detection of high incidence of K-*ras* oncogenes during human colon tumorigenesis. *Nature (London)* 32: 298, 1987.

D'Emilia, J., Bulovas, K., D'Ercole, K., Wolf, B., Steele, G., and Summerhayes, I. C. Expression of the c-*erb*B-2 gene product (p185) at different stages of neoplastic progression in the colon. *Oncogene* 4:1233, 1989.

Erisman, M. D., Rothberg, P. G., Diehl, R. E., Morse, C. C., Spandorfer, J. M., and Astrin, S. M. Deregulation of c-*myc* gene expression in human colon carcinoma is not accompanied by amplification or arrangement of the gene. *Mol. Cell. Bio.* 5:1969, 1985.

Erisman, M. D., Litwin, S., Keidan, R. D., Comis, R.L., and Astrin, S. M. Noncorrelation of the expression of the c-*myc* oncogene in colorectal carcinoma with recurrence of disease or patient survival. *Cancer Research* 48:1350, 1988.

Fearon, E. R., Cho, K. R., Nigro, J. M., Kern, S. E., Simons, J. W., Ruppert, J. M., Hamilton, S. R., Preisinger, A. C., Thomas, G. 0., Kinzler, K. W., and Vogelstein, B. Identification of a chromosome 18q gene that is altered in colorectal cancers. *Science* 247:49, 1990.

Heerdt, B. G., Halsey, H. K., Lipkin, M. and Augenlicht, L. H.. Expression of mitochondrial cytochrome *c* oxidase in human colonic cell differentiation, transformation, and risk for colonic cancer. *Cancer Research* 50:1596, 1990.

Leppert, M., Dobbs, M., Scambler, P., O'Connell, P., Nakamura, Y., Stauffer, D., Woodward, S., Burt, R., Hughes, J., Gardner, E., Lathrop, M., Wasmuth, J., Lalouel, J.-M. and White, R. The gene for familial polyposis coli maps to the long arm of chromosome 5. *Science* 238:1411, 1987.

Muto, T. , Bussey, H. J., and Morson, B. C. The evolution of cancer of the colon and rectum. *Cancer* 36:2251, 1975.

Nigro, J. M., Baker, S.J., Preisinger, A. C., Jessup, J. M., Hostetter, R., Cleary, K., Bigner, S. H., Davidson, N., Baylin, S., Devilee, P., Glover, T., Collins, F.S., Weston, A., Modali, R., Harris, C. C. and Vogelstein, B. Mutations in the p53 gene occur in diverse human tumour types. *Nature* 342:705, 1989.

Okamoto, M., Sasski,M., Sugio, K., Sato, C., Iwama, T., Ikeuchi,T., Tonomura, T., Sasazuki, T. and Miyaki, M., 1988. Loss of consitutional heterozygosity in colon carcinoma from patients with familial plyposis coli. *Nature* 331:273.

Rosen, N., Bolen, J. B., Schwartz, A. M., Cohen, P., DeSeau, V. and Israel, M. A. Analysis of $pp60^{c\text{-}src}$ protein kinase activity in human tumor cell lines and tissues. *J. Biol. Chem.* 261:13754, 1986.

Schweinfest, C. W., Henderson, K. W., Gu, J.–R., Kottaridis, S. D., Besbeas, S., Panotopoulou, E., and Papas, T. S. Subtraction hybridization cDNA libraries from colon carcinoma and hepatic cancer. *Genet. Annal. Techn. Appl.* 7:64, 1990.

Solomon, E., Voss, R., Hall, V., Bodmer, W.F., Jass, J.R., Jeffreys, A. J., Lucibello, F. C., Patel, I. and Rider, S.H. Chromosome 5 allele loss in human colorectal carcinomas. *Nature* 328:616, 1987.

Stewart, J., Evan, G., Watson, J. and Sikora, K. Detection of the c–*myc* oncogene product in colonic polyps and carcinomas. *Br. J. Cancer* 53:1, 1986.

Vogelstein, B., Fearon, E. R., Hamilton, S. R., Kern, S. E., Preisinger, A. C., Leppert, M., Nakamura, Y., White, R., Smits, A. M. M. and Bos, J. L. Genetic alterations during colorectal–tumor development. *N. Engl. J. Med.* 319:525, 1988.

Yow, H., Wong, J. M., Chen, H. S., Lee, C., Steele, G.D. and Chen, L. B. Increased mRNA expression of a laminin–binding protein in human colon carcinoma : complete sequence of a full length cDNA encoding the protein. *Proc. Natl. Acad. Sci. USA,* 85:6394.

TUMORS AND AGING: THE INFLUENCE OF AGE-ASSOCIATED IMMUNE CHANGES UPON TUMOR GROWTH AND SPREAD

William B. Ershler

Department of Medicine
University of Wisconsin
Madison, Wisconsin 53706

INTRODUCTION

There has been a clinical impression that tumors are less malignant in older people. Such has been claimed for breast, colon, prostate and lung carcinomas (Schottenfield and Robbins, 1971; Berkson *et al.*, 1957, Calabrese *et al.*, 1973; Ershler *et al.*, 1983; Pickren *et al.*, 1982; Suen *et al.*, 1974). The great heterogeneity in clinical populations, confounded by antecedent illness, medicines, exposures, and social circumstances have precluded a statistical confirmation of such age-associated changes. Nonetheless, in experimental animals, we and others have found significant differences in tumor growth and spread when the common variable is host age. Weakly immunogenic tumors such as B16 melanoma or Lewis lung carcinoma (3LL) grow more slowly in old mice, but more immunogenic tumors such as methylcholanthrene-induced fibrosarcomas grow more rapidly. We have explored a variety of proposed mechanisms for the observed differences and have concluded that the age-associated decline in immune function (immune senescence) is central to the reduced aggressiveness of weakly antigenic tumors in older hosts. This conclusion is based on the following findings:

a) Primary growth and metastases of weakly antigenic experimental tumors is less in immune-deficient mice (Yuhas *et al.*, 1974; Ershler *et al.*, 1984c). This is not true of the more highly antigenic tumors, such as those induced by methylcholanthrene or UV light.

b) The growth of B16 melanoma or 3LL correlates directly with the level of immune competence (Yuhas *et al.*, 1974; Ershler *et al.*, 1984c). Reduced immune competence is associated with slower tumor growth; restoration of immune functions is associated with more rapid growth (Ershler *et al.* , 1984b; Tsuda *et al.*, 1987). Under certain circumstances, lymphocytes, or factors therefrom, can enhance tumor cell proliferation *in vitro* (see below), and angiogenesis both *in vitro* and *in vivo* (Hadar *et al.*, 1988; Kreisle *et al.*, 1988).

c) With age, there is a well characterized immune deficiency, primarily of T-cells, and reduced production of cytokines is generally observed.

IMMUNESENESCENCE

In all mammalian species studied to date, there is an age-related decline in immune function which begins before sexual maturation and develops progressively thereafter. Extensive reports have described a wide variety of age-related abnormalities and these have been nicely reviewed by Thoman and Weigle (1989). It is generally believed that age-related immune deficiency develops coincident with the gradual involution of the thymus gland and thymic-related (or T-cell) functions are most profoundly affected (Price and Makinodan, 1972; Stutman, 1974; Weksler *et al.*, 1976). Humoral immunity is less affected, but age-associated alterations have been reported (Serge and Serge, 1976; Callard and Basten, 1977). Although less well studied, changes in monocyte/macrophage function have been observed with age but these are less in magnitude than those described for T-cell function (Antonaci *et al.*, 1984; Rabatic *et al.*, 1988). Age-related change in the production of cytokines have been reported, most notably for interleukin-2 (IL-2) (Thoman and Weigle, 1981; Thoman and Weigle, 1982; Gillis *et al.*, 1981; Chang *et al.*, 1983; Ershler *et al.*, 1985), but also for others, including the monokines IL-l (Inamizu *et al.*, 1985; Bruley-Rosset and Vergnon, 1984) and tumor necrosis factor (Bradley *et al.*, 1989). The defect in IL-2 production appears at the level of gene expression, as reduced levels of IL-2 mRNA are observed in mitogen-stimulated lymphocytes from old individuals (Fong and Makinodan, 1989; Wu *et al.*, 1986).

EXPERIMENTAL TUMORS AND AGING

The relationship between aging and the development of cancer has been extensively studied (Anisimov, 1983), but the age effect upon progression of disease (i.e., tumor growth and metastases) has been less well characterized. With certain experimental tumors, such as methylcholanthrene (MCA)-induced fibrosarcomas (Stjernsward, 1966), mammary carcinomas (Rockwell *et al.*, 1972,; Rockwell, 1981) and UV light-induced sarcomas (Urban *et al.*, 1982; Urban and Schrieber, 1984;

Flood *et al.*, 1980), older animals show more rapid tumor growth and shorter survival. In the UV light-induced sarcoma model, more aggressive disease in older mice correlates with age-related reduced tumor-specific cytolytic T-cell function (Urban *et al.*, 1982; Urban and Schrieber, 1984; Flood *et al.*, 1980). The general characteristic of experimental tumors that are more aggressive with age is that they are chemically or virally induced and are highly immunogenic. In contrast, the B16 murine melanoma arose spontaneously (Greene, 1977), and is weakly immunogenic (Bystryn, 1976; Baniyash *et al.*, 1982; Celik *et al.*, 1983; Ershler, 1988). We have shown, in the B16 model, slower tumor growth and fewer pulmonary colonies after i.v. injection. There is also longer survival after i.v. or i.p. inoculation in old mice (Ershler *et al.*, 1984a, 1984b, 1984c). We have found that this is true for other weakly antigenic tumors (see Figure 1) and other laboratories have made similar observations with respect to B16 and other weakly immunogenic tumors grown in immune-deficient hosts (Yuhas *et al.*, 1974; Fidler, 1974; Fidler *et al.*, 1977; Fidler and Nicholson, 1978; Richie *et al.*, 1981; Kubota *et al.*, 1981; Treves *et al.*, 1976; Prehn and Lappe, 1971; Prehn, 1971, Prehn, 1972; Murasko and Prehn, 1983). We examined the rate of subcutaneous (s.c.) tumor growth and experimental metastases for a number of murine tumors with the common variable being host age. Figure 1 demonstrates growth curves for B16 melanoma, 3LL, and S180 fibrosarcoma. These curves typify what we have invariably observed: weakly antigenic tumors grow more slowly and survival is longer in old mice.

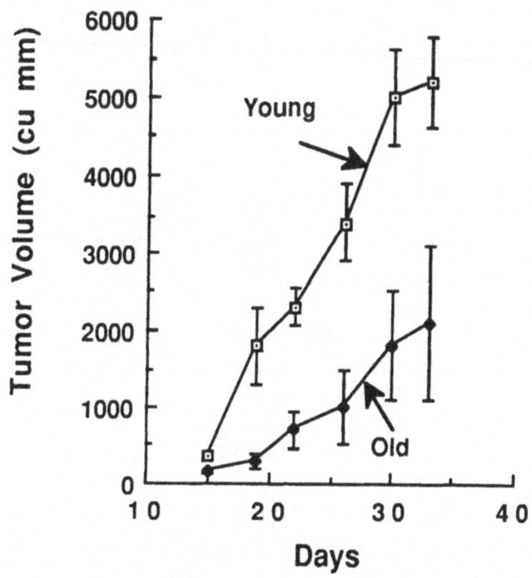

Figure 1A. *B16 Melanoma Growth (s.c.) in Young (2-4 mos) and Old (24 mos) C57Bl/6 Mice* (Ershler et al., 1984c).

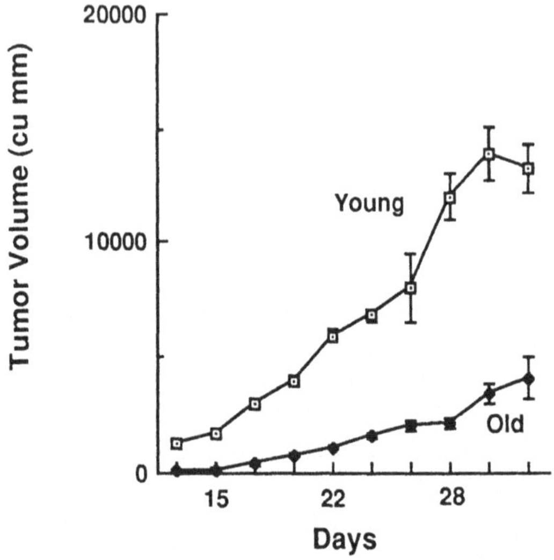

Figure 1B. *Lewis Lung Carcinoma Growth (s.c.) in Young and Old C57Bl/6 Mice* (*Ershler et al.*, 1984b).

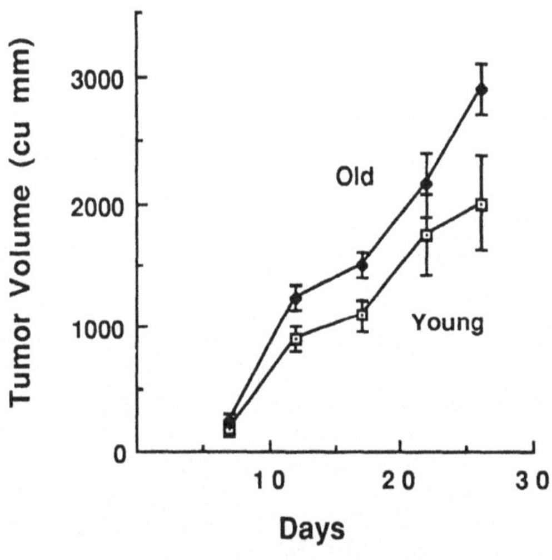

Figure 1C. *S180 Tumor Growth (s.c.) in Young (2-4 mos) and Old (24 mos) Balb/c mice.*
Unlike the weakly antigenic B16 or 3LL, there was no demonstrable "age advantage" in this highly antigenic tumor model (unpublished).

With more antigenic tumors, such as S180, there no longer is an observable age-advantage. After intravenous (i.v.) injection of B16, pulmonary colonies were also fewer in old mice (Figure 2) and survival was longer (data not shown).

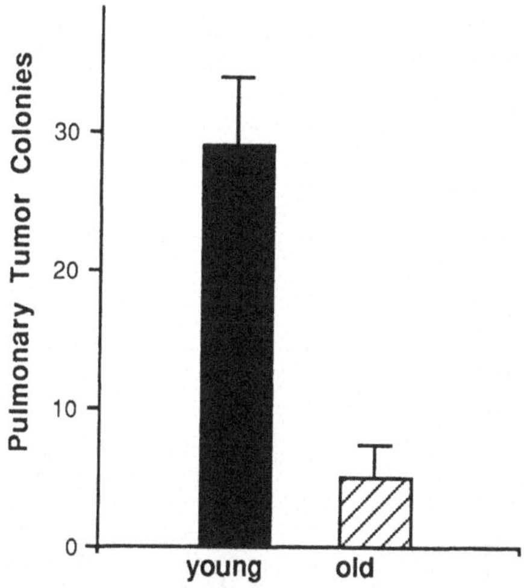

Figure 2. *Pulmonary Tumor Colonies After i.v. Injection of 10^4 B16 Fl Cells.* Young and old mice were given injections of cells into the lateral tail vein. Eighteen days later mice were sacrificed (n=10/group) and the number of colonies (± SEM) counted (Ershler *et al.,* 1984a).

PROPOSED MECHANISMS FOR THE OBSERVED "AGE-ADVANTAGE"

For the past several years we have explored a variety of mechanisms that may account for the difference in tumor behavior with age. Candidate factors were considered as those that influence tumor growth and also change with age. Accordingly, endocrine, nutritional, wound healing and angiogenesis factors were initially explored. These experiments have been previously reviewed (Kaesberg and Ershler, 1989) and results from these studies suggest the importance of immune factors.

EVIDENCE THAT IMMUNE FACTORS ARE INVOLVED

The importance of immunesenescence as an explanation of the observed age-advantage was suggested by the studies of Yuhas 3LL(1974) with the Line 1 alveolar cell murine carcinoma. They demonstrated that slow tumor growth occurs with advanced age and correlated this with the level of immune competence. They also found that growth was slower in mice after sublethal irradiation or hydrocortisone treatment. Fidler and Nicholson, using the B16 i.v. metastases model, found that tumor cell arrests in capillary beds and tumor cell survival after i.v. injection are quantitatively less in immune-deficient mice (Fidler *et al.*, 1977). These observations are consistent with the hypothesis of Prehn and colleagues (Prehn and Lappe, 1971; Prehn, 1971, Prehn, 1972; Murasko and Prehn, 1983) that host immunity may, under certain circumstances, stimulate tumor growth.

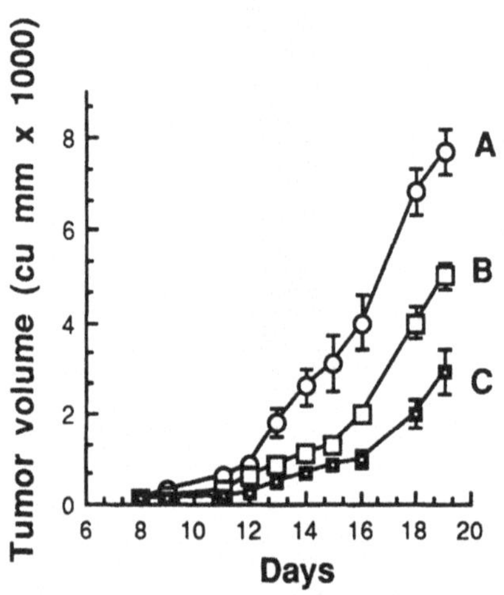

Figure 3. *The Effect of Thymectomy and Anti-theta Antiserum on The Growth of B16 Melanoma in Young Mice.*
Mice were thymectomized 8 weeks before inoculation of tumor cells (on day 0). Rabbit anti-theta antiserum was injected twice (on days -7 and -4). **A**, sham thymectomized; **B**, thymectomized; C, thymectomized and anti-theta antiserum (Tsuda *et al.*, 1988).

These earlier observations led us to the hypothesis that immunesenescence accounted for a large component of the observed reduced tumor growth with age that we were observing with B16 melanoma. In studies performed in the laboratory of Weksler and colleagues, young mice, rendered T-cell deficient (such as after thymectomy and/or treatment with anti-theta antibody) were found to have slower tumor growth (Figure 3). Furthermore, when young, thymectomized, lethally irradiated mice received bone marrow (Ershler *et al.*, 1984b) or splenocytes (Tsuda *et al.*, 1988) from old donor mice, tumor growth and donor age were inversely related (Figure 4).

AGE-SENSITIVE IMMUNE ENHANCEMENT MECHANISMS

Over the years, several "immunoenhancing" mechanisms have been described. One of these mechanisms is the immunofacilitation that results from circulating tumor antigen, antitumor antibody, or antigen-antibody complex (blocking factors), as initially described by the Hellstroms and their co-workers (Hellstrom and Hellstrom, 1977; Hellstrom *et al.*, 1969; Proctor *et al.*, 1973; Sjogren *et al.*, 1971; Tamerius *et al.*, 1976). Although it is possible that an age-related deficiency in the production of blocking factors may be associated with more effective antitumor

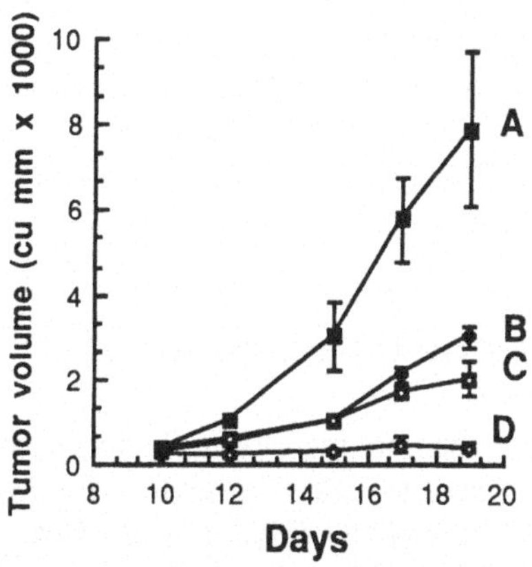

Figure 4. *B16 Melanoma Grows More Slowly in Mice Which Received Spleen Cells from Old Donors.*
Young mice were thymectomized and 8 weeks later were lethally irradiated and given i.v. injections of $8x10^6$ spleen cells from syngeneic young or old mice. Seventeen days later mice were inoculated with B16 cells s.c. (day 0). The volume of the tumors at times indicated is presented as mean ±SEM for groups of 6 mice. **A**, young controls; **B**, young, thymectomized, irradiated recipients of spleen cells from young donors; **C**, old control mice; D, young, thymectomized, irradiated recipients of spleen cells from old donors (Tsuda *et al.*, 1988).

immunity, we have elected not to pursue this hypothesis, primarily because among weakly antigenic tumors, such as B16 melanoma, 3LL and most human cancers, that are so weakly immunogenic, such a mechanism seems unlikely. Another immune tumor-enhancing mechanism is the generation of tumor-specific suppressor cells. Extensive studies in this area (reviewed by Broder and Waldmann, 1978; North, 1984) suggest that shortly after oncogenesis (or perhaps even before [Fisher and Kripke, 1977; Fisher and Kripke, 1978]), there develops in immune competent hosts, suppression of tumor specific immunity (Fisher and Kripke, 1977; Fisher and Kripke, 1978; Fujimoto *et al.*, 1976a; Fujimoto 1976b; Isakov *et al.*, 1978; Berendt and North, 1980) which results in tumor enhancement. For example, the passive transfer of splenocytes or T-cells from tumor-bearing animals to animals that had been previously immunized to MCA-induced fibrosarcoma renders that animal no longer resistant to MCA tumor cell transplants (Fujimoto *et al.*, 1976a; Fujimoto, 1976b). Furthermore, in this model, selective depletion of T-cells (by anti T-cell antisera) or of T-suppressor cells (by anti-IJ allo-antisera) abrogated tumor-enhancement by splenocyte transfusions (Greene *et al.*, 1977). Tumor induced specific immune suppression has been demonstrated in other tumor models (including UV light-induced fibrosarcomas (Fisher and Kripke, 1977; Fisher and Kripke, 1978) and the weakly immunogenic 3LL [Treves *et al.*, 1974; Isakov *et al.*, 1978; Treves *et al.*, 1976). Additionally, we have demonstrated that B16 growth is augmented when mice are simultaneously co-inoculated with spleen cells from B16 tumor-bearing mice, a finding consistent with the presence of suppressor T-cells in the spleen of these tumor bearing mice (Ershler *et al.,* 1988). Nevertheless, the importance of such a mechanism in the pathogenesis of tumors that are weakly immunogenic has yet to be established.

DIRECT ENHANCEMENT OF TUMOR GROWTH

Cells considered part of the immune system (lymphocytes, monocytes, etc.) may also produce factors that enhance tumor growth. For example, T-lymphocytes produce an angiogenesis factor (LIA) (Hadar *et al.*, 1988; Auerbach *et al.*, 1976; Sidky and Auerbach, 1976) which may augment tumor vascularization. Recently, we have identified a factor present in the supernatant of spleen cell cultures that stimulates B16 growth *in vitro*. This factor is currently being characterized in detail. Preliminary findings suggest that it is similar in activity to other factors currently under investigation in other laboratories (Table 1). Several groups have identified growth-enhancing activity in supernatants from cultured normal human mononuclear cells (Sandru *et al.*, 1988; Hamburger *et al.*, 1978; Hamburger and White, 1982) or rodent splenocyte cultures (Eijan *et al.*, 1987; Eijan *et al.*, 1989; Suzuki *et al.*, 1988) that stimulate normal or tumor cell proliferation. In working out the details for optimal *in vitro* human tumor clonogenic growth, Hamburger and colleagues have identified a factor produced by human monocytes that is heat stable, acid labile and stimulatory for tumor growth (Sandru *et al.*, 1988; Hamburger *et al.*, 1978; Hamburger and White, 1982). The tumor-stimulating and angiogenesis factors mentioned are present in cell culture supernatants prepared in a manner similar to that for the tumor enhancing factor (TEF) that we have been characterizing. The factors have been partially characterized biochemically, but not purified or examined at the molecular level, and age-related changes have not been described.

Table 1. Biochemical Characteristics of Tumor Enhancing Activity in Spleen Cell Supernatants (SCS) or Peripheral Blood Mononuclear Cell Supernatants

Variable	Our findings (unpublished)	Hamburger *et al.* (1978, 1982)	Sandru *et al.* (1988)
Heat	Activity persists despite heating SCS to 80°C for 30 minutes.	Activity persists at 56°C for 30 minutes, but lost at lOO°C for 10 minutes.	Activity partially destroyed at 56°C, and completely at 80°C.
pH	Loss of activity if pH of SCS temporarily (2 hrs.) reduced to 2.5.	Loss of activity if pH of SCS temporarily (2 hrs.) reduced to 2.5.	Loss of activity if pH of SCS temporarily (2 (2 hrs.) reduced to 2.5.
Trypsin	Results in loss of the majority of activity.	Results in approximately 90% loss of activity. ·	---
Reduction	SCS reduced by *B*-mercaptoethanol results in near complete loss of	SCS reduced by dithiothreitol (DTT) did not abolish the activity.	SCS reduced by DTT results in almost complete loss of activity.
Heparin Binding	TEF in unbound fraction.	---	---

CONCLUSIONS

In experimental models employing weakly antigenic tumors, tumor growth and spread is less in old animals. This probably reflects what is observed in humans, although for many reasons, the alterations in tumor malignant behavior are less clearly demonstrable. It is our belief that age-associated decline in immune function accounts for much of the observed "age-advantage". With weakly antigenic tumors, host anti-tumor immune mechanisms are generally ineffectual (lack of antigen), and in these situations immune competence confers no specific advantage. However, lymphocyte or monocyte-mediated facilitation of tumor growth (immune enhancement) may still occur despite the lack of tumor antigens. We believe that the most important mechanism whereby lymphocytes or monocytes augment weakly antigenic tumors is by the production of a soluble factor that stimulates cellular proliferation and/or new blood vessel formation. We further propose that the production of this factor declines with age. We seek now to systematically characterize the tumor-enhancing activity present in spleen cell culture supernatants and evaluate the changes that occur in this activity over the life span.

REFERENCES

Anisimov, V.N. Carcinogenesis and aging. *Adv. in Cancer Research* 40:365 (1983).

Antonaci, S., Jirillo, E., Ventura, M.T., Garofolo, A.R., and Bonomo, L. Non-specific immunity in aging: Deficiency of monocyte and polymorphonuclear cell mediated functions. *Mechanisms of Ageing and Development* 24:367 (1984).

Auerbach, R.A., Kubai, L. and Sidky, Y. Angiogenesis induction by tumors, embryonic tissue and lymphocytes. *Cancer Research* 36:3435 (1976).

Baniyash, M., Smorodinsky, N.I., Yaakubovicz, M., Witz, I.P. Serologically detectable MHC and tumor associated antigens on B16 melanoma variants and humoral immunity in mice bearing these tumors. *J. Immunol.* 129:1318 (1982).

Berendt, M.J. and North, R.J. T-cell mediated suppression of anti-tumor immunity. An explanation for the progressive growth of an immunogenic tumor. *J. Exp. Med.* 151:69 (1980).

Berkson, J., Harrington, S.W., Clagett, O.T., Kirklin, J.W., Dockerty, M.B. and McDonald, J.R. Mortality and survival in surgically treated cancer of the breast: A statistical summary of some experience of the Mayo Clinic. *Mayo Clin. Proc.* 32:645 (1957).

Bradley, S.F., Vibhagool, A., Kunkel, S.L., and Kauffman, C.A. Monokine secretion in aging and protein malnutrition. *J. Leukocyte Biology*. 45:510 (1989).

Broder, S. and Waldmann, T.A. The suppressor-cell network in cancer. *New Eng. J. Med.* 299:1281, 13351 (1978).

Bruley-Rosset, M. and Vergnon, I. Interleukin-1 synthesis and activity in aged mice. *Mechanisms of Ageing and Development* 24:247 (1984).

Bystryn, J.C. Release of tumor associated antigens by murine melanoma cells. *J. Immunol.* 116:1302 (1976).

Calabrese, C.T., Adam, Y.G., Volk, H. Geriatric colon cancer. *Am. J. Surgery* 125:181 (1973).

Callard, R.E. and Basten, A. Immune function in aged mice. II. B-cell function. *Cellular Immunol.* 31:26 (1977).

Celik, C., Lewis, D.A. and Goldrosen, M.H. Demonstration of immunogenicity with the poorly immunogenic B16 melanoma. *Cancer Research* 43:3507 (1983).

Chang, M.P., Makinodan, T., Peterson, W.J. and, Strehler, B.L. Role of T-cells and adherent cells in age-related decline in murine interleukin-2 production. *J. Immunol.* 129:2426 (1983).

Eijan, A.M., Jasnis, M.A., Kohan, S.S., and Oisgold-Daga, S. Nature of the spleen cell populations capable of releasing tumor-enhancing factors. *J. Surg. Oncol.* 36:161 (1987).

Eijan, A.M., Jasnis, M.A., Motta, B., and Oisgold-Daga, S. Isolated soluble fractions from spleen cell culture supernatants induce tumor-enhancement. *J. Surg. Oncol.* 41:134 (1989).

Ershler, W.B., Gamelli, R.L., Moore, A.L., Hacker, M.P., and Blow, A.J. Experimental tumors and aging: Local factors that may account for the observed age advantage in the B16 murine melanoma model. *Exp. Gerontol.* 19:367 (1984a).

Ershler, W.B., Moore, A.L., Roessner, K., and Ranges, G.E. Interleukin-2 and aging: Decreased IL-2 production in healthy older people does not correlate with reduced helper cell numbers or antibody response to influenza vaccine and is not corrected *in vitro* by Thymosin Alpha One. *Immunopharmacol.* 10:11 (1986).

Ershler, W.B., Moore, A.L., Shore, H., and Gamelli, R.L. Transfer of age-associated restrained tumor growth in mice by old to young bone marrow transplantation. *Cancer Research* 44:5677 (1984b).

Ershler, W.B., Socinski, M.A., and Greene, C.J. Bronchogenic cancer, metastases and aging. *J. Am. Ger. Soc.* 31:673 (1983).

Ershler, W.B., Stewart, J.A., Hacker, M.P., Moore, A.L. and Tindle, B.H. B16 murine melanoma and aging: Slower growth and longer survival in old mice. *J. Nat. Can. Inst.* 72:161 (1984c).

Ershler, W.B., Tuck, D., Moore, A.L., Klopp, R.G., and Kaesberg, P.R. Immunologic enhancement of growth of B16 melanoma. *Cancer* 61:1792 (1988).

Fidler, I.J., Gersten, D.M. and Riggs, C.W. Relationship of host immune status to tumor cell arrest, distribution and survival in experimental metastases. *Cancer* 40:46 (1977).

Fidler, I.J. and Nicholson, G.L. Tumor cells and host properties affecting the implantation and survival of blood-borne metastatic variants of B16 melanoma. *Israel J. Med. Sci.* 14:38 (1978).

Fidler, I.J. Immune stimulation-inhibition of experimental cancer metastases. *Cancer Research*. 34:481 (1974).

Fisher, M.S. and Kripke, M.L. Further studies on the tumor-specific suppressor cells induced by ultraviolet radiation. *J. Immunol.* 121:1139 (1978).

Fisher, M.S. and Kripke, M.L. Systemic alteration induced in mice by ultraviolet light irradiation and its relationship to ultraviolet carcinogenesis. *Proc. Nat. Acad. Sci. (USA).* 74:1688 (1977).

Flood, P.M., Urban, J.L., and Kripke, M.L., and Schreiber, H. Loss of tumor-specific and idiotype-specific immunity with age. *J. Exp. Med.* 154:275 (1980).

Fong, T.C., and Makinodan, T. *In situ* hybridization analysis of the age-associated decline in IL-2 messenger RNA expressing murine T-cells. *Cellular Immunology* 118:199 (1989).

Fujimoto, S., Greene, M.I., and Sehon, A.H. Regulation of the immune response to tumor antigens. I. Immunosuppressor cells in tumor-bearing hosts. *J. Immunol.* 116:791 (1976a).

Fujimoto, S., Greene, M.I., Sehon, A.H. Regulation of the immune response to tumor antigens. II. The nature of the immunosuppressor cells in tumor-bearing hosts. *J. Immunol.* 116:800 (1976b).

Gillis, S., Kozak, R., Durante, M., and Weksler, M.E. Immunologic studies of aging: Decreased production and response to T-cell growth factor by lymphocytes from aged humans. *J. Clin. Invest.* 67:942 (1981).

Greene, E.L. Handbook on genetically standardized JAX mice. Second ed., Bar Harbor Times Publishing Co., Bar Harbor, Maine (1977).

Greene, M.I., Dorf, M.E., Pierres, M.,and Benacerraf, B. Reduction of syngenic tumor growth by an I-J alloantiserum. *Proc. Nat. Acad. Sci. (USA)* 74:5118 (1977).

Hadar, E., Ershler, W.B., Kreisle, R.A., Ho, S.P., Volk, M.J., and Klopp, R.G. Lymphocyte induced angiogenesis factor is produced by L3T4+ murine T lymphocytes, and its production declines with age. *Cancer Immunol. Immunotherapy.* 26:31 (1988).

Hamburger, A.W., Salmon, S.E., Kim, M.B., Sochlness, B., Trent, J.M., Alberts, D.S., and Schmidt, H. Direct cloning of human ovarian carcinoma cells in agar. *Cancer Research* 38:3438 (1978).

Hamburger, A.W., White, C.P., Lurie, K., and Kaplan, R. Monocyte-derived growth factors for human tumor clonogenic cells. *J. Leukocyte Biology* 40:381 (1986).

Hamburger, A.W., White, C.P. Interactions between macrophage and human clonogenic cells. *Stem Cells* 1:209 (1982).

Hellstrom, I., Hellstrom, K.E., Evans, C.A., Heppner, G.H., Pierce, G.E., and Yang, J.P.S. Serum-mediated protection of neoplastic cells from inhibition by lymphocytes immune to their tumor specific antigens. *Proc. Nal. Acad. Sci. (USA).* 62:362 (1969).

Hellstrom, K.E.and Hellstrom I. Immunologic enhancement of tumor growth, In: Green, I., Cohen, S., McCluskey, R.T. eds. **Mechanisms of Tumor Immunity.** Wiley, New York (1977).

Inamizu, T., Chang, M.P., and Makinodan, T. Influence of age on the production and regulation of interleukin-1 in mice. *Immunology* 55:447 (1985).

Isakov, N., Segal, S., Hollander, N. and Feldman, M. An immunoregulatory factor associated with spleen cells from tumor-bearing animals. I. Effects on tumor growth and antibody production. *Int. J. Cancer* 22:465 (1978).

Kaesberg, P.R. and Ershler, W.B. The change in tumor aggressiveness with age: Lessons from experimental animals. *Seminars in Oncology* 16:28 (1989).

Kreisle, R.A. and Ershler, W.B. Investigation of tumor angiogenesis in an intradermal mouse model: Role of host-tumor interactions. *J. Nat. Cancer Inst.* 80:849 (1989).

Kubota, K., Kubota, R., Takeda, S., and Matsuzawa, T. Effect of age and sex of host mice on growth and differentiation of teratocarcinomas OTT6050. *Exp. Gerontol.* 16:371 (1981).

Murasko, D.M. and Prehn, R.T. Ability of immune reactivity to potentiate tumor growth. In: Ray, P.K. ed., **Immunobiology of Transplantation, Cancer and Pregnancy**. Pergamon Press, New York (1983).

North, R.J. The murine anti-tumor immune response and its therapeutic manipulation. *Adv. Immunol.* 35:89 (1984).

Pickren, J.W., Tsukada, Y., and Lane, W.W. Liver metastasis: Analysis of autopsy data. In: Weiss, H.J. and Gilbert, H.A. eds., **Liver Metastases.** G.K. Hall, Boston (1982).

Prehn, R.T. and Lappe, M.A. An immunostimulation theory of tumor development. *Transplant Rev.* 7:26 (1971).

Prehn, R.T. Perspectives in oncogenesis: Does immunity stimulate or inhibit neoplasia? *Res. J. Reticuloendothelial Soc.* 10:1 (1971).

Prehn, R.T. The immune reaction as a stimulator of tumor growth. *Science* 176:170 (1972).

Price, G.B. and Makinodan, T. Immunologic deficiencies in senescence. I. Characterization of intrinsic deficiencies. *J. Immunol.* 108:403 (1972).

Proctor, J.W., Rudenstam, C.M., and Alexander, P. A factor preventing the development of lung metastases in rats with sarcomas. *Nature* 242:29 (1973).

Rabatic, S., Sabioncello, A., Dekaris, D., and Kardum, I. Age-related changes in functions of peripheral blood phagocytes. *Mechanisms of Ageing and Development* 45:223 (1988).

Richie, J.P., McDonald, J., and Gittes, R.F. Resistance to intravenous tumor metastases in the athymic nude mouse: a paradoxic response. *Surgery* 90:214 (1981).

Rockwell, S.C., Kallman, R.F., and Fajardo, F. Characteristics of a serially transplanted mouse mammary tumor and its tissue-culture adapted derivative. *J. Nat. Cancer Inst.* 49:735 (1972).

Rockwell, S.C. Effect of host age on transplantation, growth and radiation response of EMT6 tumors. *Cancer Research* 41:527 (1981).

Sandru, G., Verguth, P., and Stadler, B.M. Stimulation of tumor growth in humans by a mononuclear cell-derived factor. *Cancer Research* 48:5411 (1988).

Schottenfeld, D. and Robbins, G.F. Breast cancer in elderly women. *Geriatrics* 71:121 (1971).

Serge, M. and Serge, D. Humoral immunity in aged mice. I. Age-related decline in the secondary responses to DNP of spleen cells propagated in diffusion chambers. *J. Immunol.* 116:731(1976).

Sidky, Y. and Auerbach, R.A. Lymphocyte-induced angiogenesis in tumor bearing mice. *Science* 192:1237 (1976).

Sjogren, H.O., Hellstrom, I., Bansal, S.C., and Hellstrom, K.E. Suggestive evidence that the blocking antibodies of tumor bearing individuals may be antigen-antibody complexes. *Proc. Nat. Acad. Sci.(USA)*, 68:1372 (1971).

Stjernsward, J. Age-dependent tumor host barrier and effect of carcinogen induced immunodepression on rejection of isografted methylcholanthrene-induced sarcoma cells. *J. Nat. Cancer Inst.* 37:505 (1966).

Stutman, 0. Cell-mediated immunity and aging. *Fed. Proc.* 33:2028 (1974).

Suen, K.C., Lau, L.L. and Yermakov, V. Cancer and old age. An autopsy study of 3535 patients over 65 years old. *Cancer* 33:1164 (1970).

Suzuki, T., Koga, N., Imamura, T., and Mitsui, Y. A novel growth factor in rat spleen which promotes proliferation of hepatocytes in primary culture. *Biochem. and Biophys. Research Com.* 153:1123 (1988).

Tamerius, J., Nepom, J., Hellstrom, I. and Hellstrom, K.E. Tumor associated blocking factors; isolation from sera of tumor-bearing mice. *J. Immunol.* 116:724 (1976).

Thoman, M. and Weigle, W.O. Cell mediated immunity in aged mice: An underlying lesion in IL-2 synthesis. *J. Immunol.* 128:2358 (1982).

Thoman, M. and Weigle, W.O. Lymphokines and aging: Interleukin-2 production and activity in aged animals. *J. Immunol.* 127:2102 (1981).

Thoman, M.L. and Weigle, W.O. The cellular and subcellular bases of Immunosenescence., *Advances in Immunology* 46:221 (1989).

Treves, A.J., Carnaud, C., Trainin, N., Feldman, M., and Cohen, I.R. Enhancing T-lymphocytes from tumor bearing mice suppress host resistance to a syngeneic tumor. *Eur. J. Immunol.* 4:722 (1974).

Treves, A.J., Cohen, I.R., and Feldman, M. Suppressor factor secreted by T lymphocytes from tumor bearing mice. *J. Natl. Cancer Inst.* 57:409 (1976).

Tsuda, T., Kim, Y.T., Siskind, G.W., DeBlasio, A., Schwab, R., Ershler, W.B. and Weksler, M.E. Role of the thymus and T-Cells in slow growth of B16 melanoma in old mice. *Cancer Research* 47:3097 (1987).

Urban, J.L., Burton, R.C., Holland, J.M., Kripkem M.L. and Schreiber H. Mechanisms of syngeneic tumor rejection: susceptibility of host selected progressor variants to various immunologic effector cells. *J. Exp. Med.* 155:557 (1982).

Urban, J.L. and Schreiber, H. Rescue of the tumor-specific immune response of aged mice *in vitro*. *J. Immunol.* 133:527 (1984).

Weksler, M.E., Innes, J.B., and Goldstein, G. Immunological studies of aging IV. The contribution of thymic involution to the immune deficiencies of aging mice, and reversal with thymopoietin. *J. Exp. Med.* 148:996 (1976).

Wu, W., Pahlavani, M., Cheung, H.T. and Richardson, A. The effect of aging on the expression of Interleukin-2 messenger ribonucleic acid. *Cellular Immunology.* 100:224 (1986).

Yuhas, J.M., Pazmino, N.H., Proctor, J.O., and Toya, R.E. A direct relationship between immune competence and the subcutaneous growth rate of a malignant murine lung tumor. *Cancer Research* 34:722 (1974).

T CELL DIFFERENTIATION AND FUNCTIONAL MATURATION IN AGING MICE

Marilyn L. Thoman, D. N. Ernst, M. V. Hobbs and W. O. Weigle

Department of Immunology, Research Institute of Scripps Clinic
La Jolla, CA 92037

Advancing age is accompanied by changes in immune potential, frequently characterized as declines in the capacity to mount effective cell-mediated or humoral immune responses (reviewed in 1-3). Age-related functional changes can be identified earliest in the T cell compartment, therefore understanding the impact of advancing age on T cell activity may provide the key to understanding immune senescence. The expression of effector function by T cells requires their activation to cell cycle entry. The sequence of events involved in T cell activation are affected by the aging process and result in the altered T cell reactivity demonstrated in the aged.

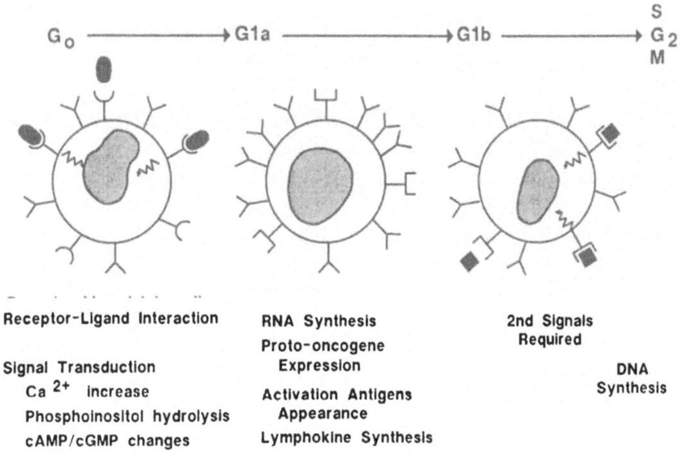

Figure 1. *T Cell Activation*

The Underlying Molecular, Cellular, and Immunological Factors in Cancer and Aging, Edited by S.S. Yang and H.R.Warner, Plenum Press, New York, 1993

As summarized in Figure 1, T cell activation is initiated by ligand binding at the T cell antigen receptor (which is mimicked by anti-T cell receptor antibodies or mitogenic lectin binding). Signal transduction pathways utilized by T lymphocytes include increases in Ca^{++} flux, activation of protein kinase C (pk-c), and accelerated phosphatidyl inositol hydrolysis (4, 5). These very early, rapid events are followed by increases in RNA synthesis, proto-oncogene expression and expression of new or greatly enhanced numbers of various cell surface receptors. Various lymphokines are also produced. Unique to the activation process of T lymphocytes is the requirement for new expression of the IL-2 receptor (IL-2R) and occupancy of this receptor for the continued progress of the cell to DNA synthesis (6).

Aged animals possess a population of T cells which is less readily induced to cell cycle entry as illustrated in Figure 2. Not only is DNA synthesis reduced (as

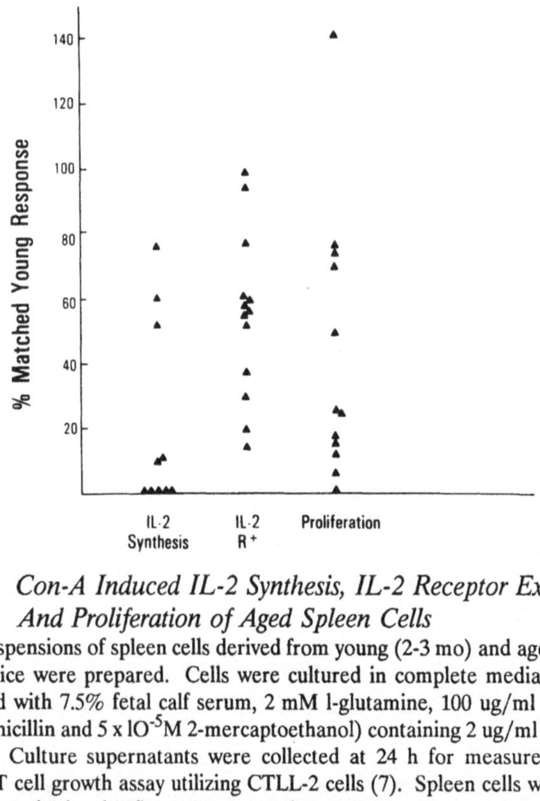

Figure 2. *Con-A Induced IL-2 Synthesis, IL-2 Receptor Expression And Proliferation of Aged Spleen Cells*

Single cell suspensions of spleen cells derived from young (2-3 mo) and aged (22-24 mo) C57BL6/J mice were prepared. Cells were cultured in complete media (RPMI 1640 supplemented with 7.5% fetal calf serum, 2 mM l-glutamine, 100 ug/ml streptomycin, 100 U/ml penicillin and 5×10^{-5}M 2-mercaptoethanol) containing 2 ug/ml Concanavalin A (Con-A). Culture supernatants were collected at 24 h for measurement of IL-2 content in a T cell growth assay utilizing CTLL-2 cells (7). Spleen cells were harvested at 48h for quantitation by flow cytometry of IL-2 receptor expression, staining with fluorescein conjugated anti-IL-2 receptor antibody (FITC-7D4). Proliferation was quantitated by ^{3}H-thymidine incorporation. Cultures were pulsed with 1 uCi/well for the final 6-8 hr of a 72 hr culture period, harvested and prepared for liquid scintillation counting. Results from individual aged mice are shown plotted as a percentage of the paired young response.

measured by ^{3}H-thymidine incorporation) but earlier activation events such as expression of IL-2 receptors and production of IL-2 are also compromised. With rare exceptions, the aged cells have been shown to be impaired in all three of these activities (7).

Other investigations have identified several age-related defects in pre-S phase T cell activation events including fewer numbers of aged murine T cells mobilizing Ca^{++} following mitogenic stimulus (8, 9), a lower degree of protein kinase C activation and translocation (10), and significantly lower phospholipid hydrolysis following stimulation (10). We have extended these observations on pre-S phase events, examining the acquisition of three G_1 phase membrane markers, the RL388 Ag, IL-2 receptors and the transferrin receptor (TfR) (11). Expression of RL388 Ag increases concurrently with T cell progression through blastogenesis and entry into G_1 phase. IL-2R expression increases with G_1 phase transit, and somewhat later transferrin receptor expression increases. Binding and uptake of both IL-2 and iron-loaded transferrin are prerequisites for S phase entry (12, 3). Detailed kinetic studies revealed that both young and aged $CD4^+$T cells showed very rapid initial increases in the expression of RL388 antigen following activation by anti-CD3 (a portion of the T cell antigen receptor complex). Although the initial cohort of cells from both aged and young animals entered G_{1a}, G_{1b} and S phases with similar kinetics, the aged population contained fewer $RL388^{hi}$, $IL\text{-}2R^+$ or TfR^+ cells (Fig. 3).

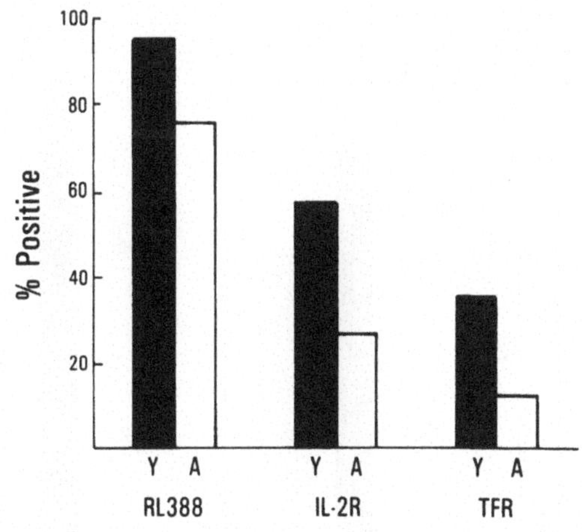

Figure 3. *Activation Antigen Expression*

Spleen cells prepared from young and aged animals were stimulated by culture with 145-2Cll (anti-CD3 [T cell antigen receptor]) for 12 hr as detailed in reference (11). Viable cells were recovered and prepared for flow cytometry. The antibodies utilized for the flow cytometry were RL388 (anti-RL388 ag), PC-61 (anti-IL-2 receptor [IL-2R]) and R17. 217 anti-transferrin receptor [TfR]). The data presented in this figure were obtained with $CD4^+$T lymphocytes, but similar observations have been made using $CD8^+$T cells (11).

These data indicate that as a population, splenic T cells derived from aged animals are poorly activated by mitogens or anti-CD3 antibodies as only a low percentage initiate cell cycle transit, display activation antigens, produce IL-2 or synthesize DNA. They further suggest that the aged population does however contain cells which are competent for cell cycle progression, but in fewer numbers than comparable population derived from young animals.

To determine whether the relatively poor activation of aged T lymphocytes to cell cycle entry and traverse is due to age associated defects previously identified in the earliest signal transduction events (8-10), experiments were designed to bypass these processes by utilizing the Ca^{++} ionophore, ionomycin, to increase Ca^{++} flux and the phorbol ester, phorbol myristate acetate (PMA) to activate pk-c. Each of these two agents was added in conjunction with Con-A to aged spleen cells which were then analyzed for IL-2 synthesis, IL-2R$^+$, and proliferation. As shown in Figure 4, the inclusion of either PMA or ionomycin can strikingly improve IL-2 synthesis and receptor expression, with ionomycin being particularly effective. These enhanced aged responses are not statistically different from the young responses. However, in contrast, ^{3}H-thymidine incorporation is not positively influenced by the inclusion of either agent.

These results suggest that the age-related decline in proliferative capacity of aged T lymphocytes is not due entirely to defects in the initial signal transduction pathways. Enhancing signal transduction with PMA or ionomycin restores the

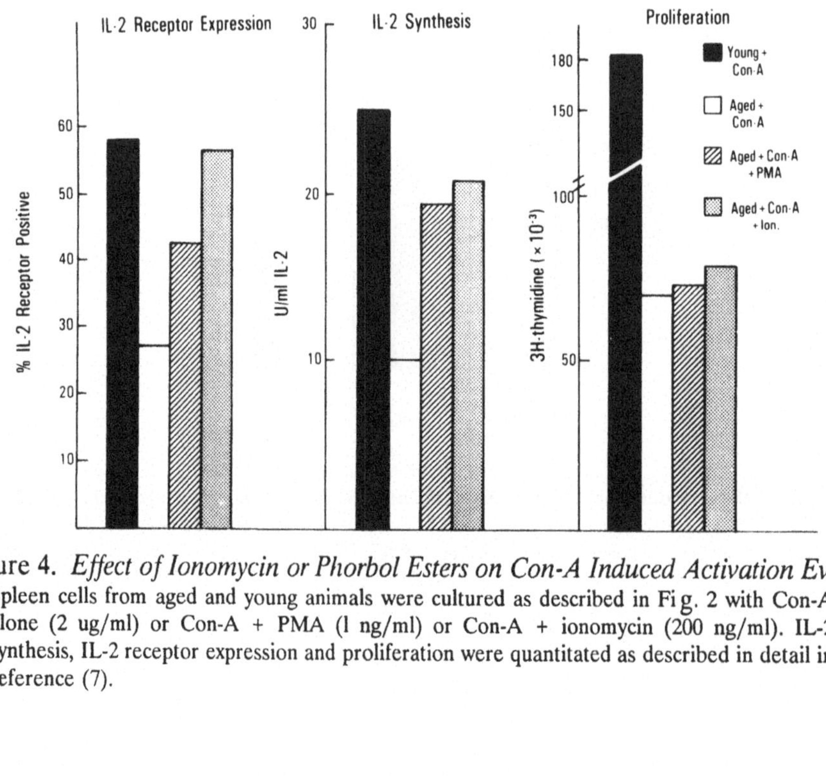

Figure 4. *Effect of Ionomycin or Phorbol Esters on Con-A Induced Activation Events*
Spleen cells from aged and young animals were cultured as described in Fig. 2 with Con-A alone (2 ug/ml) or Con-A + PMA (1 ng/ml) or Con-A + ionomycin (200 ng/ml). IL-2 synthesis, IL-2 receptor expression and proliferation were quantitated as described in detail in reference (7).

capacity for aged T cells to undergo G_1 transit. However aged T cells may also arrest at the G_{Ib}/M boundary, as demonstrated by the data presented in Figures 5 and 6. IL-2R$^+$ cells were purified by fluorescence-activated cell sorting and recultured with rIL-2 following which the growth of individual cells as well as the entire population was monitored. By sorting for T cells expressing high amounts of IL-2R$^+$ only those able to initiate blastogenesis and G_1 phase transit, therefore not displaying the "early" age-related defects, were selected. Even so, as shown in Figure 5, DNA synthesis (as measured by ^{3}H-thymidine incorporation) was diminished in the cultures of aged IL-2R$^+$ cells. Furthermore, while the growth rates of individual aged and young cells vary considerably (Figure 6), in general the average rate of growth by the aged cells is slower than that of the young. Also a higher percentage of aged IL-2R$^+$ cells are unable to undergo division in these conditions relative to IL-2R$^+$ young cells. Both major T cell subsets (CD4$^+$ and CD8$^+$) display these defects.

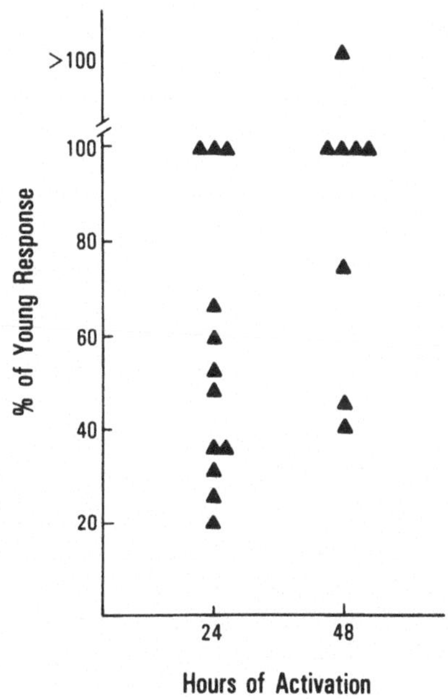

Figure 5. *Proliferation of IL-2 Receptor Bearing Lymphocytes*
Spleen cells from individual aged and young mice were cultured in complete media containing 2 ug/ml Con-A. Cells were harvested at either 24 hr or 48 hr of culture and stained with FITC-7D4 (anti-IL-2R). IL-2R$^+$ cells were purified by fluorescence activated cell sorting (FACS). IL-2R$^+$ cells were then recultured in the presence of an optimal concentration (5U/ml) of recombinant human IL-2 (rIL-2). Proliferation was quantitated by ^{3}H-thymidine incorporation 24 hr after reculture. The results are expressed as

$$\frac{\#\ \text{cpm aged cultures}}{\#\ \text{cpm young cultures}} \times 100$$

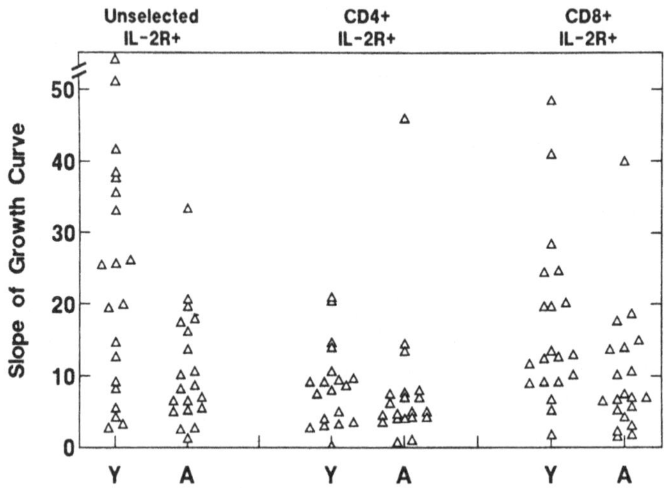

Figure 6. *Growth Rate of Individual IL-2R⁺ Cells*

IL-2R⁺ T cells were prepared as described in Fig. 4 and plated at 1-2 cells/well in media containing 5U/ml rIL-2. The number of cells/well were counted on days 1 through 5 after reculture in IL-2. The slope of the growth curves obtained for individual clones has been determined. Unselected IL-2R⁺ cells were sorted solely on the basis of IL-2 receptor expression while CD4⁺ and CD8⁺ IL-2 receptor bearing cells were purified by sorting double-stained cells which had been incubated with both FITC- 7D4 and either phycoerythrin-GK1.5 (CD4⁺) or phycoerythrin-anti-Ly-2 (CD8⁺). Y = young, A = aged.

These data reveal that, as a population, aged T splenocytes are activated to cell cycle entry at a lower frequency and may traverse through multiple rounds of cell cycle more slowly, based on the growth rate data in Figure 6, than their younger counterparts. Two alternative hypotheses have been proposed to explain these age-related changes in T cell activity: 1) That the aged T cell population is functionally mosaic comprised of "good", activable T cells and "bad" cells which are nonfunctional or 2) that the subset composition of the T cell pool changes with age, accumulating cells whose function is not optimally measured in the assays employed, nor maximally stimulated by the activation agents employed.

In general aging has not been shown to have a significant impact on the total number of T cells (14, 15), nor on their distribution into the two major subsets ($CD4^+$, $CD8^+$) (16, 17). Recently several lines of investigation have identified subdivisions of the $CD4^+$ (helper) population. Dissection of the $CD4^+$ population into two subsets has been made on the basis of the spectrum of lymphokines which each subset produces (18, 19), and two antisera (C363.16A [anti-45R] and SM3GII) appear to be useful for distinguishing these subsets phenotypically (20-23). As summarized in Table I, one subset predominately produces IL-2. Phenotypically this population is contained within the $CD45R^{hi}$ and $3GII^+$ compartment (20, 21). The other subset is characterized by a low ratio of IL-2 to IL-4 synthesis and is $CD45R^{lo}$

and 3GII⁻. The expression of both 45R and 3GII is lost upon activation. In contrast, the expression of another activation marker, Pgp-1 (recognized by the IM7.8.7 antibody), is elevated upon T cell exposure to antigen or mitogen. Thus memory $CD4^+$ T cells are Pgp-1^{hi}, $CD45R^{lo}$, and $3GII^-$, and this population is relatively enriched for IL-4 producing cells.

TABLE I. Antibodies Utilized in Subset Analyses

Antibody Designation	Antigenic Determinant	Function of Subset	Reference
RL172 GK1.5	CD4	Distinguishes "helper" class of T lymphocytes	26, 27
3.155	CD8	Distinguishes cytolytic effector T cells and suppressor T cells	28
IM7.8.1	Pgp 1	High expression distinguishes memory or activated T cells	24, 25, 29
C363.16A	CD45RB	High expression distinguishes on $CD4^+$ cells which produce IL-2, IL-3 and γ-IFN (Thl) lost from cells activated by antigen or mitogen	21, 22
SM3GII	3G II	Distinguishes $CD4^+$ cells producing IL-2 and γ-IFN (Th 1)	20

These three antisera have been employed to type the splenic $CD4^+$ T cell population resident in young and aged animals (30). The results are summarized in Figure 7. Several striking changes in subset composition are shown to occur with advancing age. A marked increase in the percentage of Pgp-$1^{hi}CD4^+$ cells is seen. Further, a decline in the percentage of the population positive for 3GII and $CD45R^{hi}$ is seen. The significance of these alterations is not completely understood, however, we suggest that they indicate an increased abundance of "memory" cells in the aged. These data are consistent with, and supportive of the suggestion that advancing age results in the accumulation of long-lived memory T cells, in part as a consequence of the decline in emigration of virgin T cells from the thymus (31). Lerner, *et al.* (32) also have described an increase in Pgp-1^{hi} T cells in aged mice and further have determined that such cells are poorly stimulated by Con-A. These data support the hypothesis that advancing age changes the subset composition of the T cell compartment which results in functional alterations.

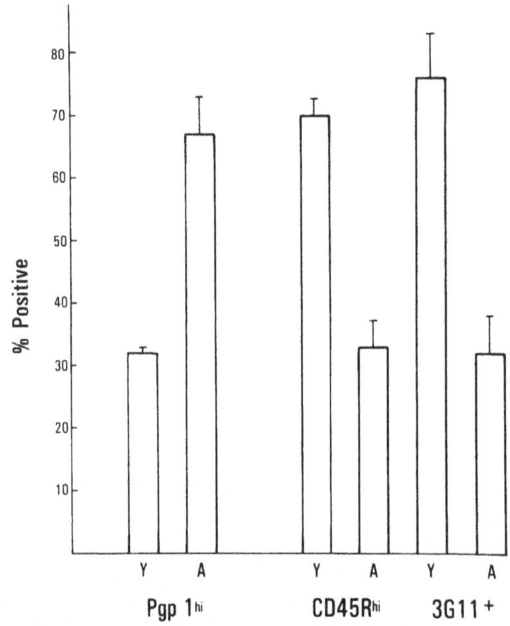

Figure 7. *Surface Marker Expression on Young And Aged CD4$^+$ T Cells.* Spleen cells from 5 young and 5 aged mice were pooled and prepared for FACS analysis as described in detail in reference (30). Antibodies used were phycoerythrin - GK1.5 (anti-CD4, fluorescein - 16A (anti-CD45RB), biotin-SM3GlI, fluorescein-IM7.8.1 (anti-Pgpl).

Clearly the loss with advancing age of the capacity for IL-2 production could significantly reduce T cell clonal expansion, and thereby diminish various T cell-mediated immune responses. It should however be possible to reconstitute such responses with IL-2, and the ability of rIL-2 to restore or improve various immune responses has been evaluated both *in vitro* and *in vivo* (33-36). Table II summarizes

TABLE II. Summary of Effects of IL-2 on In Vitro and In Vivo Immune Responses*.

In Vitro Responses	Aged Response -IL-2	(% young) +IL-2
1° Antibody	24	87
2° Antibody	20	79
MLR	23	108
Suppressor Cell	11	98
***In Vivo* Responses**		
1° CML	17	59
2° CML	8	80
IgM Antibody	4	24
IgG Antibody	16	26

***In Vitro Responses.**

Spleen cell suspensions were prepared from young or aged C57BL6/J mice and cultured as described in (33, 34) for the *in vitro* generation of various immune responses. To one half of the culture wells IL-2 was added. The results, which are described in greater detail elsewhere (33, 34) are expressed as a percentage of the control young response value.

In Vivo Responses.

Individual aged and young animals were injected intraperitoneally with allogeneic tumor cells (30 x 10^6P815) for the 1°CML, and on days 0 and 14 for the 2°CML. Other animals received 0.1 ml of a 10% solution of sheep red blood cells (SRBC) for the generation of the IgM and IgG responses. rIL-2 (250U) was administered twice daily for three days beginning the day following antigen injection. Cytolytic responses were quantitated by ^{31}Cr-release assays using ^{31}Cr-labeled P815 target cells, and peritoneal effector cells (36). The antibody response was quantitated in a plaque forming cell assay with or without an IgG developing anti-sera, using spleen cells from the SRBC-injected animals.

these results which clearly demonstrate that IL-2 can augment *in vitro* both cell-mediated and humoral responses. *In vivo* IL-2 is able to only weakly augment antibody formation. In contrast, however, cell-mediated lympholysis responses are strongly enhanced *in vivo* by IL-2 injection. These data demonstrate that, in particular cellular immune responses (mixed lymphocyte responses and cell mediated lympholysis) may be markedly enhanced in the aged by supplemental IL-2, suggesting that effector T cell function is largely limited in aged animals by diminished clonal expansion secondary to loss of IL-2 synthesizing capacity.

It has been widely assumed that in an aged individual, few if any virgin T lymphocytes are added to the peripheral compartment due to thymic involution (37, 38). However, little is known regarding the capacity of the aged thymus for reconstituting the peripheral pool. We have initiated studies in this area focusing on renewal of T cell number and function following peripheral depletion. Ultimately our goal is to determine whether T cell maturation is qualitatively as well as quantitatively altered by advancing age.

In order to address the issue of T cell renewal, animals of various ages (3-24 mo) are depleted of T cells by administration of anti-thymocyte serum, which results in the lowering of the number of peripheral blood T cells from 25% to <5%. Over the course of three to four weeks the percentage of Thy^+PBL returns to near the preinjection level in all age groups. At 4-5 weeks post-depletion animals are sacrificed and several T cell functional assays performed on the spleens. The results of several such experiments are tabulated in Table III. The extent of the recovery of Thy^+PBL is equal in all three age groups tested (3, 12 and 24 mo). However it must be noted that the percentage of Thy^+PBL does decline with age. Functional recovery (compared to age-matched, sham-injected controls) is variable. Con A induced proliferation fully recovers to control levels in all age groups. Reconstitution of the mixed lymphocyte response (MLR) is not complete in the 24 mo animals and the capacity for IL-2 synthesis is not well reconstituted even in "middle-aged" (12 mo) mice. These data suggest that as the thymus ages, not only do quantitative changes occur in mature thymocytes, but perhaps also qualitative alterations occur in the mature functional subsets. Such a possibility is being further investigated.

In conclusion, immunosenescence, the loss of immunologic vigor with advancing age, is the result of changes in T cell subset composition. The T lymphocytes which predominate in the aged appear to be those which are "memory" cells and of a subset which produces little IL-2, but greater amounts of IL-4. T cell subset compositional alterations may occur not only as a consequence of antigenic exposure but also because of quantitative and qualitative changes in intrathymic T cell maturation. These changes would significantly alter the nature of the immunologic responses triggered in the aged versus young individual and their ability to respond to new antigenic challenge.

TABLE III. Recovery of T Cells After Peripheral Depletion

	Age of Mice		
	2 mo	12 mo	24 mo
Number of Thy^+ PBL	65%	50%	93%
Mitogen Proliferation	85%	78%	80%
Mixed Lymphocyte Response	77%	69%	58%
IL-2 Synthesis	111%	48%	---

*Responses expressed as percent of age-matched sham-depleted control cells. Individual animals of various ages were depleted of peripheral T cells by intraperitoneal injection of anti-thymocyte sera. The effectiveness of this treatment was monitored by FACS analysis of peripheral blood lymphocytes stained with an anti-Thy reagent. Thirty-five days following depletion, animals were sacrificed and the peripheral blood prepared for FACS analysis of the percentage of Thy^+ cells. Functional analyses involved the culture of spleen cells with Con-A (2 ug/ml) or irradiated allogeneic cells. Culture supernatants from Con-A activated cells were collected and tested for IL-2 content 24 hr after culture initiation (7). ^{3}H-thymidine (1 uCi/well) was added to other Con-A containing or allogeneic cell-containing wells at 72 hr to quantitate proliferation. Following a 6-8 hr pulse these wells were harvested and prepared for liquid scintillation counting.

REFERENCES

1. Nagel, J.E. *Rev. Biol. Res. Aging* 1: 103 (1983).

2. Miller, R. A. The cell biology of aging: immunological models. *J. Geron.* 44: B4 (1989).

3. Thoman, M. L. and Weigle, W. 0. The cellular and subcellular bases of immunosenescence. *Adv. Immunol.* 46: 221 (1989).

4. Isakov, N., Mally, M. I., Scholz, W. and Altman, A. T-lymphocyte activation: The role of protein kinase C and the bifurcating inositol phospholipid signal transduction pathway. *Immunol. Rev.* 95: 89 (1989).

5. Linch, D. C., Wallace, D. L. and O'Flynn, K. Signal transduction in human T lymphocytes. *Immunol. Rev.* 95: 137 (1987).

6. Cantrell, D. and Smith, K. A. The interleukin-2 T-cell system:A new cell growth model. *Science* 224: 1312 (1984).

7. Thoman, M. L. and Weigle, W. 0. Partial restoration of ConA-induced proliferation, IL-2 receptor expression and IL-2 synthesis in aged murine lymphocytes by phorbol myristate acetate and ionomycin. *Cell. Immunol.* 114: 1 (1988).

8. Miller, R. A., Jacobson, B., Weil, G. and Simons, E. R. Diminished calcium in-flux in lectin stimulated T cells from old mice. *J. Cell. Physiol.* 132: 337 (1987).

9. Lerner, A., Philosophe, B. and Miller, R. Defective calcium influx and preserved inositol phosphate generation in T cells from old mice. *Aging: Imunol. Infect. Dis.* 1: 149 (1988).

10. Prouse, J., Filburn, C., Harrison, S., Bucholz, N. and Nordin, A. Age-related defect in signal transduction during lectin activation of murine T lymphocytes. *J. Immunol.* 139: 1472 (1987).

11. Ernst, D.N., Weigle, W.0., McQuitty, D.N., Rothermel, A.L. and Hobbs, M.V. Stimulation of murine T cell subsets with anti-CD3 antibody. Age-related fects in the expression of early activation molecules. *J. Immunol.* 142:1413 (1989).

12. Neckers, L. M. and Cossman, J. Transferrin receptor induction in mitogen-stimulated human T lymphocytes is required for DNA synthesis and cell division and is regulated by interleukin 2. *Proc. Natl. Acad. Sci. USA.* 80: 3493 (1983).

13. Herzberg, V. L. and Smith, K. A. T cell growth without serum. *J. Immunol.* 139: 998 (1987).

14. Stutman, O. Lymphocyte subpopulations in NZB mice: Deficit of thymus-dependent lymphocytes. *J. Immunol.* 109: 602 (1972).

15. Callard, R. E. and Basten, A. Immune function in aged mice. I. T-cell responsiveness using phytohaemagglutinin as a functional probe. *Cell. Immunol.* 31: 13 (1977).

16. O'Leary, J. J., Fox, R., Bergh, N., Rodysill, K. and Hallgren, H. M. Expression of the human T cell antigen receptor complex in advanced age. *Mech. Age. Dev.* 45: 239 (1988).

17. Sidman, C. L., Luther, E. A., Marshall, J. D., Nguyen, K. A., Roopenian, D. C. and Worthen, S. M. Increased expression of major histocompatibility complex antigens on lymphocytes from aged mice. *Proc. Natl. Acad. Sci. USA.* 84: 7624 (1987).

18. Mosmann, T., Cherwinski, H., Bond, M., Giedlin, M. and Coffman, R. Two types of murine helper T cell clone 1. Definition according to profiles of lymphokine activities and secreted proteins. *J. Immunol.* 136: 2348 (1986).

19. Mosmann, T. and Coffman, R. Heterogeneity of cytokine secretion patterns and function of helper T cells. *Adv. Immunol.* 46: 111 (1989).

20. Hayakawa, K. and Hardy, R. Murine $CD4^{+}T$ cell subsets defined. *J. Exp. Med.* 168: 1825 (1988).

21. Bottomley, K., Lugman, M., Greenbaum, L., Carding, S., West, J., Pasqualini, T. and Murphy, D. A monoclonal antibody to murine CD45R distinguishes $CD4^{+}T$ cell populations that produce different cytokines. *Eur. J. Immunol.* 19: 617 (1989).

22. Birkeland, M. L., Johnson, P., Trowbridge, I. S. and Pure, E. Changes in CD45 isoform expression accompany antigen-induced murine T-cell activation. *Proc. Natl. Acad. Sci. USA.* 86: 6734 (1989).

23. Lee, W. T., Yin, X. M. and Vitetta, E. S. Functional ontogenetic analysis of murine $CD45R^{hi}$ and $CD45R^{lo}CD4^{+}T$ cells. *J. Immunol.* 144: 3288 (1990).

24. Butterfield, K., Fathman, G. and Budd, R. A subset of memory $CD4^{+}$ helper T lymphocytes identified by expression of Pgp-l. J. Exp. Med. 169: 1461 (1989).

25. MacDonald, H. R., Budd, R. C. and Cerotini, J.-C. Pgp-l (Ly24) as a marker of murine memory T lymphocytes. *Curr. Top. Microbiol. Immunol.* 159: 97 (1990).

26. Ceredig, R., Lowenthal, J., Nabholz, M. and MacDonald, H. Expression of interleukin 2 receptors as a differentiation marker on intrathymic stem cells. *Nature* 314: 98 (1985).

27. Dialynas, D. P., Wilde, D. B., Marrack, P., Pierres, A., Wall, K. A., Havran, W., Otten, G., Loken, M. R., Pierres, M., Kappler, J. and Fitch, F. W. Characterization of the murine antigenic determinant designated L_3T_{4A}, recognized by monoclonal antibody GK1.5:expression of L_3T_{4A}, by functional T cell clones appears to correlate primarily with class II MHC antigen-reactivity. Immunol. Rev. 74: 1983 (1983).

28. Sarimento, M., Glasebrook, A. and Fitch, F. W. IgG or IgM monoclonal antibodies reactive with different determinants of the molecular complex bearing Lyt 2 antigen block T cell-mediated cytolysis in the absence of complement. *J. Immunol.* 125: 2665 (1980).

29. Trowbridge, I. S., Lesley, J., Schulte, R., Hyman, R. and Trotter, J. Biochemical characterizaton and cellular distribution of a polymorphic murine cell-surface glycoprotein expressed on lymphoid cells. *Immunogenetics* 15: 299 (1982).

30. Ernst, D. N., Hobbs, M. V., Torbett, B. E., Glasebrook, A. L., Rehse, M. A., Bottomly, K., Hayakawa, K., Hardy, R. A. and Weigle, W. 0. Differences in the expression profiles of CD45RB, Pgp-l, and 3Gll membrane antigens and in the patterns of lymphokine secretion by splenic $CD4^+$T cells from young and aged mice. *J. Immunol.* in press (1990).

31. Scollay, R., Butcher, E. and Weissman, I. Thymus cell migration. Quantitative aspects of cellular traffic from the thymus to the periphery in mice. *Eur. J. Immunol.* 10: 210 (1980).

32. Lerner, A., Yamada, T., Miller, R. Pgp-l^{hi} T lymphocytes accumulate with age in mice and respond poorly to concanavalin A. *Eur. J. Immunol.* 19: 977 (1989).

33. Thoman, M. L. and Weigle, W. 0. Lymphokines and aging:lnterleukin-2 production and activity in aged animals. *J. Immunol.* 127: 2102 (1981).

34. Thoman, M. L. and Weigle, W. 0. Cell-mediated immunity in aged mice: an underlying lesion in IL-2 synthesis. *J. Immunol.* 128: 2358 (1982).

35. Thoman, M. L. and Weigle, W. 0. Deficiency in suppressor T cell activity in aged animals. Reconstitution of this activity by Interleukin 2. *J. Exp. Med.* 157: 2184 (1983).

36. Thoman, M. L. and Weigle, W. 0. Reconstitution of *in vivo* cell-mediated lympholysis responses in aged mice with Interleukin 2. *J. Immunol.* 134: 949 (1985).

37. Tosi, P., Kraft, R., Luzi, P., Cintorino, M., Fankhauser, G., Hess, M. and Coltier, H. Involution patterns of the human thymus. I. Size of the cortical area as a function of age. *Clin. Exp. Immunol.* 47: 497 (1982).

38. Weksler, M. The thymus gland and aging. *Ann. Intern. Med.* 98: 105 (1988).

CYTOGENETICS AND CLINICAL CORRELATIONS IN BREAST CANCER

Julia C. Emerson, Sydney E. Salmon, William Dalton, Daniel L. McGee, Jin-Ming Yang, Floyd H. Thompson, and Jeffrey M. Trent*

Arizona Cancer Center
University of Arizona
Tucson, Arizona 85724

*University of Michigan Cancer Center
Ann Arbor, Michigan 48109

ABSTRACT

We describe an ongoing study examining the relevance of cytogenetic changes in primary and metastatic breast cancer. Tumors samples from breast cancer patients are karyotype using G-banding techniques, and all chromosomal findings, including the presence of structural and numeric clonal abnormalities, are documented in a dynamic patient data base. Information on essential clinical characteristics is collected, and patients are followed longitudinally for disease recurrence, progression, and survival. Statistical analyses will examine potential correlations between specific abnormalities and clinical features of the disease, and survival differences between patients will be examined as a function of karyotypic differences. We anticipate that this research will provide insights on the natural history of breast cancer and help direct the search for the underlying molecular mechanisms of tumor genesis and progression.

INTRODUCTION

Breast cancer is the most common neoplasm occurring among U.S. women. In 1990 it is estimated that 150,000 new cases will be diagnosed, accounting for 29%

The Underlying Molecular, Cellular, and Immunological Factors in Cancer and Aging, Edited by S.S. Yang and H.R.Warner, Plenum Press, New York, 1993

of all new cancers in women.[1] The risk of breast cancer increases with age throughout a woman's lifespan,[2] with an estimated 70% of cases occurring in women over the age of 50.[3] It is thus apparent that the major impact of breast cancer is in older women. Breast cancer incidence rates in this country have been increasing over the past decade, which may reflect better and earlier disease detection. However, even if breast cancer incidence rates remain relatively stable over the coming decades, the number of new cases each year is expected to rise as the current U.S. population ages, and the numbers of women in older age groups increases.

In the current investigation chromosomal abnormalities in breast cancer are being identified and correlated with clinical and biological features of the disease. We anticipate that such cytogenetic correlations have the potential to provide significant information regarding the natural history of breast cancer, as has been true for cytogenetic studies of the leukemias and lymphomas. Furthermore, it is the detection of non-random chromosomal abnormalities that can guide efforts to identify the underlying molecular mechanism of tumor development and progression.

Breast Cancer Cytogenetics

The cytogenetic examination of human solid tumor, including breast carcinoma, has lagged significantly behind cytogenetic studies of the human leukemias and lymphomas,[5] despite the fact that solid tumors contribute significantly more to morbidity and mortality. The paucity of studies and information on chromosomal changes in solid tumors is attributable in part to the technical difficulties in obtaining analyzable chromosomal preparations. Among these difficulties are the inherently low mitotic activity of most tumors, low yields of viable cells in tissue culture, and the infiltration of tumor tissue by normal stromal cells.[6] However, recent methodological advances now make it possible to systematically study the cytogenetic changes in solid tumors.[7]

The majority of breast cancer cases examined to date by cytogenetic techniques were studied prior to the advent of modern chromosome banding techniques, which allow for individual chromosomes to be unequivocally identified.[8] Thus, these pre-banding studies are primarily of historical interest, although several common chromosomal features from these early studies can be identified. Most breast cancers studied pre-banding were metastatic tumors, and most demonstrated aneuploidy, often with numerous structural chromosome alterations (e.g., marker chromosomes).[9-11]

Far fewer breast tumors have been studied using modern banding techniques; however, in the banded cases features common to the majority of unbanded preparations continue to be observed. In particular, banded studies of breast tumors continue to reveal that the majority of cases are aneuploid with structural changes frequently found. Findings from most studies suggest that specific chromosomes are commonly altered in breast cancer.[12-22] Abnormalities involving chromosome 1 have been reported frequently, with the long arm of chromosome 1 often involved in translocations; however, the translocation breakpoints and translocation partners have been observed to be highly variable, which given the ubiquitous nature of chromosome 1 alterations in solid tumors, suggests that these changes may represent secondary events perhaps associated with tumor progression. Other chromosomes frequently found to be altered in banded studies of breast cancer include chromosomes 6, 7, and 11; in particular, alterations of 6q, 7p, and 11q have often been identified.

The current investigation is designed to further elucidate the nature of recurring, non-random chromosomal abnormalities in breast cancer and to establish whether these specific cytogenetic changes have clinical and biologic significance.

MATERIALS AND METHODS

The present study is a prospective follow-up study of women presenting with primary or metastatic breast cancer. For the purposes of this study, primary breast cancer designates the initial presentation with the disease, while metastatic breast cancer refers to disease recurrence subsequent to the initial diagnosis. The referral population of the Arizona Cancer Center serves as the source population for such cases, who are included if there is histologic confirmation of the diagnosis and if there is sufficient tumor sample available for cytogenetic analysis. Clinical data and follow-up information for each subject are obtained from the primary physician or medical record review. Clinical variables being collected include characteristics of the tumor at the time of presentation (e.g., histology, stage, size, nodal involvement, presence of distant metastases, and hormone receptor content), other clinical factors (e.g., age, menopausal status, and family history), and information related to treatment, disease progression, and patient survival. All clinical and laboratory data are entered into a dynamic patient data base from which relevant data can be extracted at the time of data analysis.

Cytogenetic studies are performed on all samples according to a standard protocol for short-term culture. Harvesting and banding techniques have been described previously.[23] Following G-banding of metaphase cells, chromosomes are examined for the presence of structural and numeric abnormalities and classified according to the International System for Human Cytogenetic Nomenclature.[24] Structural abnormalities are considered to represent clonal change if at least two cells are observed with the same structural rearrangement. Numeric abnormalities are regarded as being of clonal origin if at least three cells are observed with the same abnormality.

Statistical methods to be used will not he detailed in this setting, other than a brief discussion (see below) of the types of analyses to be performed.

RESULTS

Because of the ongoing accrual of subjects and the longitudinal nature of this study, only very preliminary results can be documented at present. To date, cytogenetic studies have been performed and clinical data obtained for 83 primary breast cancer cases and 49 metastatic breast cancer cases. Table I summarizes key characteristics of the patients. Table Ia shows that the majority of primary breast cases studied to date were 50 years of age or older at the time of their diagnosis. Almost a quarter of the patients reported a positive family history of breast cancer in a first degree relative. Estrogen receptors were positive in 61% of the tumors, and estrogen receptor positivity was significantly more frequent in women over the age of 50 ($p < 0.05$). Positive axillary nodes were present in 46% of these women at the time of surgery. Approximately 20% had Stage I, close to 60% Stage II, and the remainder Stage III or IV breast cancer at the time of primary surgery.

Table I. Clinical Characteristics of Primary and Metastatic Breast Cancer Patients Whose Biopsies Were Submitted for Cytogenetic Analysis.

a. **Primary Breast Cancer Cases (N = 83)**

	No. with characteristic
Age $\geq$ 50 at diagnosis	54 (.65)
Post-menopausal	56 (.08)
Positive family history	20 (.24)
Estrogen receptor positivity	51 (.61)
Positive nodes	38 (.46)

b. **Metastatic Breast Cancer Cases (N = 49)**

	No. with characteristic
Age $\geq$ 50 at biopsy	35 (.71)
Five years or less since 1st diagnosis	28 (.57)
Positive nodes at 1st diagnosis	30 (.61)
Received adjuvant chemotherapy	28 (.57)
Received adjuvant hormonal therapy	11 (.22)
Received adjuvant radiotherapy	11 (.22)

Of the metastatic breast patients (Table I b), the majority of the women studied to date were 50 years of age or older at the time of positive biopsy for metastatic cancer. In 57% of these patients the time interval from the initial diagnosis of breast cancer to the appearance of distant metastasis was less than 5 years. Sixty-one percent of patients with metastatic breast cancer presented with positive axillary nodes at the time of original diagnosis, and over half of the patients received adjuvant chemotherapy for their primary tumor, with far fewer receiving either adjuvant hormonal or radiation treatment.

Table II. Cytogenetic Findings in Primary and Metastatic Breast Cancer Cases Studied.

	Primary Disease (N = 83)	Metastatic Disease (N= 49)
Karyotyping successful:		
No*	27 (.33)	5 (.10)
Yes	56 (.67)	44 (.90)
Results of karyotyping:		
Normal	29 (.52)	17 (.39)
Abnormal	27 (.48)	27 (.61)
Abnormalities Detected:		
Structural abnormalities	14 (.52)	26 (.06)
Numeric abnormalities	17 (.63)	20 (.77)

*Cells did not grow in culture or no metaphases were detected.

Cytogenetic results for the 83 primary breast cancer patients are summarized in Table II. No mitoses were obtained in 27 of the samples (33% of cases). Karyotyping was possible for the remaining 56 cases from which mitoses were obtained. Examination of the demographic and initial characteristics of those patients in whom mitoses were obtained and those with no mitoses did not reveal any significant differences between these groups.

Among the 56 cases of primary breast cancer successfully karyotyped, approximately half were found to have normal karyotypes, and approximately half were found to have abnormal karyotypes. Among the 27 patients with abnormal karyotypes, 14 patients demonstrated one or more structural clonal abnormalities, and 17 patients demonstrated one or more numeric clonal abnormalities. These categories are not mutually exclusive with a number of patients demonstrating both structural and numeric abnormalities.

The frequency with which specific chromosomes were involved in structural clonal abnormalities is illustrated in Figure 1. Structural abnormalities were detected most frequently in chromosomes 1, 2, 3, 6, 7, and 11; a variety of abnormalities were observed including translocation, deletions, inversions, and insertions. As can be appreciated from the Figure, the vast majority of numeric chromosomal abnormalities detected thus far in this series of primary breast cancers have been losses of normal chromosome homolog. Those chromosomes showing loss most frequently have been chromosomes 8, 9, 10, 11, 16, 17, and 19.

Results of the cytogenetic studies on the 49 metastatic breast cancer cases are also summarized in Table II. No mitoses were obtained in 5 of the 49 cases, with mitoses obtained in the remaining 44 cases. Karyotypes of these 44 cases were normal in 17 of the cases and abnormal in 27 of the cases. Among those patients having abnormal karyotypes, 26 demonstrated one or more structural clonal abnormalities, and 20 demonstrated one or more numeric clonal abnormalities. The structural abnormalities that we have observed in metastatic breast cancer are shown in Figure 2, with chromosomes 1, 3, 7, and 11 most frequently involved. Numeric abnormalities in metastatic breast cancer are also summarized in Figure 2 and show a somewhat different pattern from that observed in primary breast cancer. The metastatic cases evidence an abundance of chromosomal gain as well as loss.

Because of statistical constraints, meaningful correlations between the clinical data and specific cytogenetic changes cannot be made until a larger number of cases have been successfully karyotyped. Likewise, analyses related to patient survival also require accrual of a larger sample size and longer follow-up.

DISCUSSION

We are currently studying the relevance of cytogenetic changes in breast cancer within a clinical framework; this investigation is of particular importance because no systematic, large-scale study of the clinical implications of cytogenetic abnormalities in breast cancer has been reported previously. Preliminary examination of the clinical data indicates that the patients available for study represent a diversity of disease presentations, and thus the eventual correlation of specific chromosomal abnormalities with clinical parameters should offer an

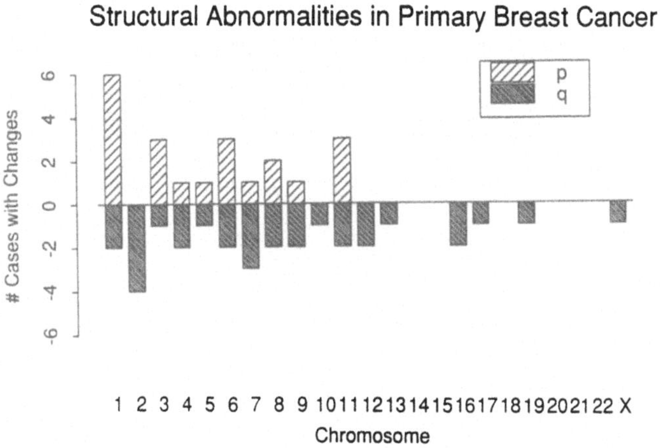

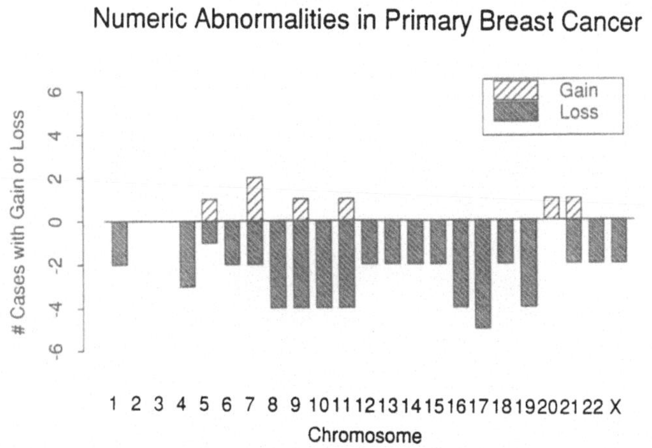

Figure 1. *Frequency of Structural and Numeric Chromosomal Abnormalities Detected among Primary Breast Cancer Cases.*

Structural Abnormalities are plotted according to chromosome arm involved (p = short arm, q = long arm); numeric abnormalities are plotted according to whether gain or loss was detected.

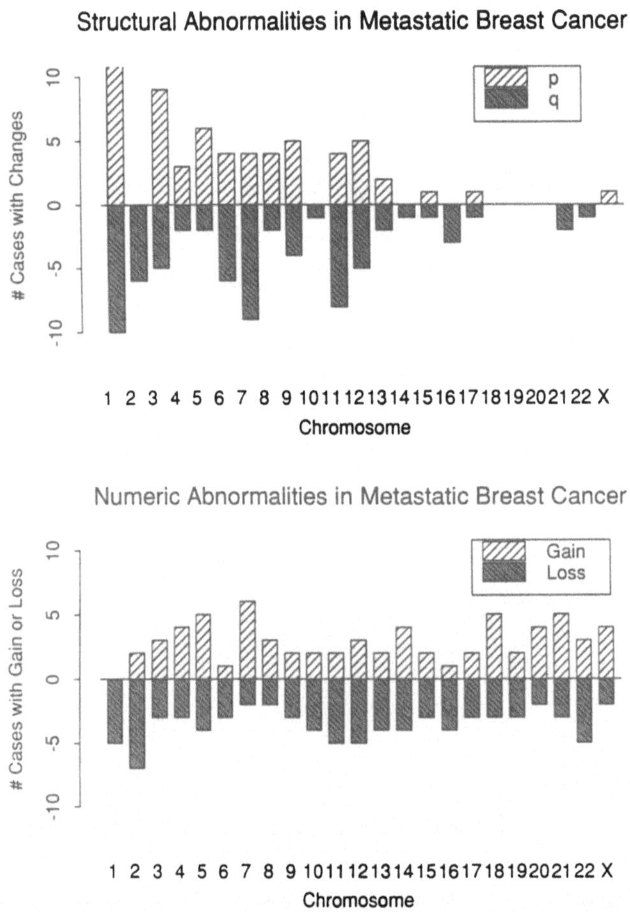

Figure 2. *Frequency of Structural and Numerical Chromosomal Abnormalities Detected among Metastatic Breast Cancer Cases.* Plotting conventions as in Figure 1.

excellent opportunity to better characterize the clinical relevance of cytogenetic changes. Preliminary cytogenetic findings demonstrate that abnormal karyotypes are a frequent finding in breast cancer. Among cases successfully karyotyped thus far, we have observed cytogenetic abnormalities in approximately half of the primary breast cancers and almost two thirds of the metastatic breast cancers.

Long-term plans call for the accrual and cytogenetic examination of a substantially larger number of cases, with longitudinal follow-up for the observation of endpoints. A hierarchy of statistical analyses will then be conducted. Initially, the distributions of observed cytogenetic abnormalities will be examined to identify statistically significant, non-random abnormalities. As reported by Brodeur, Tsiatis, *et al.*, computer simulations will be used to generate expected distributions of numeric and structural abnormalities.[25] The expected distribution will then be compared to the observed distribution of abnormalities to identify non-random involvement of a particular chromosome, arm, or region. As an example from our primary breast cancer studies discussed above, it seems apparent that more cases are observed with structural abnormalities of the short arm of chromosome 1 than would be expected due to chance alone; however, distinguishing which of the other chromosome arms are non-randomly involved is more difficult. The methods to be used will allow for chromosome length to be accounted for when testing for non-random involvement with structural abnormalities.

Recurring, non-random abnormalities thus identified will then be correlated with clinical parameters to determine the relationship of particular chromosomal changes to features of the disease. Multivariate survival methods will also be used to compare the survival of patients with and without specific abnormalities adjusting for such covariates that are known to affect outcome, such as age, treatment, and initial stage of disease. Endpoints will include time to relapse for primary breast cancer and time to death for metastatic breast cancer.

The strengths and limitations of this particular type of study deserve comment. Strengths of the study include that it involves a relatively well-defined population from whom complete data regarding disease characteristics and outcomes should be available. Our study is designed to answer questions regarding the nature of recurring, non-random chromosomal abnormalities in breast cancer, but also can potentially define the clinical significance of such cytogenetic changes.

Potential limitations of this or any other study of solid tumor cytogenetics include both technical and sample size limitations. Technical issues which must be considered include insuring a high success rate for growth of tumor cells in short-term culture. Also, methods need to be developed to assure that the actual cells being karyotyped are tumor cell. From a statistical standpoint, sample size constraints are a major concern. A large enough sample of cases must be examined in order to allow for analyses of how particular chromosomal abnormalities might be related to the clinical parameters; in particular, the use of multivariate models to describe such relationships will require a substantially larger number of cases.

It seems apparent that recurring site of chromosomal change in human tumors may represent markers of molecular events involved in tumor generation or progression. We have described a study in progress in which we hope to identify the most frequently occurring sites of chromosomal change in primary and metastatic breast cancer and deter:nine the relationship of such changes to the natural history of this disease. We anticipate that the recognition, and ultimately, the molecular understanding of these abnormalities will provide further insights into the neoplastic process and enhance our understanding of the biologic mechanism underlying the clinical features of breast cancer.

ACKNOWLEDGEMENTS

These studies were supported by grants CA41183 and CA23074. We acknowledge the outstanding technical assistance of Ann Burgess.

REFERENCES

1. Silverberg, E., Boring, C.C. and Squires, T.S. Cancer Statistics *CA* 40:9 (1990).

2. Kelsey, J.L. and Berkowitz, G.S. Breast cancer epidemioLogy. *Cancer Research* 48:5615 (1988).

3. Stewart, J.A. and Foster, R.S. Breast cancer and aging. *Seminars Oncol.* 16:41 (1989).

4. **"Cancer Statistics Review 1973-1987"** U.S. department of Health and Human Services, NIH Publication No. 90-2789 (1988).

5. Mitelman, F. *"Catalog of Chromosome Aberrations in Cancer, Ed. 3".* Alan R. Liss, Inc., New York (1988).

6. Teyssier, J.R. The chromosomal analysis of human solid tumors: a triple challenge. *Cancer Genet Cytogenet* 37:103 (1989).

7. Trent, J. Crickard, K., Gibas, Z., Goodacre, A., Pathak, S., Sandberg, A.A., Thompson, F.H., Whang-Peng, J., and Wolman, S. Methodologic advances in the cytogenetic analysis of human solid tumors. *Cancer Genet Cytogenet* 19:57 (1986).

8. Sandberg, A.A. "**The Chromosomes in Human Cancer and Leukemia**" Elsevier, New York (1980).

9 Trent, J.M. Cytogenetic and molecular biologic alterations in human breast cancer: a review. *Breast Cancer Res Treat* 5:221 (1985).

10. Cervenka, J. and Koulischer, L. "**Chromosomes in Human Cancer**", R. Gorlin, ed., Charles Thomas Publishers, Springfield, Illinois (1973).

11. Atkin, N.B. "**Cytogenetic Aspects of Malignant Transformation**", S. Karger, Basel, Switzerland (1976).

12. Mark, J. Two pseudodiploid human breast carcinomas studied with G-band technique. *Eur J Cancer* 11:815 (1975).

13. Kovacs, G. Preferential involvement of chromosome 1q in a primary breast carcinoma. *Cancer Genet Cytogen* 3:125 (1981).

14. Rogers, C.S., Hill, S.M. and Hulten, M.A. Cytogenetic analysis in human breast carcinoma. I. Nine cases in the diploid range investigated using direct preparations. *Cancer Genet Cytogenet* 13:95 (1984).

15. Gebhart, E., Bruderlein, S., Augustus, M., Siebert, E., Feldner, J. and Schmidt, W. Cytogenetic studies on human breast carcinomas. *Breast Cancer Res Treat* 8:125 (1986).

16. Ferti-Passantonopoulou, A.D. and Panani, A.D. Common cytogenetic findings in primary breast cancer. *Cancer Genet Cytogenet* 27:289 (1987).

17. Gerbault-Seureau, M, Vielh, P. Zafrani, P., Salmon, R., Dutrillaux, B. Cytogenetic study of twelve near-diploid breast cancers with chromosomal changes. *Ann Genet* 30:138 (1987).

18. Hill, S. M., Rodgers, C.S. and Hulten, M.A. Cytogenetic analysis in human breast carcinoma. II. Seven cases in the triploid/tetraploid range investigated using direct preparations. *Cancer Genet Cytogenet* 24:45 (1987).

19. Trent, J.M. Yang, J.M. Thompson, F.H., Leibovitz, A., Villar, H.V. and Dalton, W.S. Chromosome alterations in human breast cancer. In: "**Oncogenes and Hormones in Breast Cancer**", M. Sluyser, ed., Ellis Horwood Ltd., Amtersdam (1987).

20. Bello, M.J. and Rey, J.A. Cytogenetic analysis of metastatic effusions from breast tumors. *Neoplasma* 36:71 (1989).

21. Trent, J.M., Kaneko, Y. and Mitelman, F. Report of the committee on structural chromosome changes in neoplasia. Human Gene Mapping 10 (1989): Tenth International Workshop on Human Gene Mapping. *Cytogenet Cell Genet* 51:533 (1989).

22. Zhang, R., Wiley, J., Howard, S.P., Meisner, L.F., and Gould, M.N. Rare clonal karyotypic variants in primary cultures of human breast carcinoma. *Cancer Res* 49:444 (1989).

23. Trent, J.M. and Thompson, F.H. In: "Methods for chromosome banding of human and experimental tumor *in vitro*", ed. by Gottesman, M. Academic Press, New York (1987).

24. International System for Human Cytogenetic Nomenclature (ISCN). *Cancer Genet Cytogenet* 21:1 (1985).

25. Brodeur, G.M., Tsiatis, A.A., Willians, D.L., Luthardt, F.W. and Green, A.A. Statistical analysis of cytogenetic abnormalities in human cancer cells. *Cancer Genet Cytogenet* 7:137 (1982).

BREAST CANCER: INFLUENCE OF ENDOCRINE HORMONES, GROWTH FACTORS AND GENETIC ALTERATIONS

Robert B. Dickson, Michael D. Johnson, Dorraya El-Ashry, Yenian Eric Shi, Mozeena Bano, Gerhard Zugmaier, Barbara Ziff, Marc E. Lippman, and Susan Chrysogelos

Vincent T. Lombardi Cancer Center
Georgetown University Hospital
3900 Reservoir Road N.W.
Washington, D.C. 20007

BREAST CANCER: AGE AND HORMONAL DEPENDENCE

Breast cancer is a disease whose frequency as well as pathologic characteristics vary markedly with age and sex. Women develop breast cancer with an incidence of approximately 1 in 10 in the United States, about 100 times the frequency in men. In women, the incidence of breast cancer increases with increasing age, but the rate of increase drops off sharply at the age of menopause (Pike *et al.*, 1981). Breast cancer is more likely in postmenopausal than in premenopausal women to be positive for the receptor for estrogen (Ottman *et al.*, 1981). Estrogen receptor positive breast cancer, whether postmenopausal or premenopausal, is associated with better prognosis than receptor negative breast cancer (Sunderland and McGuire, 1990). These statistics have contributed to the view that exposure of the mammary gland to ovarian estrogens (and progestins) is critical to onset and malignant progression of breast cancer. Indeed, perimenarchal loss of ovarian function can result in a decrease in breast cancer risk by a factor of 100 to about that found in men (Brown, 1981). Furthermore, ovariectomy and/or antiestrogenic and antiprogestational drugs have been successfully used in treatment of breast cancer (Iino *et al.*, 1990).

Though ovarian steroids appear to be critical in the onset of breast cancer and the growth of premenopausal disease, other growth regulatory mechanisms must come into play after loss of ovarian function during menopause. In addition to endocrine

The Underlying Molecular, Cellular, and Immunological Factors in Cancer and Aging, Edited by S.S. Yang and H.R.Warner, Plenum Press, New York, 1993

hormonal factors, a genetic factor(s) is thought to influence breast cancer risk. It has been estimated that 5-10% of breast cancer in women under 50 years of age is highly associated with a familial propensity for the disease. The epidemiology of breast cancer in these families fits a model of an inherited autosomal dominant gene accounting for a much higher proportion of premenopausal than postmenopausal cancers (Ponder, 1990). The identity of this gene remains unknown, as does its function at the cellular level. It is also not clear whether any biochemical mechanism relating to inherited tendencies for premenopausal breast cancer might have some relationship biochemically to postmenopausal mechanisms of tumorigenesis. For instance, it may be that, like retinoblastoma, the predisposing gene is inherited as a heterozygous deletion and sporadically mutated to yield a very early onset disease. To pursue this hypothetical analogy, if two spontaneous mutations of a specific locus are required in breast cancer, as in the sporadic form of retinoblastoma, then onset would be later in life than in familial breast cancer (Weinberg, 1990). It is also possible that in the heterozygous condition, a predisposing mutation might have some other type of impact on developing breast cancer (Ponder, 1990).

HORMONAL CONTROL OF MAMMARY PROLIFERATION

The regulation of normal breast development, breast carcinogenesis, and growth and progression of breast cancer seems to depend upon response to hormonal factors. Historically, the most well-defined hormonal factors are the endocrine steroids and peptides produced by the glandular epithelium of the ovaries, pituitary, endocrine pancreas, and adrenal cortex. More recently the ability of both normal and malignant tissue to synthesize locally acting hormones has been recognized. One class is that of the paracrine hormones, factors released by one cell type which then modulate the function of neighboring cells of the same or a different tissue. A second class is that of the autocrine hormones, factors released by one cell type that act back on the same cell type through surface receptors. In the mammary gland, it appears likely that stromal, myoepithelial, and epithelial cells communicate by paracrine hormones and that additional autocrine mechanisms may also exist, particularly for epithelial cells.

The now classical observations of Beatson in the 1890's (Beatson, 1896) established the fact that endocrine influences are important in growth control of breast cancer. More recent studies have implicated ovarian estrogens as the primary endocrine influence. In contrast, proliferation of normal mammary epithelium appears to require both of the ovarian steroids: estrogen and progesterone. Cellular mitoses occur predominantly in the luteal phase of the menstrual cycle, when progesterone is in highest abundance. This is in clear contrast to the endometrium, in which cellular mitoses occur predominantly in the follicular phase, when estrogen is "unopposed" by progesterone (Anderson *et al.*, 1988; Longacre and Bartow, 1986). In rodent models of carcinogen induced mammary cancer, it has been shown that both progesterone and estrogen are able to support initial tumor formation and early tumor growth (Welsch, 1985; Jabara *et al.*, 1973; Robinson and Jordan, 1987). It has also been shown that administration of sustained, high doses of a synthetic progestin (medroxy progesterone acetates MPA) to adult BALB/c mice with intact ovaries leads to development of malignant mammary tumors (Molinolo *et al.*, 1987). Presumably, the mechanism of interaction of estrogen and progesterone in normal and malignant rodent and human breast is based on the requirement of estrogen to induce expression of progesterone receptor. However, other mechanisms of interaction are possible (Clarke and Sutherland, 1990). Current controversy also surrounds both estrogen and progestin components of the oral contraceptive as risk factors in developing breast cancer (Anderson *et al.*, 1988; McCarty, 1989). Estrogen and progesterone receptors have been localized to a luminal subpopulation of ductal and lobular epithelial cells in women and rodents. Receptors appear to be absent from terminal end bud epithelial cells. Thus, estrogen and progesterone receptors appear to be present in at least partially differentiated epithelium. It is not yet clear whether these steroid receptor positive cells are precursors to breast cancer, although circumstantial evidence suggests the possibility (Daniel *et al.*, 1989; Dulbecco, 1990). Hormonal responsiveness persists in about one third of breast cancers. In human breast cancer treatment, antihormonal therapy as well as high dose estrogen or progestin have been used successfully to control metastatic disease.

GROWTH FACTORS: REGULATION OF PROLIFERATION AND INTERACTION WITH ESTROGEN AND PROGESTERONE

Recent studies have begun to address the mechanisms of action of estrogen and progesterone in the promotion and growth of malignancy. Many investigators are examining defective or overexpressed growth regulatory genes (oncogenes) and locally acting polypeptide hormones (growth factors) as mediators and modulators of steroid action (Dulbecco, 1990; Paul and Schmidt, 1989; Heldin and Westermark, 1984). One class of growth factors includes the transforming growth factors which derive their name from their ability to reversibly induce the transformed phenotype (initially defined as the capacity for anchorage independent growth) in certain rodent fibroblasts. They are polypeptides which were initially found to be synthesized and secreted by a variety of retrovirally, chemically, or oncogene-transformed human and rodent cell lines (Heldin and Westermark, 1984; Goustin *et al.*, 1986; Sporn and Roberts, 1986).

Two major classes of structurally and functionally distinct transforming growth factors are TGFα and TGFß. TGFα and TGFα-like peptides are members of a multiple species family ranging from apparent molecular masses of 6 to 30 kDa. They compete with the EGF for binding to the same receptor Bates *et al.*, 1988; Massaque, 1983; Derynk, 1988). The TGFß family consists of at least three related gene products, each forming 25 kDa dimeric species (Cheifetz *et al.*, 1988). There appears to be a complex pattern of interaction of these species with the TGFß receptors, which have been described as three different molecular weight species. TGFß, and more recently TGFα, have been found in the urine and pleural and peritoneal effusions of cancer patients (Stromberg *et al.*, 1987; Artega *et al.*, 1988a; Sairenji *et al.*, 1987). These growth factors have also been observed in some normal tissues (Heldin and Westermark, 1984; Goustin *et al.*, 1986; Sporn and Roberts, 1986; Bates *et al.*, 1988; Derynck, 1988). Treatment of both normal and malignant epithelial tissue with TGFβ of all subtypes generally has a growth inhibitory and sometimes differentiating effect.

At least two other classes of monomeric, but disulfide-linked, growth factors are also relevant: insulin-like growth factors (IGF I and IGF II, and their binding proteins) and fibroblast growth factors (FGF, a family of at least seven members) (Heldin and Westermark, 1984; Goustin, 1986; Sporn and Roberts, 1986). A more recently described growth factor, mammary derived growth factor 1 (MDGF1) has been found in human milk and in conditioned medium from human breast cancer cell lines (Bano *et al.*, 1990a; Bano *et al.*, 1985; Bano *et al.*, 1990b). This glycosylated, monomeric and non-disulfide linked 62kDa growth factor may also play a role in growth regulation of normal and malignant human mammary epithelium. It has been hypothesized that transformation of cells from normal to malignant may directly result from increased production of growth stimulatory factors or decreased production of growth inhibitory substances, or altered responsiveness to either or both of transforming groups of growth factors (Sporn and Roberts, 1986).

An important perspective in understanding pathways of growth control in human neoplastic cells is a knowledge of growth regulation of the normal cells from which the cancer derived. To date, this area of investigation in epithelial cells has lagged behind studies of the influence of growth factors in cancer due to the difficulties involved in culture of normal epithelial cells. However, the recent development of specialized serum-free culture conditions has facilitated the study of growth regulation in normal human keratinocytes (Coffey *et al.*, 1987), normal human bronchial epithelial cells (Masui *et al.*, 1986), and normal human mammary epithelial cells (Stampfer and Bartley, 1985; Hammond *et al.*, 1984). Though human mammary epithelial cells may now be cultured *in vitro*, it is not yet clear that the cultured subtype is of the lineage or differentiation type(s) which would give rise to breast cancer in a woman. For example, receptors for estrogen and progesterone have not been demonstrated in these cells, and they appear to have a basal epithelial "stem cell" character (Stempfer and Bartley, 1985; Hammond *et al.*, 1984).

Studies on steroid-growth factor interactions in human mammary tissue have been restricted to the malignant epithelium. In hormone responsive human breast cancer cells, growth stimulation by estrogen is accompanied by an increase in growth stimulatory TGFα production (Bates *et al.*, 1988; Perroteau *et al.*, 1986; King *et al.*, 1989), whereas growth inhibition of hormone responsive breast cancer cell lines by an antiestrogen is paralleled by augmented secretion of growth inhibitory TGFß (Knabbe *et al.*, 1987). Similar effects have been observed with progestins, TGFα, EGF and the EGF receptor being induced, while TGFβ was inhibited (antiprogestins having the opposite effect) (Murphy *et al.*, 1986; Murphy *et al.*, 1988; Murphy *et al.*, 1989). In hormone independent breast cancer cell lines, however, both of these growth factors, as well as many other growth regulatory peptides, are constitutively produced (Bates *et al.*, 1986; Artega *et al.*, 1988a; Dickson and Lippman, 1988). These results are consistent with, but do not prove, a role for growth factors in the expression of a more malignant phenotype and escape from normal hormonal control. It is of special note that milk, the natural secretory product of the mammary epithelial cell, is an extraordinarily rich source of growth factors (Salomon and Kidwell, 1988).

MULTIPLE ROLES FOR TGFα AND EGF IN MAMMARY PROLIFERATION, CARCINOGENESIS AND TUMOR GROWTH

EGF appears to be an important regulator both of the proliferation and differentiation of the mouse mammary gland *in vivo* and of mouse mammary explan *in vitro* (Vonderhaar, 1988; Oka *et al.*, 1988). EGF is also a required supplement for the clonal anchorage dependent growth, *in vitro*, of normal human mammary epithelial cells (Stampfer, 1985). However, although human breast cancer cells do not require exogenous EGF for continuous growth, many breast cancer cell lines retain receptors and growth stimulatory responses to EGF (Osborne *et al.*, 1980; Davidson *et al.*, 1987). Mouse salivary gland-derived EGF appears to be necessary for spontaneous mammary tumor formation in the mouse model (Kurachi *et al.*, 1985) as well as for growth of the tumors once they are formed. EGF can also partially replace estrogen to promote limited tumor growth of a human breast cancer cell line (MCF-7) implanted in nude mice (Dickson *et al.*, 1986b). TGFα, a structural and functional homolog of EGF, can produce essentially the same biological effects in mouse mammary explants and cultured human and mouse mammary epithelial cell lines as EGF (Vonderhaar, 1988; Salomon *et al.*, 1987), but its role in normal or malignant mammary development has not been fully defined. It is of interest that TGFα mRNA has been detected in mammary epithelium by *in situ* hybridization during the proliferative, lobuloalveolar development state of rodent and human pregnancy (Liscia *et al.*, 1990). TGFα mRNA and protein and EGF receptor are detected *in vitro* in proliferating human mammary epithelium, but are very low in resting organoids (Bates *et al.*, 1990; Shoyab *et al.*, 1989). The TGFα acts as an autocrine growth factor in normal human mammary epithelial cells in mass culture; an anti-EGF receptor antibody reversibly inhibits proliferation (Salomon *et al.*, 1987). A new member of this growth factor family, termed amphiregulin (Shoyab *et al.*, 1989), has also been discovered in a breast cancer cell line treated with a tumor promoter, but its exact physiological role in normal and malignant proliferation remains to be determined. It appears to inhibit breast tumor cells, but not normal cells *in vitro* (Plowman *et al.*, 1990).

TGFα has been directly implicated as a modulator of cellular transformation in a number of studies. Overexpression of TGFα following transfection of a human TGFα cDNA expression vector into the immortal, but non-tumorigenic, mouse mammary epithelial cell line NOG-8 led to its capacity for anchorage-independent growth (Shankar *et al.*, 1989). Another study utilized MCF-10, a newly described, spontaneously immortalized human breast ductal epithelial cell line, as recipient for the TGFα gene. This cell line, which is negative for estrogen and progesterone receptors but contains a high level of EGF receptors, was also transformed by TGFα transfection (Ciardiello *et al.*, 1990). In contrast TGFα transfection into MCF-7 cells which have low levels of EGF receptor does not confer a significant growth advantage *in vitro* or *in vivo* (Clarke *et al.*, 1989). In two of three studies using rodent fibroblasts as recipients for human or rat TGFα cDNA, transformation to full tumorigenicity was also achieved (Rosenthal *et al.*, 1986; Watanabe *et al.*, 1987). In contrast, in the third study, TGFα transfection induced increased proliferation but not full malignant progression to tumorigenicity

(Finzi *et al.*, 1987). EGF can also act as a transformation-inducing agent (an oncogene) when transfected and overexpressed in rodent fibroblasts (Stern *et al.*, 1987).

There is also evidence to suggest that the level of secretion of TGFα in breast cancer is associated with oncogene expression. A direct correlation among TGFα production, *ras* oncogene expression, and malignant transformation has been demonstrated in a recent study utilizing a glucocorticoid-inducible point-mutated c-Ha-*ras* construct transfected into immortal mouse mammary epithelial cells (Ciardiello *et al.*, 1988). As c-Ha-*ras* was induced with glucocoorticoid the cells became transformed and secreted TGFα. However, in this study, transformation of cells was observed with a more rapid time course than induction of TGFα synthesis, suggesting that production of the growth factor might be a secondary response to growth rather than an essential mediator of growth. This same group has also observed that in the MCF-10 cell line, v-*ras*^{H}-induced transformation is accompanied by TGFα induction, and here it was possible to block the transformed phenotype with antisera to TGFα (Ciardiello *et al.*, 1990). The relationships among expression of oncogenes, TGFα and TGFα function are probably dependent upon the cell type in question. In studies of human breast cancer biopsies, TGFα mRNA and protein were detected in 70% or more of the specimens (Bates *et al.*, 1988; Gregory *et al.*, 1989) and in approximately 30% of benign breast lesions (Travers *et al.*, 1988). Immunoreactive TGFα has been found in fibroadenomas and 25-50% of primary human mammary carcinomas (Perroteau *et al.*, 1986; Macias *et al.*, 1987) and an EGF related protein of 43kDa has been recently isolated from breast cancer patient urine (Eckert *et al.*, 1990). Perhaps detection of TGF α/EGF in tumor biopsies serum or urine will eventually be found useful in determining prognosis or tumor burden.

A very recent group of studies has addressed the effect of TGFα overexpression (with MMTV or metalothionine promoters) in the mammary glands of transgenic mice. In one study using outbread mice, the gland was hyperproliferative, but exhibited delayed penetration of the epithelial ducts into the stromal fat pad (Jhappan *et al.*, 1990). Such a delayed penetration has also been observed with local mammary implants of EGF (Coleman and Daniel, 1990). Two other TGFα transgenic mouse studies using inbred strains have also shown the mammary glands to be hyperproliferative, sometimes resulting in mammary cancer after multiple pregnancies (Sandgren *et al.*, 1990; Matsui *et al.*, 1990). The significance of the different results with outbred versus inbred strains is not yet clear.

In human breast cancer cell lines *in vitro*, clear evidence of significant autocrine growth control by the TGFα-EGF receptor system has only been seen in the MDA-MB-468 cell line, a line with high TGFα expression and an amplified EGF receptor (Ennis *et al.*, 1989). Such studies would appear to have clear implications for developing novel therapeutic strategies. However, it seems likely that excepting the few percent of breast cancers overexpressing EGF receptor by such a gene amplification, that this growth factor receptor system will not be of primary importance in autocrine growth regulation of malignant and metastatic disease. It seems more likely that the EGF receptor-TGFα system may be much more critical in normal gland growth and early stages of breast tumorigenesis. Therapeutic strategies employing EGF receptor ligands or antibodies coupled to toxins or therapeutic drugs could conceivably find future therapeutic utility, since a large portion of hormone independent breast cancers express significant levels of this receptor even though a direct function of this receptor has not been proven (Dickson and Lippman, 1988; Davidson *et al.*, 1987).

THE EGF/TGFα RECEPTOR, c-*erb*B_2 and c-*erb*B_3

The potential roles of TGFα or EGF in transformation may also involve alterations in the expression and function of their receptor, the EGF receptor. Clinical evidence for an association of increased expression of the EGF receptor, and its structurally related homolog c-*erb*B_2, with more aggressive and hormone unresponsive breast cancer has accumulated in recent years (Sainsbury *et al.*, 1987; Perez *et al.*, 1984; Slamon *et al.*, 1989; Paik *et al.*, 1990). This is also supported by studies of *in vitro* cultured primary human breast cancer biopsies (Spitzer *et al.*, 1987) and in established human breast cancer cell lines (Davidson *et al.*, 1987). EGF receptor expression (but not c-*erb*B_2 expression) appears to be inversely correlated with expression of the estrogen receptor (Sainsbury *et al.*, 1987). In contrast to transfections of breast cells with mutated c-Ha-*ras* oncogene which induces TGFα, transfection with the oncogenic counterpart of c-*erb*B_2 (or *neu*) does not induce TGFα (Ciardiello *et al.*, 1989). Thus TGFα overexpression is coupled to transformation in some but not all cases. In transfection studies on rodent fibroblasts, overexpression of the EGF receptor can predispose cells to expression of the transformed phenotype upon stimulation by EGF (Velu *et al.*, 1987; Di Fiore *et al.*, 1987; Riedel *et al.*, 1988). Likewise, transfection of rodent fibroblasts with c-*erb*B_2, structurally related to the EGF receptor but lacking EGF binding capacity, results in transformation (Hudziak *et al.*, 1987; Di Fiore *et al.*, 1987. A new family member, c-*erb*B_3 has also been recently identified in breast cancer (Kraus *et al.*, 1989), however, its implications for breast cancer biology or prognosis are unknown at present.

Until recently, no ligands for c-*erb*B_2 have been identified. A TGFα-related species of aapproximately 30 kDa has been isolated from the conditioned medium of the hormone independent MDA-MB-231 breast cancer cell line (and identified in some other hormone dependent and independent breast cancer cell lines (Bates *et al.*, 1988; King *et al.*, 1989; Dickson *et al.*, 1987; Dickson *et al.*, 1986a; Lupu *et al.*, 1989). When tested on cells containing EGF receptor, such as fibroblasts, normal mammary epithelial cells, and hormone dependent breast cancer cells, the growth factor purified from MDA-MB-231 cells is stimulatory. However, on cells expressing high levels of c-*erb*B_2 in addition to the EGF receptor, the growth factor derived from MDA-MB-231 cells is inhibitory (Lupu *et al.*, 1990). It is not yet clear if inhibition can be obtained *in vivo* or if the 30kDa growth factor from other breast cancer cell lines has this characteristic. The TGFα-like molecule from MDA-MB-231 cells is capable of displacing the monoclonal antibody 4D5 from its epitope on c-*erb*B_2, and appears to be the first candidate ligand for c-*erb*B_2 receptor (Lupu *et al.*, 1989). The relationship between the gene for this protein and TGFα remains to be determined since sequencing has not been reported.

OTHER GROWTH FACTOR-RECEPTOR SYSTEMS IN BREAST CANCER

TGFα may not be the only stimulatory growth factor produced by the mammary epithelium. A new growth factor termed mammary derived growth factor 1 (MDGF1) has been recently purified to apparent homogeneity from human milk. The factor has an apparent molecular mass of 62 kDa and a pI of 4.8. An apparently identical factor has been isolated from primary breast cancer and human mammary tumor cells suggesting that MDGF1 might be an autocrine or paracrine growth factor for breast cancer cells (Bano *et al.*, 1990; Bano *et al.*, 1985; Bano *et al.*, 1990b). It has been reported that human mammary epithelial cell lines possess receptors specific for MDGF1 of 120-140 kDa in size (Bano *et al.*, 1990). Recent studies have demonstrated that upon ligand stimulation, a protein of approximately 185kDa in size becomes rapidly phosphorylated on tyrosine residue(s). The relationship between the binding protein and phosphoprotein remains to be determined, but it seems possible that the MDGF1 receptor has tyrosine kinase activity which is ligand-activated Bano *et al.*, 1990b).

The FGFs and IGFs may also play a role in mammary proliferation and cancer. Although FGF receptors are detected in normal mammary epithelial cells, they have not been reported in breast cancer. It is unknown whether FGF receptor expression is lost during transformation, or whether breast cancer is derived from a normal cell type devoid of receptors. Expression of IGF-I receptor is correlated with good prognosis in hormone dependent breast cancer (Kozma *et al.*, 1988). Basic and acidic FGF as well as FGF-5 are produced by normal mammary stromal fibroblasts, as is IGF-I (Valverius *et al.*, 1990; Cullen *et al.*, 1990). Normal mammary epithelial cells are stimulated by these growth factors, while mammary epithelial cells partially transformed with c-*myc* or SV40T have a transforming growth response to the FGFs (Valverius *et al.*, 1990). Stroma of breast cancer patients produces IGF II (Yee *et al.*, 1988). Breast cancer cell lines also have been shown to produce mRNA for all members of the FGF family as well as IGF related molecules and IGF binding proteins (Foekens *et al.*, 1989; Huff *et al.*, 1986; Yee *et al.*, 1990). IGF and FGF related growth factors may contribute to paracrine communication in tumors. Perhaps the major function of FGFs released by breast cancer is in promoting tumor angiogenesis (Folkman and Klagsbrun, 1987).

TGFβ FAMILY, MAMMASTATATIN, AND MDGI: GROWTH INHIBITORY FACTORS

Growth stimulatory factors appear to be important in proliferation of normal and malignant breast epithelium, but locally acting growth inhibitory factors almost certainly play an equally essential role. Among the best known is the TGFβ family of three genes. The homodimeric forms are known as TGFβ, TGFβ_2 and TGFβ_3. TGFβ is a potent local inhibitor of mammary end bud development when implanted in the developing gland (Silberstein and Daniel, 1987). Inhibition is associated with epithelium-dependent synthesis of type I collagen, glycosaminoglycan, and chondroitin sulfate matrix components (Silberstein *et al.*, 1990). Both TGFβ and TGFβ_2 are effective inhibitors *in vitro* of breast cancer cell lines (Knabbe *et al.*, 1987; Artega *et al.*, 1988b; Zugmaier *et al.*, 1989; Arrick *et al.*, 1990) and normal mammary epithelial cells in culture (Valverius *et al.*, 1989). TGFβ_3 has not been available for study to date. Inhibition of normal mammary epithelial cells by TGFβ is associated with multiple effects: profound morphological alterations, differentiation, as evidenced by induction of milk fat globule antigen (Walker-Jones *et al.*, 1989) and rapid induction of c-*sis* protooncogene (Bronzert *et al.*, 1990). Normal mammary epithelial cells produce TGFβ, while breast cancer cell lines make all three family members (Knabbe *et al.*, 1987; Arrick *et al.*, 1990). In hormone dependent breast cancer cell lines, estrogen suppresses and antiestrogen induces growth inhibitory TGFβ (Knabbe *et al.*, 1987); however, the relevance *in vivo* of these observations is not yet certain.

A second growth inhibitory molecule called mammastatin has also been isolated from conditioned medium of normal breast epithelial cells in culture. A monoclonal antibody has been produced which blocks the effect of this inhibitor. Release of the inhibitor is increased by treatment of cells with high dose, cytostatic levels of estrogen, and it is inhibitory for breast cancer cells in culture (Ervin *et al.*, 1989). The relevance of these observations *in vivo* is not known.

Finally, another growth inhibitor, MDGI (mammary derived growth inhibitor) has been isolated from lactating bovine mammary glands and milk fat globule membranes (Bohmer *et al.*, 1987). This 13kDa inhibitor has been sequenced and cloned, and antibodies have been prepared. MDG1 shares sequence homology with a family of proteins which bind hydrophobic ligands such as retinoic acid or fatty acids. The growth inhibitor is synthesized in developing lobuloalveolar structures, and is particularly abundant in proximal parts of the terminally differentiated gland (Kurtz *et al.*, 1990). This molecule also reversibly inhibits proliferation of normal and malignant mammary epithelial cells *in vitro* (Bohmer *et al.*, 1987), but observations *in vivo* are lacking.

THE *RAS, MYC, FOS, AND JUN* ONCOGENES IN BREAST CANCER: THEIR INTERACTIONS WITH ESTROGEN AND GROWTH FACTORS

In the classical studies of rodent fibroblasts transformed by Harvey, Kirsten or Maloney murine sarcoma viruses (Sporn and Todaro, 1980; Anzano *et al.*, 1985; Anzano *et al.*, 1983), increased production of "sarcoma growth factor" (SGF) was demonstrated. SGF was later characterized as consisting of the two growth factors, TGFα and TGFß. Similarly, increased production of TGFα has been reported following transfection of MCF-7 human breast cancer cells with v-Ha-*ras* (the oncogene of Harvey sarcoma virus) or of mouse mammary epithelial cells by a point-mutated human c-Ha-*ras* gene (Salomon *et al.*, 1987; Ciardiello *et al.*, 1988; Dickson, *et al.* 1987). The actual incidence of point-mutations of the c-Ha-*ras* and c-Ki-*ras* proto-oncogenes in breast cancer appears to be low; they have been observed so far in only two hormone independent human breast cancer cell lines (Kraus *et al.*, 1984; Kozma *et al.*, 1988). However, the role of unmutated but overexpressed c-Ha-*ras* protooncogene in clinical cases of human breast cancer has not yet been fully clarified. One study indicates a positive correlation between expression of p21 *ras* protein and malignant progression of human breast cancer (Clair *et al.*, 1987). In another study, no such correlation was observed, although malignant and dysplastic breast lesions did have elevated levels of p21 *ras* protein compared to normal tissues (Horan-Hand, 1987). Neither of these studies addressed the state of mutational activation of the *ras* gene, but studies by several other groups indicate that *ras* activation along with some additional event(s) are necessary for neoplastic transformation, at least of rodent cells (Medina, 1988), making the role of *ras* problematic in human breast cancer.

The nuclear protooncogenes, c-*myc*, c-*fos*, and c-*jun*, are also of interest in breast cancer. c-*myc* protooncogene can confer immortality to fibroblasts (Kelekar and Cole, 1987) and alter fibroblast responsiveness to growth factors (Leof *et al.*, 1987; Stern *et al.*, 1986). In human primary breast cancer, c-*myc* amplification and overexpression have been reported in 15% to 40% of tumors (Escot *et al.*, 1986; Bonilla *et al.*, 1988; Cline *et al.*, 1987; Varley *et al.*, 1987). Though not found to be associated with clinical staging or other known prognostic variables, c-*myc* amplification was found to correlate with poor prognosis (Varlay *et al.*, 1987). Expression of the c-*myc* protooncogene under control of the mammary lactation specific whey acidic protein (WAP)-promoter in transgenic mice gave rise to mammary tumors in more than 80% of the animals after pregnancy (Schoenberger *et al.*, 1988). Similar results were obtained with activated c-Ha-*ras* under a mammary specific promoter (Andrea *et al.*, 1987), and dramatic synergism was observed with simultaneous expression of c-Ha-*ras* and c-*myc* in mammary tumorigenesis (Sinn *et al.*, 1987). *In vitro* studies have also introduced the c-*myc* gene into immortalized human mammary epithelial cells using an amphotropic retroviral vector. In immortalized mammary epithelial cells transfected either with c-*myc* or SV40T (but not v-*ras*^{H}) it was observed that the cells could be stimulated to grow in soft agar by either bFGF, aFGF, EGF, or TGFα (Valverius *et al.*, 1990). These data suggest that c-*myc* might function in early breast cancer lesions to allow growth factors or hormones to act to drive aberrant transformed growth. The nuclear protooncogenes are also induced when human breast cancer cell lines are stimulated to proliferate in monolayer culture *in vitro* by estrogen (Weisz *et al.*, 1990; Musgrove and Sutherland, 1990; Dubik *et al.*, 1987). Estrogen induces c-*fos* and c-*jun* within one-half hour and c-*myc* within one hour of treatment. It is not yet clear whether these nuclear protooncogenes are necessary or sufficient for estrogen action. c-*myc* protooncogene may also have a special relationship to breast cancer in older women. Increased amplification of c-*myc* has been observed that in human breast cancer tissue in postmenopausal patients. It is possible that this reflects cumulative proliferation and/or contributes to aberrant mitogenic responses in postmenopausal breast cancer (Escot *et al.*, 1986).

Rb, nm23, p53 AND THROMBOSPONDIN AS MALIGNANCY SUPPRESSING GENES

A recently emerging concept in malignant progression is that loss of expression of tumor repressor genes cooperates with acquisition of expression of oncogenes (Mikkelsen and Cavenee, 1990). In addition, it has been suggested that loss of expression of tumor suppressor genes may sensitize cells to the transforming effects of growth factors (Koi *et al.*, 1989). The study of tumor suppressors is a very young field in breast cancer, but at least three promising leads have been established. The most extensively studied suppressor gene is the retinoblastoma or Rb gene (on chromosome 13). Its alleles both are lost in some breast cancer lines like MDA-MB-468, and reexpression of the gene by gene transfer suppresses the malignant phenotype (Lee *et al.*, 1990). It is not yet clear what proportion of breast tumors lose Rb during their progression nor what is the effect on cancer prognosis or tumor biology of Rb loss. An interesting connection has been observed between TGFβ and the Rb protein: TGFβ treatment of cells maintains Rb in the unphosphorylated, active form (Laiho *et al.*, 1990). A more recently studied tumor suppressor is the p53 gene (chromosome 17). When mutated, this gene may also act as an oncogene. A high proportion of breast cancer cell lines appear to have mutations in the p53 gene (Nigro *et al.*, 1989), but again, the prognostic implications are unclear. The abnormal proliferation phenotype may not be the only tumor characteristic held in check by suppressor genes. The nm 23 gene has been shown to correlate inversely with axillary lymph node metastases and survival in breast cancer. The nm23 gene product may act to suppress the metastatic phenotype in breast cancer based on gene transfer studies with melanoma (Steeg *et al.*, 1988). Thrombospondin is another protein which appears to suppress the process of angiogenesis in other cancers (Rastinejad *et al.*, 1989), however, it has not been studied in breast cancer yet. The full biological and prognostic significance of all of these putative tumor suppressors in breast cancer is a promising area for future study.

Clearly, the steroidal endocrine effectors of mammary proliferation, carcinogenesis and tumor growth interact with a host of other influences in breast tumor progression. Both stromal and epithelial components appear to be important in this process. Future studies should address the mechanisms behind steroid regulation of growth and inhibitory factors, and the underlying biological significance of expression of positive and negative acting growth factors and of oncogenes and tumor suppressors in breast cancer. Perhaps new therapeutic strategies will also emerge from such studies as well.

REFERENCES

Anderson, T.J., Battersby, S. and Macintyre, C.C.A. Proliferative and secretory activity in human breast during natural and artificial menstrual cycles. *American J. of Pathology*, 130:193-204, 1988.

Andrea, A.C., Schoenberger, C.A., Grover, B., Hennighauser, L, LeMaur, M. and Gerlinger, P. Ha-*ras* oncogene expression directed by a milk protein gene promoter: tissue specificity, hormonal regulation and tumor incidence in transgenic mice. *Proc. Nat'l. Acad. Sci. USA*. 84:1299-1303, 1987.

Anzano, M.A., Roberts, A.B., De Larco, J.E., Wakefield, L.M., Assoian, R.K., Roche, N.S., Smith, J.M., Lazarus, J.E. and Sporn, M.B. Increased secretion of type ß transforming growth factor accompanies viral transformation of cells. *Mol. Cell. Biol.* 5:242-250, 1985.

Anzano, M.A., Roberts, A.B., Smith, J.M., Sporn, M.B. and DeLarco, J.E. Sarcoma growth factor from conditioned medium of virally transformed cells is composed of both type α and type ß transforming growth factors. *Proc. Natl. Acad. Sci. (U.S.A.)* 80:6264-6268, 1983.

Arrick, B.A., Korc, M. and Derynck, R. Differential regulation of three transforming growth factor β species in human breast cancer cell lines by estradiol. *Cancer Res.*, 50:299-303, 1990.

Artega, C.L., Hanauske, A.R., Clark, G.M., Osborne, C.K., Hazarika, P., Pardue, R.L., Tio, F. and Von Hoff, D.D. Immunoreactive alpha transforming growth factor (IrαTGF) activity in effusions from cancer patients: a marker of tumor burden and patient prognosis. *Cancer Res.* 48:5023-5028, 1988a .

Artega, C.L., Tandon, A.K., Von Hoff, D.D. and Osborne, C.K. Transforming growth factor ß: potential autocrine growth inhibitor of estrogen receptor-negative human breast cancer cells. *Cancer Res.*, 48:3898-3903, 1988b.

Bano, M., Kidwell, W.R., Lippman, M.E. and Dickson, R.B. Characterization of MDGF-1 receptor in human mammary epithelial cell liver. *J. Biol. Chem.*, 265:1874-1880, 1990a.

Bano, M., Lupu, R., Kidwell, W.R., Lippman, M.E. and Dickson, R.B. Characterization of MDGF1 and its receptor in human breast cancer cells. *Proceedings of the American Association for Cancer Research*, Washington, D.C., 1990b.

Bano, M., Solomon, D.S. and Kidwell, W.R. Purification of mammary derived growth factor 1 (MDGF 1) from human milk and mammary tumors. *J. Biol. Chem.* 260:5745-5752, 1985.

Bates, S.E., Davidson, N.E., Valverius, E.M., Dickson, R.B., Freter, C.E., Tam, J.P., Kudlow, J.E., Lippman, M.E. and Salomon, D.S. Expression of transforming growth factor alpha and its mRNA in human breast cancer: its regulation by estrogen and its possible functional significance. *Mol. Endo.* 2:543-555, 1988.

Bates, S.E., McManaway, M.E., Lippman, M.E. and Dickson, R.B. Characterization of estrogen responsive transforming activity in human breast cancer cell lines. *Cancer Res.* 46:1707-1713, 1986.

Bates, S.E., Valverius, E.M., Ennis, B.W., Bronzert, D.A., Sheridan, J.P., Stampfer, M.R., Mendelsohn, S., Lippman, M.E. and Dickson, R.B. Expression of the transforming growth factor α/Epidermal growth factor receptor pathway in normal human breast epithelial cells. *Endocrinology* 126:596-607, 1990.

Beatson, G.T. On the treatment of inoperable cases of carcinoma of the mamma: suggestion for a new method of treatment, with illustrative cases. *Lancet* 2:104-107, 1986.

Bohmer, F.D., Kraft, R., Otto, A., Wernstedt, C., Hellman, U., Kurtz, A., Mullen, T., Rohde, K., Etzold, G., Lehmann, W., Langen, P., Heldin, C.H. and Grosse, R. Identification of a polypeptide growth inhibitor from bovine mammary gland. *J. Biol. Chem.* 262:15137-15143, 1987.

Bonilla, M., Ramirez, M., Lopez-Cuento, J., and Gariglio, P. In vivo amplification and rearrangements of c-*myc* oncogene in human breast tumors. *J. Nat'l. Cancer Inst.*, 80:665-671, 1988.

Bronzert, D.A., Bates, S.E., Sheridan, J.A., Lindsay, R., Valverius, E.M., Stampfer, M.R., Lippman, M.E. and Dickson, R.B. TGFβ induces PDGF mRNA and PDGF secretion while inhibiting growth in normal human mammary epithelial cells. *Molec. Endocrinol.* 4:981-989, 1990.

Brown, J.B. Hormone profiles in young women at risk for breast cancer: A study of ovarian function during thelarch, menarche and menopause and after childbirth. In: Banbury Report 8: Hormones and Cancer. Edited by Pike, M.C., Siiteri, P.K. and Welsch, C.W. Cold Spring Harbor Laboratory, pp. 33-56, 1981.

Cheifetz, S., Bassols, A., Stanley, K., Ohta, M., Greenberger, J. and Massague, J. Heterodimeric Transforming Growth Factor ß. *J. Biol. Chem.* 263:10783-10790, 1988.

Ciardiello, F., Hynes, N., Kim, N., Valverius, E.M., Lippman, M.E. and Salomon, D.S. Transformation of mouse mammary epithelial cells with the Ha-ras but not the neu oncogene results in a gene dosage-dependant increase in transforming growth factor α production. *FEBS Letters* 250:474-478, 1989.

Ciardiello, F., Kim, N., Hynes, N., Jaggo, R., Redmond, S., Liscia, D.S., Sanfilippo, B., Marlo, G., Callahan, R., Kidwell, W.R. and Salomon, D.S. Induction of transforming growth factor α expression in mouse mammary epithelial cells after transformation with a point-mutated c-Ha-ras protooncogene. *Mol. Endocrinol* 2:1202-1216, 1988.

Ciardiello, F., McGready, M., Kim, N., Basalo, F., Hynes, N., Langton, B.C., Yokozaki, H., Sucki, T., Elliot, J.W., Masui, H., Mendelsohn, J., Soule, H., Russo, J. and Salomon, D. TGFα expression is enhanced in human mammary epithelial cells transformed by an activated c-Ha-ras but not by the c-neu protooncogene and over-expression of the TGFα cDNA leads to transformation. *Cell Growth and Differentiation* 1:407-420, 1990.

Clair, T., Miller, W.R. and Cho-Chung, Y.S. Prognostic significance of the expression of a ras protein with a molecular weight of 21,000 by human breast cancer. *Cancer Res.*, 47:5290-5296, 1987.

Clarke, R., Brunner, N., Katz, D., Glanz, P. Dickson, R.B., Lippman, M.E. and Kern, F. The effects of a constitutive production of TGFα on the growth of MCF-7 human breast cancer cells in vitro and *in vivo*. *Mol. Endocrinol.*, 3:372-380, 1989.

Clarke, C.L. and Sutherland, R.L. Progestin regulation of cellular proliferation. *Endocrine Reviews* 11:266-301, 1990.

Cline, M., Battifora, H. and Yokota, J.J. Protooncogene abnormal-ities in human breast cancer: Correlations with anatomic features and clinical course of diagnosis. *J. Clin. Oncol.* 5:999-1006, 1987.

Coffey, R.J., Derynck, R., Wilcox, J.N., Bringman, T.S., Goustin, A.S., Moses, H.L. and Pittelkow, M.R. Production and auto-induction of transforming growth factor-α in human keratinocytes. *Nature* 328:817-820, 1987.

Coleman, S. and Daniel, C.W. Inhibition of mouse mammary ductal morphogenesis and down regulation of the EGF receptor by epidermal growth factor. *Developmental Biology* 137:425-433, 1990.

Cullen, K.J., Hill, S., Paik, S., Smith, H.S., Lippman, M. and Rosen, N. Growth factor mRNA expression by human breast fibroblasts from benign and malignant lesions. *Proc. Am. Ass. Cancer Res.* 1990

Daniel, C.W., Silberstein, G.A. and Strickland, P. Direct action of 17β estradiol in mouse mammary ducts analyzed by sustained release implants and steroid autoradiography. *Cancer Research* 47: 6052-6057, 1987.

Davidson, N.E., Gelmann, E.P., Lippman, M.E. and Dickson, R.B. Epidermal growth factor receptor gene expression in estrogen receptor-positive and negative human breast cancer cell lines. *Mol. Endocrinol.* 1:216-223, 1987.

Derynck, R. Transforming growth factor α. *Cell* 54:593-595, 1988.

Dickson, R.B., Huff, K.K., Spencer, E.M. and Lippman, M.E. Induction of epidermal growth factor-related polypeptides by estradiol in MCF-7 human breast cancer cells. *Endocrinology* 118: 138-142, 1986a.

Dickson, R.B., Kasid, A., Huff, K.K., Bates, S., Knabbe, C., Bronzert, D., Gelmann, E.P. and Lippman, M.E. Activation of growth factor secretion in tumorigenic states of breast cancer induced by 17-ß-estradiol or v-ras^H oncogene. *Proc. Nat'l. Acad. Sci. (U.S.A.)* 84: 837-841, 1987.

Dickson, R.B. and Lippman, M.E. Control of human breast cancer by estrogen. growth factors, and oncogenes. In: Breast Cancer: Cellular and Molecular Biology edited by M.E. Lippman and R.B. Dickson, Kluwer Press, Boston, pp. 119-166, 1988.

Dickson, R.B., McManaway and M.E., Lippman, M.E. Estrogen-induced factors of breast cancer cells partially replace estrogen to promote tumor growth. *Science* 232:1540-1543, 1986b.

Di Fiore, P.P., Pierce, J.H., Fleming, T.P., Hazan, R., Ullrich, A., King, C.R., Schlessinger, J. and Aaronson, S.A. Overexpression of the human EGF receptor confers an EGF-dependent transformed phenotype to NIH 3T3 cells. *Cell* 51:1063-1070, 1987.

Di Fiore, P.P., Pierce, J.H., Kraus, M.H., Segatto, O., King, C.R. and Aaronson, S.A. erbB-2 is a potent oncogene when overexpressed in NIH/3T3 cells. *Science* 237:178-182, 1987.

Dubik, D., Dembinski, T.C. and Shiu, R.P.C. Stimulation of c-myc oncogene expression associated with estrogen-induced proliferation of human breast cancer cells. *Cancer Research* 47:6517-6521, 1987.

Dulbecco, R. Experimental studies in mammary development and cancer: relevance to human cancer. *Advances in Oncology* 5:3-6, 1990.

Eckert, K., Granetzny, A., Fischer, J., Nexo, E. and Grosse, R. An Mr 43,000 epidermal growth-factor related protein purified from the urine of breast cancer patients. *Cancer Research* 50:642-647, 1990.

Ennis, B.W., Valverius, E.M., Lippman, M.E., Bellot, F., Kris, R., Schlessinger, J., Masui, H., Goldberg, A., Mendelsohn, J. and Dickson, R.B. Anti EGF receptor antibodies inhibit the autocrine stimulated growth of MDA-MB-468 breast cancer cells. *Mol. Endocrinol.* 3:1830-1838, 1989.

Ervin, P.R., Kaminski, R.C., Cody, R.C. and Wicha, M.S. Production of mammastatin, a tissue specific growth inhibitor, by normal human mammary epithelial cells. *Science* 244:1585-1587, 1989.

Escot, C., Theillet, C., Lidereau, R., Spyratos, F., Champeme, M.H., Gest, J. and Callahan, R. Geneticalteration of the c-myc proto-oncogene in human primary breast carcinomas. *Proc. Nat'l. Acad. Sci. (U.S.A.)* 83:4834-4838, 1986.

Finzi, E., Fleming, T., Segatto O., Pennington, C.Y., Bringman, T.S., Derynck, R. and Aaronson, S.A. The human transforming growth factor type α coding sequence is not a direct-acting oncogene when overexpressed in NIH 3T3 cells. *Proc. Nat'l. Acad. Sci. (U.S.A.)* 84:3733-3737, 1987.

Foekens, J.A., Portengen, M., Janssen, M. and Klijn, J.G.M. Insulin-like growth factor I receptors and insulin-like growth factor I activity in primary human breast cancer. *Cancer* 63:2139-2147, 1989.

Folkman, J. and Klagsbrun, M. Angiogenic Factors. *Science* 235: 442-447, 1987.

Goustin, A.S., Leof, E.B., Shipley, G.D. and Moses, H.L. Growth factors and cancer. *Cancer Res.* 46:1015-1029, 1986.

Gregory, H., Thomas, C.E., Willshire, I.R., Young, J.A., Anderson, H., Baildan, A. and Howell, A. Epidermal and transforming growth factor α in patients with breast tumors. *British J. Cancer* 59:605-609, 1989.

Hammond, S.L., Ham, R.G. and Stampfer, M.R. Serum-free growth of human mammary epithelial cells: rapid clonal growth in defined medium and extended serial passage with pituitary extract. *Proc. Nat'l. Acad. Sci.* (U.S.A.), 81:5435-5439, 1984.

Heldin, C.H. and Westermark, B. Growth factors: mechanism of action and relations to oncogenes. *Cell* 37:9-20, 1984.

Horan-Hand, P., Vilase, V., Thor, A., Ohuchi, N. and Schlom, J. Quantitation of Harvey ras p21 enhanced expression in human breast and colon carcinomas. *J. Nat'l. Cancer Inst.* 79:59-65, 1987.

Hudziak, R.M., Schlessinger, J. and Ullrich, A. Increased expression of the putative growth factor receptor $p185^{HER2}$ causes transformation and tumorigenesis of NIH 3T3 cells. *Proc. Nat'l. Acad. Sci. (U.S.A.)* 84:7159-7162, 1987.

Huff, K.K., Lippman, M.E., Spencer, E.M. and Dickson, R.B. Secretion of an insulin-like growth factor I-related polypeptide by human breast cancer cells. *Cancer Res.* 46:4613-4619, 1986.

Iino, Y., Gibson, D.F.C. and Jordan, V.C. Antiestrogen therapy for breast cancer: Current strategies and potential causes for therapeutic failure, in: Regulatory Mechanisms in Breast Cancer edited by Lippman, M.E. and Dickson, R.B., Kluwer Academic Publishers, Norwell, Massachusetts, pp. 221-238, 1990.

Jabara, A.G., Toyne, P.H., Harcourt, A.G. Effects of time and duration of progesterone administration on mammary tumors induced by DMBA in Sprague Dawley rats. *Br. J. Cancer* 27:63-71, 1973.

Jhappan, C., Stahle, C., Harkins, R.N., Fausto, N., Smith, G.H. and Merlino, G.T. TGFα overexpression in transgenic mice induces liver neoplasia and abnormal development of the mammary gland and pancreas. *Cell* 61:1137-1146, 1990.

Kelekar, A. and Cole, M.D. Immortalization by c-myc, H-ras, and Ela oncogenes induces differential cellular gene expression and growth factor responses. *Mol. Cell Biol.* 7:3899-3907, 1987.

King, R.J.B., Wang, D.Y., Daley, R.J. and Darbre, P.D. Approaches to studying the role of growth factors in the progression of breast tumors from the steroid sensitive to insensitive state. *J. Steroid Biochem.* 34:133-138, 1989.

Knabbe, C., Wakefield, L., Flanders, K., Kasid, A., Derynck, R., Lippman, M.E. and Dickson, R.B. Evidence that TGF beta is a hormonally regulated negative growth factor in human breast cancer. *Cell* 48:417-428, 1987.

Koi, M., Afshari, C.A., Annab, L.A. and Barrett, J.C. Role of a tumor-suppressor gene in the negative control of anchorage-independent growth of Syrian hamster cells. *Proc. Nat'l. Acad. Sci. U.S.A.* 86:8773-8777, 1989.

Kozma, S.C., Bogaard, M.E., Buser, K., Saurer, S.M., Bos, J.L., Groner, B. and Hynes, N.E. The human c-Kirsten ras gene is activated by a novel mutation in codon 13 in the breast carcinoma cell line MDA-MB 231. *Nucleic Acids Research* 15:5963-5971, 1988.

Kraus, M.H., Issing, W., Miki, T., Popescu, N.C. and Aaronson, S.A. Isolation and characterization of ERBB3, a third member of the ERB/epidermal growth factor receptor family: evidence for overexpression in a subset of human mammary tumors. *Proc. Nat'l. Acad. Sci. U.S.A.* 86:9193-9197, 1989.

Kraus, M.H., Yuspa, Y. and Aaronson, S.A. A position 12-activated H-ras oncogene in all Hs578T mammary carcinosarcoma cells but not normal mammary cells of the same patient. *Proc. Nat'l. Acad. Sci. U.S.A.* 81:5384-5388, 1984.

Kurachi, H., Okamoto, S. and Oka, T. Evidence for the involvement of the submandibular gland epidermal growth factor in mouse mammary tumorigenesis. *Proc. Nat'l. Acad. Sci. U.S.A.* 81:5940-5943, 1985.

Kurtz, A., Vogel, F., Funa, K., Heldin, C.H. and Grosse, R. Developmental regulation of mammary-derived growth inhibitor expression in bovine mammary tissue. *J. Cell Biol.* 110:1779-1789, 1990.

Laiho, M., DeCaprio, J.A., Ludlow, J.W., Livingston, D.M. and Massague, J. Growth inhibition by TGFβ linked to suppression of retinoblastoma protein phosphorylation. *Cell* 62:175-185, 1990.

Lee, E., Bookstein, R. and Lee, W-H. Role of the retinoblastoma gene in the oncogenesis of human breast carcinoma. In: Regulation of Breast Cancer edited by M.E. Lippman and R.B. Dickson, Kluwer Press, Boston, pp. 23-44, 1990.

Leof, E.B., Proper, J.A. and Moses, H.L. Modulation of transforming growth factor type β action by activated ras and c-*myc*. *Mol. Cell Biol.* 7:2649-2652, 1987.

Liscia, D.S., Merlo, G., Ciardiello, F., Kim, N., Smith, G.H., Callahan, R.H., and Salomon, D.S. Transforming growth factor-α messenger RNA localization in the developing adult rat and human mammary gland by in situ hybridization. *Developmental Biology* 140: 123-131, 1990.

Longacre, T.A. and Bartow, S.A. A correlative morphologic study of human breast and endometrium in the menstrual cycle. *Am. J. Surg. Path.* 10:382-393, 1986.

Lupu, R., Colomer, R., Zugmaier, G., Slamon, D. and Lippman, M.E. A ligand for the $erbB_2$oncogene product interacts directly with both the EGF rerceptor and $erbB_2$ *Science* 249:1552-1554, 1990.

Lupu, R., Dickson, R.B. and Lippman, M.E. Biologically active glycosylated TGFα released by estrogen receptor negative human breast cancer cell line. *UCLA Symposium on Growth Regulation of Cancer* (abstract) 1989.

Macias, A., Perez, R., Hägerström, T. and Skoog, L. Identification of transforming growth factoralpha in human primary breast carcinomas. *Anticancer Research* 7:1271-1280, 1987.

Massague, J. Epidermal growth factor-like transforming growth factor. *J. Biol. Chem.* 258:13606-13613, 1983.

Masui, T., Wakefield, L.M., Lechner, J.F., La Veck, M.A., Sporn, M.B. and Harris, C.C., Type ß transforming growth factor is the primary differentiation-inducing serum factor for normal human bronchial epithelial cells. *Proc. Nat'l. Acad. Sci. U.S.A.* 83:2438-2442, 1986.

Matsui, Y., Halter, S.A., Holt, J.T., Hogan, B.L.M. and Coffey, R. Development of mammary hyperplasia and neoplasia in MMTV-TGFα transgenic mice. *Cell* 61:1147-1155, 1990.

McCarty, K.S. Proliferative stimuli in the normal breast: estrogens or progestins. *Human Pathology* 20:1137-1138, 1989.

Medina, D. The preneoplastic state in mouse mammary tumorigenesis. *Carcinogenesis* 9:1113-1120, 1988.

Mikkelsen, T. and Cavenee, W. Suppressors of the malignant phenotype. *Cell Growth and Differentiation* 1:201-207, 1990.

Molinolo, A.A., Lanari, C., Charreau, E.H., Sanjuan, N. and Pasquilini, C.D. Mouse mammary tumors induced by medrony progesterone acetate: immunohistochemistry and hormonal receptors. *J. Natl. Cancer Inst.* 79:1341-1350, 1987.

Murphy, L.C. and Dotzlau, H. Regulation of transforming growth factor β messenger ribonucleic acid abundance in T47D, human breast cancer cells. *Mol. Endocrinol.* 3:611-617, 1989.

Murphy, L.C., Murphy, L.J., Dubik, D., Bell, G.I. and Shiu, R.P.C. Epidermal growth factor gene expression in human breast cancer cells: regulation of expression by progestins. *Cancer Res.* 48:4555-4560, 1988.

Murphy, L.J., Sutherland, R.L., Steed, B., Murphy, L.C. and Lazarus, L. Progestin regulation of epidermal growth factor receptor in human mammary carcinoma cells. *Mol. Endocrinol.* 46:728-734, 1986.

Musgrove, E.A. and Sutherland, R.L. Steroids, growth factors and cell cycle controls in breast cancer. In: Regulation of Breast Cancer edited by Lippman, M.E. and Dickson, R.B. Kluwer Academic Publishers, Norwell, Massachusetts, pp. 305-331, 1990.

Nigro, J.M., Baker, S.J., Preisinger, A.C., Jessup, J.M., Hostetter, R., Cleary, K., Bigner, S.H., Davidson, N., Baylin, S., Devilee, P., Glover, T., Collins, F.S., Westin, A., Modali, R., Harris, C.C. and Vogelstein, B. Mutations of the p53 gene occur in diverse tumor types. *Nature* 232:705-708, 1989.

Oka, T., Tsutsumi, O., Kurachi, H., and Okamoto, S. The role of epidermal growth factor in normal and neoplastic growth of mouse mammary epithelial cells. In: Breast Cancer: Cellular and Molecular Biology edited by M.E. Lippman and R.B. Dickson. Kluwer Press, Boston, pp. 343-362, 1988.

Osborne, C.K., Hamilton, B., Titus, G., Livingston, R.B. Epidermal growth factor stimulation of human breast cancer cells in culture. *Cancer Res.* 40:2361-2366, 1980.

Ottman, R., Hoffman, P.G., and Siiteri, P.K. Estrogen receptor assays in familial and non-familial breast cancer. In: Banbury Report 8: Hormones and Breast Cancer (Pike, M.C., Siiteri, P.K. and Welsch, C.W., eds.), Cold Spring Harbor Laboratory, pp. 191-211, 1981.

Paik, S., Hazan, R., Fisher, E.R., Sass, R.E., Fisher, B., Redmond, C., Schlessinger, J., Lippman, M.E. and King, C.R. Pathologic findings from the National Surgical Adjuvant breast and bowel project: prognostic significance of $erbB_2$ protein overexpression in primary breast cancer. *J. Clin. Oncol.* 8:103-112, 1990.

Paul, D. and Schmidt, G.H. Immortalization and malignant transformation of differentiated cells by oncogenes *in vitro* and in transgenic mice, Critical Reviews in Oncogenesis. 1:307-321, 1989.

Perez, R., Pascual, M., Macias, A. and Lage, A. Epidermal growth factor receptors in human breast cancer. *Breast Cancer Reg. Treat.* 4: 189-193, 1984.

Perroteau, I., Salomon, D., DeBortoli, M., Kidwell, W., Hazarika, P., Pardue, R., Dedman, J. and Tam, J. Immunological detection and quantitation of alpha transforming growth factors in human breast carcinoma cells. *Breast Cancer Res. Treat.* 7:201-210, 1986.

Pike, M.D., Henderson, B.E., and Casagrande, J.T. The epidemiology of breast cancer as it relates to menarche pregnancy and menopause. In: Banbury Report 8: Hormones and Breast Cancer (Pike, M.C., Siiteri, P.K. and Welsch, C.W., eds.), Cold Spring Harbor Laboratory, pp. 3-21, 1981.

Plowman, G.D., Green, J.M., McDonald, V.C., Neubauer, M.G., Disteche, C.M., Todaro, G.J. and Shoyab, M. The amphiregulin gene encodes a novel epidermal growth factor-related protein with tumor inhibitory activity. *Molecular and Cellular Biology* 10:1969-1981, 1990.

Ponder, B.A.J. Inherited predisposition to cancer. *Trends in Genetics* 6:213-218, 1990.

Rastinejad, F., Polverini, P.J. and Bouck, N.P. Regulation of the activity of a new inhibitor of angiogenesis by a cancer suppressor gene. *Cell* 56:345-355, 1989.

Riedel, H., Massoglia, S., Schlessinger, J. and Ullrich, A. Ligand activation of overexpressed epidermal growth factor receptors transforms NIH 3T3 mouse fibroblasts. *Proc. Nat'l. Acad. Sci. (U.S.A.)* 85:1477-1482, 1988.

Robinson, S.P., and Jordan, V.C. Reversal of the antitumor effects of tamoxifen by progesterone in the DMBA-induced rat mammary carcinoma model, Cancer Research. 47:5386-5390, 1987.

Rosenthal, A., Lindquist, P.B., Bringman, T.S., Goeddel, D.V. and Derynck, R. Expression in rat fibroblasts of a human transforming growth factor-α cDNA results in transformation. *Cell* 46:301-309, 1986.

Sainsbury, J.R., Farndon, J.R., Needham, G.K., Malcolm, A.J. and Harris, A.L. Epidermal-growth-factor receptor status as predictor of early recurrence of and death from breast cancer. *Lancet* i:1398-1402, 1987.

Sairenji, M., Suzuki, K., Murakami, K., Motohashi, H., Okamoto, T. and Umeda, M. Transforming growth factor activity in pleural and peritoneal effusions from cancer and non-cancer patients. *Jpn. J. Cancer Res. (Gann)* 78:814-820, 1987.

Salomon, D.S. and Kidwell, W.R. Tumor associated growth factors in malignant rodent and human mammary epithelial cells. In: Breast Cancer: Cellular and Molecular Biology edited by M.E. Lippman and R.B. Dickson. Kluwer Press, Boston, pp. 363-390, 1988.

Salomon, D.S., Perroteau, I., Kidwell, W.R., Tam, J. and Derynck, R. Loss of growth responsiveness to epidermal growth factor and enhanced production of alpha-transforming growth factors in ras-transformed mouse mammary epithelial cells. *J. Cell. Physiol.* 130: 397-409, 1987.

Sandgren, E.P., Luetteke, N.C., Palmiter, R.D., Brinster, R.L. and Lee, D.C. Overexpression of TGFα in transgenic mice: induction of epithelial hyperplasia, pancreatic metaplasia and carcinoma of the breast. *Cell* 61:1121-1135, 1990.

Schoenberger, C.A., Andres, A.C., Groner, B., van der Valk, M., LeMeur, M. and Gerlinger, P. Targeted c-myc gene expression in mammary glands of transgenic mice induces mammary tumors with constitutive mild protein gene transcription. *EMBO J.*, 7:169-175, 1988.

Shankar, V., Ciardiello, F., Kim, N., Derynck, R., Liscia, D.S., Merlo, G., Langton, B.C., Sheer, D., Callahan, R., Bassin, R.H., Lippman, M.E., Hynes, N. and Salomon, D.S., 1989, Transformation of normal mouse mammary epithelial cells following transfection with a human transforming growth factor alpha cDNA. *Mol. Carcinogen.* 2:1-11, 1989.

Shoyab, M., Plowman, G.D., McDonald, V.L., Bradley, J.G. and Todaro, G.J. Structure and function of human amphiregulin: a member of the epidermal growth factor family. *Science* 243:1074-1076, 1989.

Silberstein, G.B. and Daniel, C.W. Reversible inhibition of mammary gland growth by transforming growth factor-β. *Science* 237:291-293, 1987.

Silberstein, G.B., Strickland, P., Coleman, S. and Daniel, C.W. Epithelium-dependent extracellular matrix sytheses in transforming growth factor β1-growth inhibited mouse mammary gland. *J. Cell Biol.* 110:2209-2219, 1990.

Sinn, E., Mullen, W., Pattengale, P., Tepler, I., Wallace, R. and Leder, P. Coexpression of MMTV/v-Ha-*ras* and MMTV/c-*myc genes in transgenic mice: synergistic action of oncogenes in vivo. Cell* 49: 465-475, 1987.

Slamon, D.J., Godulphin, W., Jones, L.A., Holt, J.A., Wong, S.G., Keith, D.E., Levin, W.J., Stuart, S.G., Udove, J., Ullrich, A. and Press, M.J. Studies of the HER-2/*neu* protooncogene in human breast and ovarian cancer. *Science* 244:621-624, 1989.

Spitzer, E., Grosse, R., Kunde, D. and Schmidt, H.E. Growth of mammary epithelial cells in breast-cancer biopsies correlates with EGF binding. *Int. J. Cancer* 39:279-282, 1987.

Sporn, M.B. and Roberts, A.B. Peptide growth factors and inflammation, tissue repair, and cancer. *J. Clin. Inv.* 78:329-332, 1986.

Sporn, M.B. and Todaro, G.J. Autocrine secretion and malignant transformation of cells. *N. Engl. J. Med.* 303:878-880, 1980.

Stampfer, M.R. Isolation and growth of human mammary epithelial cells. *J. Tiss. Cult. Meth.* 9:107-115, 1985.

Stampfer, M.R. and Bartley, J.C. Induction of transformation and continuous cell lines from normal human mammary epithelial cells after exposure to benzo-*a*-pyrene. *Proc. Nat'l. Acad. Sci. (U.S.A.)* 82:2394-2398, 1985.

Steeg, P.S., Bevilacqua, G., Rosengard, A.M., Croce, V. and Liotta, L.A. Altered expression of Nm23, a gene associated with low tumor metastatic potential, during adenovirus 2 E1a inhibition of experimental metastases. *Cancer Res.* 48:6550-6554, 1988.

Stern, D.F., Hare, D.L., Cecchini, M.A. and Weinberg, R.A. Construction of a novel oncogene based on synthetic sequences encoding epidermal growth factor. *Science* 235:321-324, 1987.

Stern, D.F., Roberts, A.B., Roche, N.S., Sporn, M.B. and Weinberg, R.A. Differential responsiveness of *myc- and ras*-transfected cells to growth factors: selective stimulation of *myc*-transfected cells by epidermal growth factor. *Mol. Cell. Biol.* 6:870-877, 1986.

Stromberg, K., Hudgins, R. and Orth, D.N. Urinary TGFs in neoplasia: immunoreactive TGF-α in the urine of patients with disseminated breast carcinoma. *Biochem. Biophys. Res. Comm.* 144:1059-1067, 1987.

Sunderland, M.C. and McGuire, W.L. Oncogenes as clinical prognostic indicators. *In*: Regulatory Mechanisms in Breast Cancer, (Lippman, M.E. and Dickson, R.B., eds.), Kluwer Academic Publishers, Norwell, Massachusetts, pp. 3-22, 1990.

Travers, M.R., Barrett-Lee, P.J., Berger, U., Luqmani, Y.A., Gazet, J-C., Powles, T.J. and Coombes, R.C. Growth factor expression in normal, benign, and malignant breast tissue. *Brit. Med. J.* 296:1621-1630, 1988.

Valverius, E.M., Bates, S.E., Stampfer, M.R., Clarke, R., McCormick, F., Salomon, D.S., Lippman, M.E. and Dickson, R.B. Transforming growth factor alpha production and EGF receptor expression in normal and oncogene transformed human mammary epithelial cells. *Mol. Endocrinol.* 3:203-214, 1989.

Valverius, E.M., Ciardiello, F., Heldin, N.E., Blondel, B., Merlo, G., Smith, G., McGready, M., Stampfer, M.R., Lippman, M.E., Dickson, R.B. and Salomon, D.S. Stromal influences on transformation of human mammary epithelial cells expressing c-*myc* and SV40T. *J. Cellular Physiol.* 145:207-216,1990.

Valverius, E.M., Walker-Jones, D., Bates, S.E., Stampfer, M.R., Clarke, R., McCormick, F., Dickson, R.B. and Lippman, M.E. Production and responsiveness to transforming growth factor β in normal and oncogene transformed human mammary epithelial cells. *Cancer Res.* 49:6269-6274, 1989.

Varlay, J.M., Swallow, J.E., Brammer, V.J., Wittaker, J.L., and Waekor, R.A. Alterations to either c-*erb*B_2 (*neu*) or c-*myc* protooncogenes in breast carcinomas correlate with short term prognosis. *Oncogene* 1:423-430, 1987.

Velu, T.J., Beguinot, L., Vass, W.C., Willingham, M.C., Merlino, G.T., Pastan, I. and Lowy, D.R. pidermal growth factor-dependent transformation by a human EGF receptor proto-oncogene. *Science* 238:1408-1450, 1987.

Vonderhaar, B.K. Regulation of development of the normal mammary gland by hormones and growth factors. *In*: Breast Cancer: Cellular and Molecular Biology (Edited by M.E. Lippman and R.B. Dickson), Kluwer Press, Boston, pp. 251-266, 1988.

Walker-Jones, D., Valverius, E.M., Stampfer, M.R., Lippman, M.E. and Dickson, R.B. Transforming growth factor β (TGFβ) stimulates expression of epithelial membrane antigen in normal and oncogene transformed human mammary epithelial cells. *Cancer Res.* 49:6407-6411, 1989.

Watanabe, S., Lazar, E. and Sporn, M.B. Transformation of normal rat kidney (NRK) cells by an infectious retrovirus carrying a synthetic rat type α transforming growth factor gene. *Proc. Nat'l. Acad. Sci. (U.S.A.)* 84:1258-1262, 1987.

Weinberg, R.A. The retinoblastoma gene and cell growth control. *Trends in Biochem. Sci.* 18:199-202, 1990.

Weisz, A., Cicatiello, L., Perisco, E., Scalona, M., and Bresciani, ?? Estrogen stimulates transcription of *c-jun* protooncogene. *Mol. Endocrinol.* 4:1041-1050,1990.

Welsch, C.W. Host factors affecting the growth of carcinogen-induced rat mammary carcinomas: a review and tribute to Charles Brenton Huggins, *Cancer Research* 45:3415-3443, 1985.

Yee, D., Cullen, K.J., Paik, S., Perdue, J.F., Hampton, B., Schwartz, A., Lippman, M.E. and Rosen, N. Insulin-like growth factor II mRNA expression in human breast cancer. *Cancer Res.* 48:6691-6696, 1988.

Yee, D., Rosen, N., Favoni, R. and Cullen, K.J. The insulin-like growth factors, their receptors and their binding proteins in breast cancer. In: Regulation of Breast Cancer Edited by M.E. Lippman and R.B. Dickson, Kluwer Press, Boston, pp. 93-106, 1990.

Zugmaier, G., Knabbe, C., Deschauer, B., Lippman, M.E. and Dickson, R.B. Inhibition of anchorage independent growth of estrogen receptor positive and estrogen receptor negative human breast cancer cell lines by TGFβ and TGFβ_2, *J. Cell Physiol.,* 141:353-361, 1989.

REGULATION OF ESTROGEN RECEPTOR EXPRESSION IN BREAST CANCER

Mary Beth Martin, Miguel Saceda, and Ralph K. Lindsey

Lombardi Cancer Research Center
Georgetown University
Washington, DC 20007

ABSTRACT

One of the most prevalent of cancers, breast cancer, is characterized by hormonal control of its growth. Expression of the estrogen receptor (ER) in MCF-7 breast cancer cells appears to be a complex process involving multiple steps subject to hormonal regulation by estrogen. Treatment of MCF-7 cells with estradiol results in the suppression of estrogen receptor protein. By 6 hours, the receptor protein declined by about 60% from a level of approximately 3.6 to 1.2 fmol/ug DNA and remained suppressed for 24-48 hours. Similar results were obtained with an estrogen receptor binding assay. Estrogen treatment also resulted in a decrease of receptor mRNA to approximately 10% of control values by 6 hours. Estrogen receptor remained at the suppressed level for up to 48 hours. Transcription run-on experiments demonstrated a transient decrease of about 90% in receptor gene transcription after 1 hour. By 3-6 hours transcription increased approximately 2-fold and remained elevated for at least 48 hours. These data suggest that estrogen suppresses ER mRNA by inhibition of ER gene transcription at early times and by a post-transcriptional effect on receptor mRNA at later times. To determine whether post-transcriptional regulation of ER gene expression is mediated by an ER-dependent mechanism independent of protein synthesis, we used the competitive estrogen antagonist, 4-hydroxytamoxifen, and the inhibitor of protein synthesis, cycloheximide, to study the regulation of ER mRNA by estradiol. 4-Hydroxytamoxifen had no effect on the steady-state level of receptor mRNA and

The Underlying Molecular, Cellular, and Immunological Factors in Cancer and Aging, Edited by S.S. Yang and H.R.Warner, Plenum Press, New York, 1993

effectively blocked the suppression of ER mRNA by estradiol. The metabolic inhibitor, cycloheximide, was unable to prevent the estrogen induced decrease in ER mRNA. These data provide evidence that the post-transcriptional suppression of ER expression through estradiol is mediated through the ER independent of protein synthesis.

INTRODUCTION

One of the most prevalent of all cancers, breast cancer, is characterized by hormonal control of its growth. It is estimated that by the year 2000 the number of new cases diagnosed each year may exceed 1,000,000. Epidemiological studies show that the age-specific incidence rates for breast cancer increases dramatically up to the age of menopause. At the time of menopause, however, the rate of incidence slows. Endocrine status is an important underlying factor in the incidence of breast cancer and may account for the differential rates of incidence in pre- and post- menopausal women. Consequently, it is important to understand the molecular mechanisms of action of steroid hormones and the regulation of estrogen receptor gene expression. Expression of the ER in human breast cancer appears to be a complex process involving multiple steps subject to hormonal regulation by estrogen.

The purpose of the present study was to determine the mechanism by which estrogen regulates the expression of its cognate receptor in MCF-7 cells. To achieve this goal, the relationship between ER protein concentration and binding capacity, the steady state levels of receptor mRNA, and the level of ER gene transcription was examined simultaneously (1). To determine whether post-transcriptional regulation of ER gene expression is mediated by a receptor-dependent mechanism independent of protein synthesis, we have used the competitive estrogen antagonist, 4-hydroxytamoxifen, and the inhibitor of protein synthesis, cycloheximide, to study the regulation of ER mRNA by estradiol. In addition we have studied the site of post-transcriptional regulation (2).

RESULTS

Effect of estrogen treatment on the level of estrogen receptor protein and binding

To determine the level of estrogen receptor protein, an enzymeimmunoassay was employed. The data presented in Fig. 1 show that estrogen treatment, 10^{-9} M, resulted in a decline in total receptor protein of about 60% from a level of approximately 3.64 fmol/ug DNA (422.4 fmol/mg protein) in control cells to approximately 1.2 fmol/ug DNA (205 fmol/mg protein) in treated cells. The level of receptor decreased by 6 hr and remained depressed for up to 48 hr. These data are in good agreement with previously reported results (3-6).

To confirm that the decreased level of estrogen receptor protein, as measured by the enzymeimmunoassay, corresponded to a decreased level of estrogen binding sites, a competition assay was employed. In response to estradiol treatment, the number of estrogen binding sites decreased from 3.64 fmol/ug DNA in control cells to 1.24 fmol/ug DNA in 24 hr treated cells. The level of binding decreased in a manner similar to the decline in receptor protein. These results strongly suggest a suppression of the estrogen receptor by estradiol.

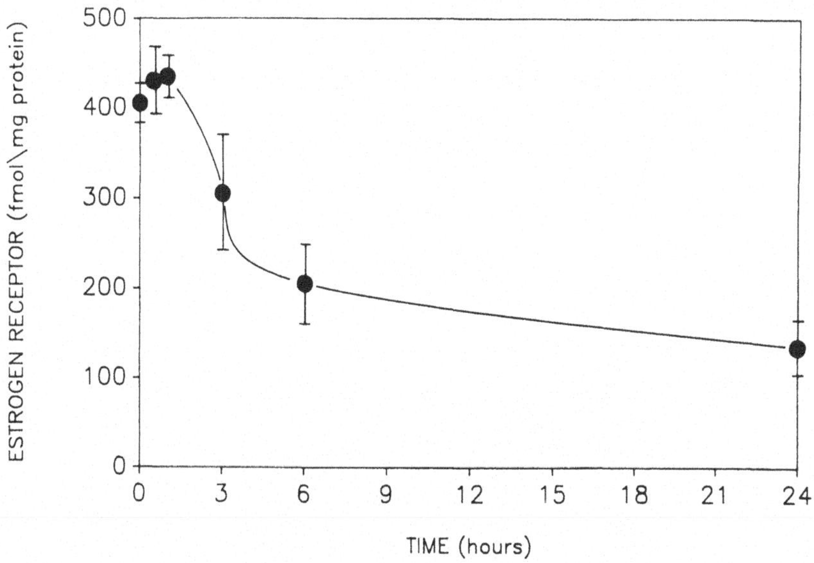

Figure 1. *Effect of estrogen on the steady-state level of estrogen receptor protein.* MCF-7 cells were grown in IMEM medium supplemented with 5% CCS. At approximately 80% confluence, the medium was replaced with phenol red-free IMEM containing 5% CCS. After two days, cells were treated with estradiol, 10^{-9} M, or ethanol for various times. Cells were washed, harvested, and homo- genized by sonication. Total estrogen receptor was determined with an enzyme immunoassay kit from Abbott Laboratories using D547 and H222 monoclonal antibodies. Results are presented as fmol of estrogen receptor per milligram of protein. Each point is the mean of several experiments.

Effect of estrogen treatment on the level of estrogen receptor mRNA

An RNase protection assay was employed to examine the effects of hormone treatment on the steady-state level of estrogen receptor mRNA. In these experiments, the level of receptor mRNA was normalized to the level of 36B4 mRNA, which is constitutively expressed in the presence of estradiol (7). Fig. 2 is a typical autoradiograph of an RNase protection assay showing the effect of estrogen treatment on the level of receptor mRNA. Changes in estrogen receptor mRNA were quantified by scanning densitometry (Fig. 3). In this study estradiol treatment (10^{-9} M) resulted in a maximum suppression of mRNA by 6 hr to approximately 10% of control values which remained at the suppressed level for up to 48 hr. These data demonstrate a close correspondence between the level of receptor protein and mRNA. Similar results were obtained if these results were normalized for total DNA in each sample. A decrease in the level of steroid receptor mRNA in response to their target hormone has been found for the glucocorticoid receptor (8, 9).

Effect of estrogen treatment on the level of estrogen receptor gene transcription

The effects of estrogen on receptor gene transcription were analyzed with

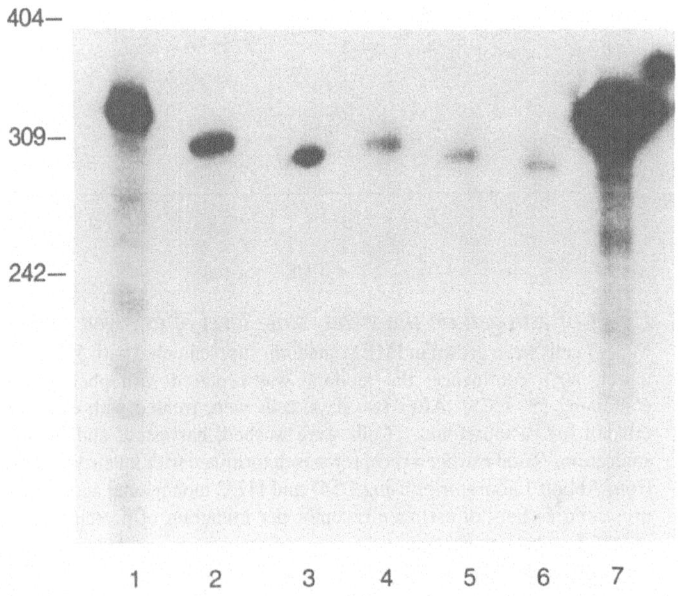

Figure 2. *Effect of estrogen on estrogen receptor mRNA.*
MCF-7 cells were treated as described in the legend to Fig. 1. Total RNA was isolated by the guanidinum isothiocynate method. 60 ug of total RNA was analyzed using an RNase protection assay. A 300 bp fragment of the ER mRNA was protected against RNase A degradation by hybridization of total RNA with ^{32}P-labeled antisense mRNA. Following hybridization, total RNA was digested with RNase A. The protected bands were separated on 6% PAGE gels and visualized by autoradiography. Lane 1, control; 2, 1 hr; 3, 3 hr; 4, 6 hr; 5, 24 hr; 6, 48 hr; and 7, probe.

a nuclear transcription run-on assay using nuclei isolated from MCF-7 cells treated with estradiol. The estrogen receptor probes included exon 1 and pOR3, a cDNA of the 3' end of the estrogen receptor (10,11). pS2 was employed as a positive inducible control. To control for artifacts due to the mitogenic nature of estrogen, 36B4 transcription was used as an internal control and the relative changes in estrogen receptor transcription were normalized to the signal obtained for 36B4. Similar results were obtained when either pOR3 or exon 1 was used as a probe. There was no significant difference in the results when the data were normalized for the number of nuclei. The progesterone and glucocorticoid receptors were also included to control for cross-hybridization of the estrogen receptor with other steroid hormone receptors.

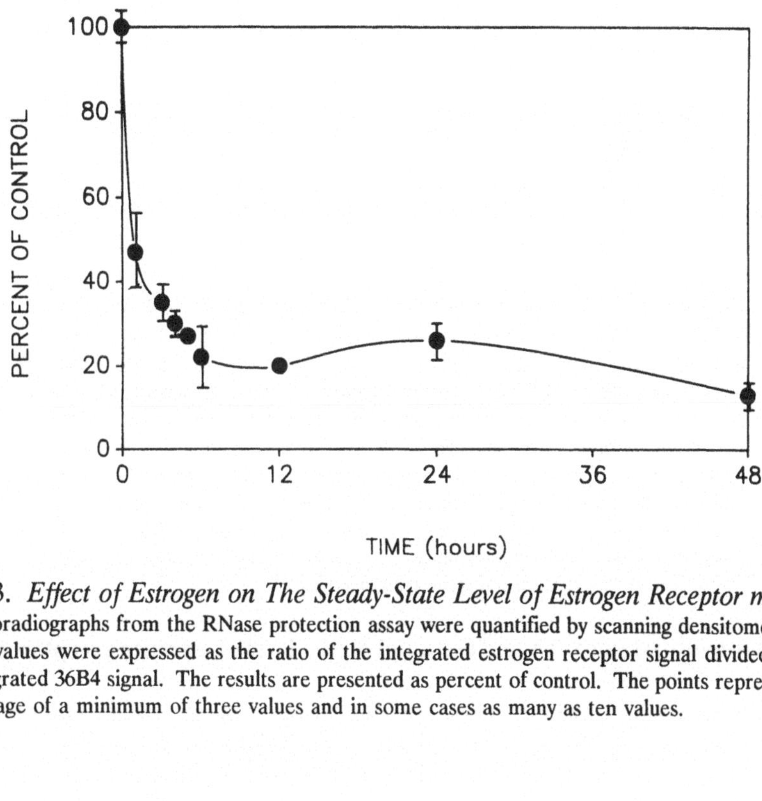

Fig. 3. *Effect of Estrogen on The Steady-State Level of Estrogen Receptor mRNA.* Autoradiographs from the RNase protection assay were quantified by scanning densitometry and the values were expressed as the ratio of the integrated estrogen receptor signal divided by the integrated 36B4 signal. The results are presented as percent of control. The points represent the average of a minimum of three values and in some cases as many as ten values.

The data in Fig. 4 indicate that there is a transient (1 hr) decrease in estrogen receptor transcription following estrogen treatment to approximately 90% of control values. This decrease is not due to a non-specific toxic response as indicated by the constitutive transcription of 36B4 and a 4- to 5-fold increase in transcription of pS2 by 30 min (Fig. 4, inset). Following this decrease, transcription increased to a level higher than that observed in control nuclei. Although estrogen treatment results in a transient suppression of estrogen receptor transcription, it is improbable that this drop is responsible for the prolonged suppression of estrogen receptor mRNA. The data suggest that the predominant mechanism suppressing estrogen receptor expression is a post-transcriptional event.

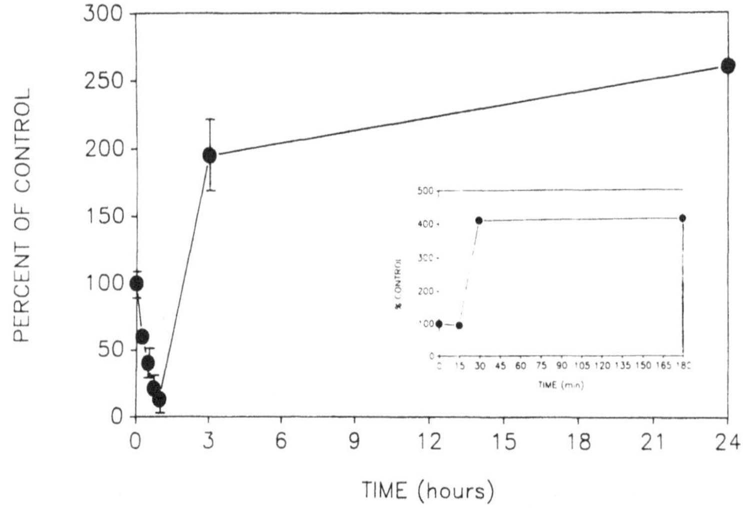

Fig. 4. *Effect of estrogen on estrogen receptor gene transcription.* MCF-7 cells were treated as described in the legend to Fig. 1. Nuclei were isolated at the indicated time points by homogenization in 1.5 M sucrose buffer containing 0.1% Brij 58; elongation of nascent transcripts was performed in a reaction buffer containing ^{32}P-UTP. Newly synthesized transcripts were isolated and hybridized to filters containing an excess of plasmid DNA. The level of transcription was determined by autoradiography and quantified by scanning densitometry. The level of transcription was expressed as the ratio of the integrated estrogen receptor signal divided by the integrated 36B4 signal. The results are presented as percent of control. Inset: The effect of estrogen on pS2 gene transcription.

Effect of 4-hydroxytamoxifen and estradiol on the level of estrogen receptor mRNA

The effect of 4-hydroxytamoxifen and estrogen on the steady-state level of estrogen receptor mRNA was determined by an RNase protection assay and the results presented in Fig 5. In this study, estradiol, 10^{-9} M, resulted in a maximum suppression of ER mRNA by 6 hr. 4-Hydroxytamoxifen, 5 x 10^{-7} M, had no significant effect on the steady-state level of estrogen receptor mRNA. When the cells were simultaneously treated with estradiol and 4-hydroxytamoxifen the suppression of ER mRNA was almost completely reversed suggesting that the post-transcriptional suppression of ER mRNA is an estrogen receptor mediated phenomenon.

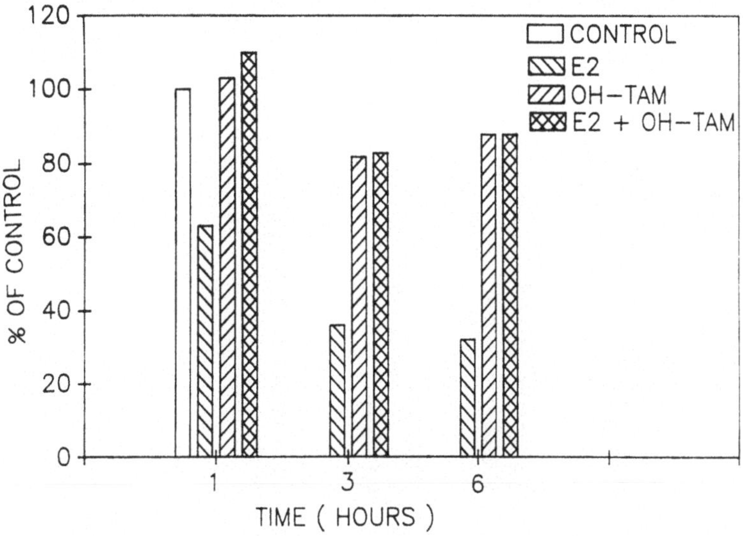

Fig. 5. *Effect of estrogen and hydroxytamoxifen on the steady-state level of estrogen receptor mRNA.*
Autoradiographs from the RNase protection assay were analyzed as described in the legend to Fig. 3.

Effect of cycloheximide and estradiol treatment on the level of estrogen receptor mRNA

The effect of 10^{-9} M estradiol, 10 ug/ml cycloheximide, or both on the steady-state level of estrogen receptor mRNA are presented in Fig 6. In this study, estradiol treatment resulted in a maximum suppression of ER mRNA by 6 hr. Cycloheximide had no significant effect on ER mRNA during this time and did not abolish the effect of estradiol suggesting that post-transcriptional suppression of ER mRNA is a primary effect of the estrogen receptor. However, other possibilities have not been ruled out such as the estrogen receptor mediated effect is through the induction of an RNA species or the estrogen receptor interacts directly with ER mRNA to alter its stability or processing.

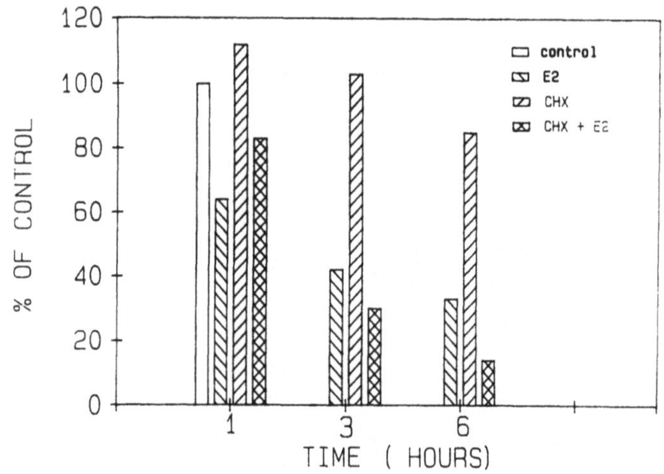

Fig. 6. *Effect of estrogen and cycloheximide on the steady-state level of estrogen receptor mRNA.*
Autoradiographs from the RNase protection assay were analyzed as described in Figure 3.

Effect of estradiol treatment on the steady-state level of nuclear and cytoplasmic ER mRNA

The effect of estradiol treatment on the steady-state level of nuclear and cytoplasmic ER mRNA was examined using the RNase protection assay. In this study, estrogen treatment resulted in a maximum suppression of nuclear ER mRNA (60%) which was sustained by 6 hr (Fig 7). There was a parallel but greater (90%) decrease in the level of cytoplasmic ER mRNA (Fig 8). These data suggest that the post-transcriptional suppression of ER mRNA is a nuclear event.

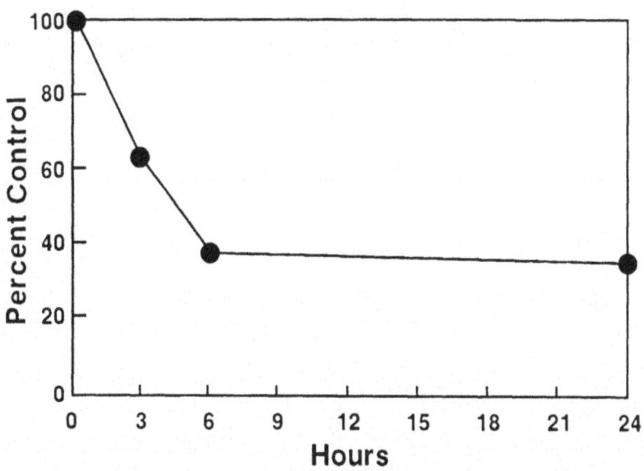

Fig. 7. *Effect of estrogen on nuclear estrogen receptor mRNA.*
MCF-7 cells were treated as described in the legend to Fig. 1. Nuclei were first isolated in 5% citric acid and homogenized in a buffer containing guanidinum isothiocynate. Nuclear RNA was isolated by centrifugation and the level of ER mRNA was determined by RNase protection as previously described in Fig. 3.

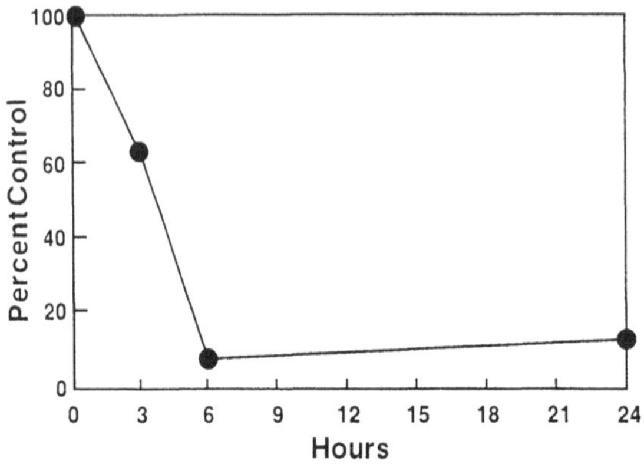

Fig. 8. *Effect of estrogen on cytoplasmic estrogen receptor mRNA.*
MCF-7 cells were treated as described in the legend to Fig. 1. Cytoplasmic RNA was isolated by the NP40 method. The level of ER mRNA was determined by RNase protection as described in Fig. 3.

CONCLUSION

The present study demonstrates that estrogen regulates its cognate receptor through suppression of receptor mRNA. The data suggest that the level of mRNA is regulated almost exclusively by a post-transcriptional event. It appears that the post-transcriptional regulation of ER mRNA is mediated by the classical estrogen receptor independent of protein synthesis. It is possible that estrogen alters mRNA stability, however, estrogen may effect other processing events such as splicing or nuclear transport. Further studies will be necessary to determine the nature of the post-transcriptional event.

REFERENCES

1. Saceda, M., Lippman, M.E., Chambon, P., Lindsey, R.K., Puente, M., and Martin, M.B. Regulation of the Estrogen Receptor in MCF-7 cells by Estradiol. *Mol. Endo.* 2: 1157-1162, 1988.

2. Saceda, M., Lippman, M.E., Lindsey, R.K., Puente, M., Martin, M.B. Role of an estrogen receptor-dependent mechanism in the regulation of estrogen receptor mRNA in MCF-7 cells. *Mol. Endocrin.* 3: 1782-1787, 1989.

3. Horwitz, K.B., and McGuire, W.L. Actinomycin D prevents nuclear processing of estrogen receptor. *J. Biol. Chem.* 253: 6319-6322, 1978.

4. Horwitz, K.B., and McGuire, W.L. Nuclear estrogen receptors. *J. Biol. Chem.* 255: 9699-9705, 1980.

5. Kaisd, A., Strobl, J.S., Huff, K., Greene, G.L., and Lippman, M.E. A novel nuclear form of estradiol receptor in MCF-7 human breast cancer cells. *Science* 225: 1162-1165, 1984.

6. Monsa, F.J.Jr., Katzenellenbogen, B.S., Miller, M.A., Ziegler, Y.S., and Katzenellenbogen, J.A. Characterization of the estrogen receptor and its dynamics in MCF-7 human breast cancer cells using a covalently attaching antiestrogen. *Endo.* 115: 143-152, 1984.

7. Masiakowski, P., Breathnach, R., Bloch, J., Gannon, F., Krust, A., and Chambon, P. Cloning of cDNA sequences of hormone-regulated genes from MCF-7 human breast cancer cell line. *Nucl. Acids Res.* 10: 7895-7903, 1982.

8. Okert, S., Poellinger, L., Dong, Y., and Gustafsson, J.-A. Down-regulation of glucocorticoid receptor mRNA by glucocorticoid hormones and recognition by the receptor of a specific binding sequence within a receptor cDNA clone. *Proc. Natl. Acad. Sci., USA* 83: 5899-5903, 1986.

9. Kalinyak, J.A., Dorin, R.I., Hoffman, A.R., Perlman, A.J. Tissue-specific regulation of glucocorticoid receptor mRNA by dexamethasone. *J. Biol. Chem.* 262: 10441-10444, 1987.

10. Green, S., Walter, P., Kumar, V., Krust, A., Bornert, J.-M., Argos, P., and Chambon, P. Human oestrogen receptor cDNA: sequence, expression, and homology to v-erb-A. *Nature* 320: 134-139, 1986.

11. Greene, G.L., Gilna, P., Waterfield, M., Baker, A., Hort, Y., and Shine, J. Sequence and expression of human estrogen receptor complementry DNA. *Science* 231: 1150-1154, 1986.

AGING AND DEVELOPMENT OF OVARIAN EPITHELIAL CARCINOMA: THE RELEVANCE OF CHANGES IN OVARIAN STROMAL ANDROGEN PRODUCTION

Margaret A. Thompson and Mark D. Adelson

Department of Obstetrics and Gynecology
S.U.N.Y. Health Science Center, Syracuse, NY 13210

ABSTRACT

There are three types of ovarian neoplasms: (1) Those which arise from the surface epithelium covering the ovary. (2) Those which are derived from the cortical mesenchymal stroma. (3) Those which develop from germ cells. Our laboratory has concentrated its effort on solid tumors in women of the first type, epithelial, which has the highest incidence and is the most lethal. Development of these tumors is correlated with aging in the ovary. They form primarily during the perimenopause. Among women, 64% of the total ovarian cancer cases are diagnosed between ages 41 and 60 years[1]. Our approach has been to establish stable tumor cell lines from patient specimens for use as *in vitro* models. We have investigated the response of these cells to steroid hormones because we hypothesized that these tumors retain some metabolic characteristics which are specific to the ovary. Our data demonstrate that testosterone and androstenedione, but not cortisol, inhibited proliferation of ovarian tumor cells *in vitro* by a mechanism which was independent of steroid receptors. These androgens are routinely synthesized and secreted by human ovary, and in the menopausal ovary the primary source of androgen is the stromal cell compartment. Because a relatively high local concentration of ovarian androgen exists *in vivo*, it is possible that androgen may suppress ovarian epithelial carcinoma in women as well. If it does, then development of this carcinoma may be facilitated when the postmenopausal ovary fails to produce adequate androgen during postreproductive years.

INTRODUCTION

Ovarian epithelial cancer is the leading cause of death from gynecologic

The Underlying Molecular, Cellular, and Immunological Factors in Cancer and Aging, Edited by S.S. Yang and H.R.Warner, Plenum Press, New York, 1993

neoplasm[2]. In 1989 ovarian cancer accounted for 4% of total cancer diagnosed in women, compared to breast cancer which accounted for 28%. In spite of its lower incidence rate compared to that for breast cancer in women, the annual number of deaths is high for patients with ovarian cancer. Data collected in 1986 reported 19,000 new cases of ovarian cancer with 11,600 deaths (61% of the total reported cases), and 123,000 new cases of breast cancer with 39,000 deaths (32% of the total reported cases). This disease presents a unique challenge in that even small tumors, early in their development, form metastasis and implant throughout the peritoneal cavity[3] while patients are yet without symptoms[4]. The wide and often spider-web-like dissemination produces surgically incurable tumors, and the primary approach has become one of cytoreduction of the tumor mass to enhance effectiveness of chemotherapy agents[5,6]. However, even with the advent of multiagent chemotherapy, median duration of survival is only 15 months[7]. Individuals commonly respond differently to any choice of chemotherapeutic agents. Furthermore ovarian cancer cells are noted for rapid development of primary drug resistance and a broad cross resistance[8, 9].

Epithelial tumors account for more than 60% of all ovarian neoplasms, and they are primarily diagnosed in adults, with the malignant forms appearing later in life[1]. Only 14% of these patients are under 41 years of age, and 4% are older than 70. This disease occurs at menopause when steroid synthetic pathways in the ovary are switching from primarily estrogen production to androgen production. Histologically these tumors are classified into three groups: benign tumor, borderline tumor, and malignant tumor. The differential diagnosis includes absence of stromal invasion for borderline tumors and its presence for carcinoma[1]. Five year survival for patients with borderline tumors is 95%, and for patients with carcinoma is 10 to 50% depending upon the stage at surgery. Therefore stromal-epithelial interaction, at least at the level of histology, is correlated with malignancy. Whether this interaction has functional significance has not yet been determined.

ENDOCRINE PARAMETERS OF OVARIAN CARCINOMA

For thirty years it has been debated whether ovarian epithelial carcinoma is an endocrine or nonendocrine tissue. Clinically these tumors are considered nonendocrine because there is no large increase in plasma levels of ovarian steroids. Smaller changes in ovarian steroid secretion would, of course, be masked by the fact that the women are perimenopausal and experience erratic residual cyclicity. Forty to sixty percent of tumor specimens contain estrogen and progesterone receptors[10, 11], and 90% to 95% have androgen receptor[12]. Yet these receptors are seldom reported for cell lines cultured from tumor specimens, even at early passage. It is possible that steroid receptors exist primarily in the stromal component of the tumor, which is left out when the epithelial cells are selectively cultured. The importance of hormones to this carcinoma has not been tested *in vivo*, primarily because the disease presents at late stage and survival is short. Hormonal therapy for these patients has been palliative, following escape of the disease from chemotherapy regimens, just prior to patient death.

Aromatase enzymatic activity, the enzyme which converts androgen to estrogen, has been reported in tumor microsomal preparations and in stable epithelial cell lines cultured from these tumors[13, 14, 15, 16]. In 1988, our laboratory characterized biochemically, for the first time, estrogen synthetic activity in three stable cell lines cultured from patients with ovarian carcinoma. The apparent K_m for conversion of testosterone to estradiol in whole cell, ranged from 4 μMolar to 59 μMolar, with a V_{max} 20 to 150 pmoles/h/mg cell protein. Similar results, apparent K_m 7-10 μMolar and V_{max} 100 to 600 pmoles/h/mg protein, were obtained with androstenedione as substrate and estrone product. We have since demonstrated comparable aromatase enzymatic activity in three additional cell lines (unpublished data). The enzymatic reaction appeared to be first order, i.e., the half time was independent of the initial concentration of substrate. The molecular activity, turnover rate (V_{max}/molecular weight), appeared similar to that of ovarian granulosa cells. Aromatization of testosterone produced 100% estradiol, and of androstenedione 90% estrone and 10% estradiol in culture medium.

These studies led us to question the implications of endocrine phenotype to development of ovarian carcinoma, and ovarian cancer's correlation with onset of menopause. It seems unlikely that these tumor cells synthesize androgen from plasma cholesterol, as this disease is rarely associated with endocrine disorders. However, if the source of androgen for tumor aromatase is not plasma cholesterol, another must be proposed. The stromal component of the primary tumor presents a plausible possibility. There are reports in old literature, between 1940 and 1958, which describe "leuteinization" of the stromal component of primary epithelial ovarian tumors[17]. A later paper by Plotz *et al.*, 1966[15] demonstrated conversion of radiolabeled progesterone to testosterone and androstenedione in a microsomal preparation from tumor tissue. Subsequently, they[16] expanded their studies and also showed aromatization of steroid precursors by whole tissue homogenates of two of six tumors measured. If tumor aromatase depends upon stroma of the primary site for androgen substrate, then the bulk of disseminated tumor would not be expected to produce estrogen, and gross endocrine disorders would be absent, consistent with clinical observations for these patients.

Androgen production is a normal feature of ovarian steroid secretion in women. Ovaries of reproductive age women secrete significant quantity of androstenedione and testosterone[18] in addition to estrogen and progesterone. Even after menopause, normal patients present data suggesting a spectrum of ovarian function. Concentration gradients across the ovary have been shown for testosterone, androstenedione, estradiol and estrone[19]. In young women the principal ovarian androgen is androstenedione[20]. The postmenopausal ovary secretes more testosterone than the premenopausal ovary[20]. However, functional importance of ovarian androgen secretion in women has not yet been defined.

As a first step in our attempt to evaluate steroid responsiveness of ovarian carcinoma to androgen, we analyzed cell proliferation of several ovarian cancer cell lines *in vitro* to increasing concentration of androgen in the growth medium. Data presented here is from one such line, 2774, which does not contain receptors for these steroids. Data from this cell line was consistent with that from our other lines, and we chose it for presentation because androgen effects via receptors need not be considered in our interpretation of these experimental results. For comparison we also included data from an endometrial cancer cell line, SW1748. We found that micromolar concentrations of androgen, but not cortisol, inhibited cell proliferation, probably by a toxic mechanism.

EXPERIMENTAL DESIGN

Data presented in this paper was obtained from two cell lines, one from an ovarian cancer and one from an endometrial cancer. Establishment and characterization of the ovarian cancer cell line, 2774, has been described in detail elsewhere[13,14]. The cells were obtained January 1976 from malignant ascites of a patient with an untreated ovarian carcinoma of endometrioid type. The endometrial cancer cell line, SW1748, was kindly supplied by Dr. R. S. Freedman, M.D. Anderson Hospital and Tumor Institute, Houston, TX.

Cells were cultured in either Leibovitz L-15 medium, 2774, or RPMI-1640, SW1748, supplemented with 5% fetal calf serum (Hyclone, Logan, UT), ITS: insulin (5 mg/liter): transferrin (5 mg/liter): selenium (5 μg/liter) (Collaborative Research, Inc., Lexington, MA), 500 units of penicillin, streptomycin (50 μg/ml (Gibco) and 2 mM L-glutamine (Gibco). Cells were maintained at 37°C in humidified air made 5% CO_2.

For experimentation cells were seeded in 6 well tissue culture plates, 3 x 10^4 cells per well. Cells were counted in triplicate at each time point to demonstrate a proliferation curve with a log growth portion. Quantization was done with a hemocytometer in the presence of trypan blue, and only cells excluding trypan blue, viable cells, were included.

Data analysis was done by two way analysis of variance, ANOVA, with post hoc t-tests to determine significance of treatment dose.

RESULTS

For clarity only two time points from each growth curve are presented in figures, one from early log growth and one from late log growth. Androstenedione was added at either 1 μMolar, 10 μMolar or 100 μMolar to 2774 cell cultures 24 h after seeding (Figure 1). Neither 1 uMolar nor 10 uMolar androstenedione had an effect on cell proliferation during log growth. However, 100 μMolar androstenedione slowed cell division drastically compared to control. Even early in log growth, at day 6, there was a significant difference between control and androstenedione treated wells. Doubling time of control cultures between day 4 and 6 was 21 h, compared to 29 h for steroid treated. Cultures with 100 μMolar androstenedione contained a large quantity of dead cell debris. The slower doubling time of the culture may, therefore, have reflected a toxic rather than a cell regulatory effect of the hormone.

Ovarian cancer cells were more sensitive to testosterone than to androstenedione (Figure 2). Ten μM testosterone inhibited log growth of treated cells significantly by day 7. Cells cultured in 100 μM testosterone did not advance beyond the number seeded. Again, cell debris was observed in the culture medium. Similar results were obtained with two other ovarian cancer cell lines, OV166 and OV1225, initiated and characterized by our laboratory[13] (data not shown).

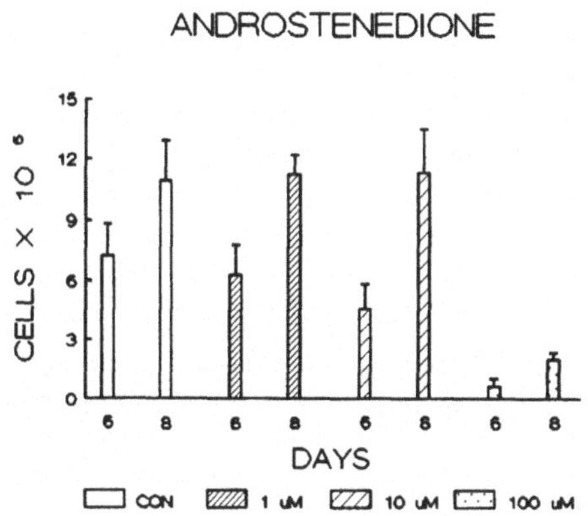

Figure 1. *The Effect of Androstenedione on Log Growth of Ovarian Cancer Cell Line 2774 at Three Concentrations.*

Analogous experiments with cortisol added to growth medium demonstrated that the androgen induced inhibition of ovarian cancer cell proliferation was specific. Experiments were conducted with the same ovarian cancer cell line 2774, and cortisol was substituted for androgen at 1 μMolar, 10 μMolar and 100 μMolar (Figure 3). For clarity results are presented for only two points from each growth curve, consisting of five time points at each dose. Analysis of variance for all twenty points, performed in triplicate, indicated there were no differences between cortisol treated and control cells during log growth.

The dose of androgen required to inhibit log growth of ovarian cancer cells was in the range of the K_m determined for the whole cell aromatase enzymatic activity[13]. That, combined with knowledge that *in situ* concentration of androgen in the ovary can also reach the micromolar range[18], led us to speculate that the mechanism underlying the effect of androgen on these cells involves the cellular cytochrome P450 enzymes. The lack of a response to cortisol might be explained by determining which

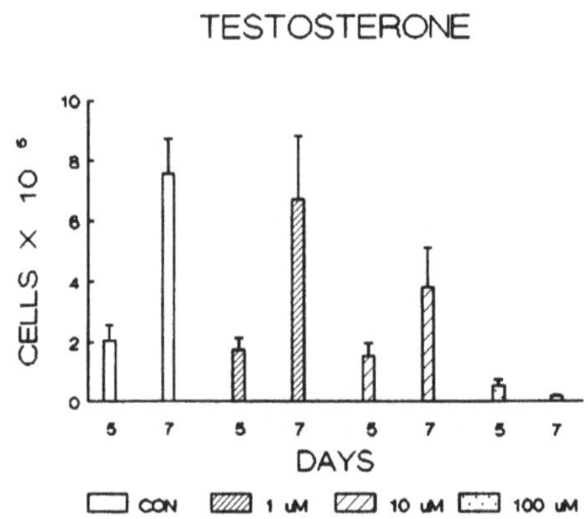

Figure 2. *The Effect of Testosterone on Log Growth of Ovarian Cancer Cell Line 2774 at Three Concentrations.*

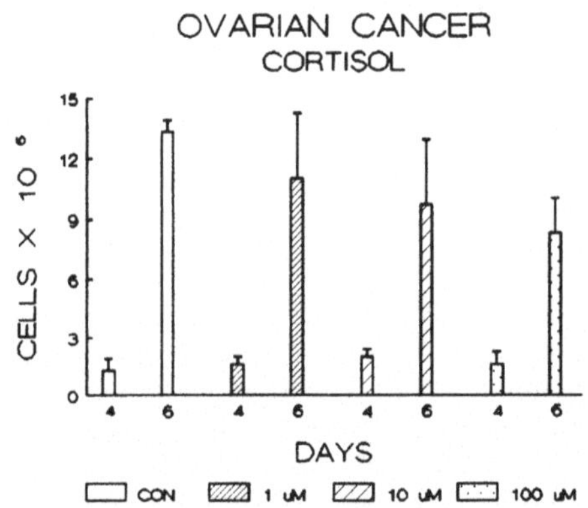

Figure 3. *The Effect of Cortisol on Log Growth of Ovarian Cancer Cell Line 2774 at Three Concentrations*

steroidogenic enzymes are present in the tumor. The extended time required to observe an effect of androgen on cell proliferation, 4 to 7 days, suggests that enzymatic production of a toxic product, which accumulates within the cell, might account for the observed phenomenon. Another human gynecologic tumor reported to contain aromatase is endometrial cancer[22]. Figure 4 shows data obtained with the endometrial cancer cell line SW1748 which was consistent with that obtained with the ovarian cancer cells. Testosterone at 100 μMolar, inhibited cell proliferation during log growth but cortisol at 100 μMolar, did not.

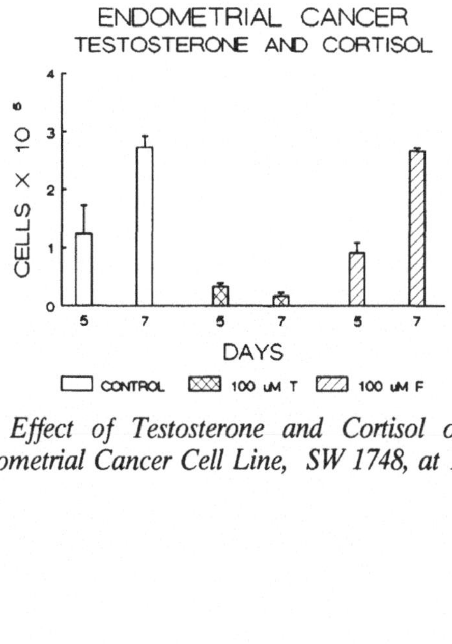

Figure 4. *The Effect of Testosterone and Cortisol on Log Growth of Endometrial Cancer Cell Line, SW 1748, at 100 μMolar*

DISCUSSION

Our laboratory has established a long term commitment to continue assessment of endocrine properties of ovarian carcinoma. We shall proceed with cell culture as our model system. Our plan is to design investigations which determine the *in vivo* source of androgen substrate for tumor aromatase. We shall ask if the ovarian stromal cell compartment produces androgen and whether the amount produced would be sufficient to inhibit tumor growth. Steroid metabolism by cancer cells will be examined to resolve which parts of the steroidogenic enzyme path they include. We shall also construct experiments to elucidate the molecular mechanism by which androgen inhibits proliferation of ovarian tumor cells.

Adequate resources are available for these studies. Five epithelial cell lines are currently available in our laboratory for construction of an *in vitro* model of the *in vivo* situation. In liquid nitrogen storage we currently have an additional 30 cultures at passages 2 to 10. Also in liquid nitrogen inventory is a stromal cell culture from an ovarian tumor. Using selective culture techniques more cultures of the nonepithelial component of primary tumors will be derived. The Department of Obstetrics and Gynecology, S.U.N.Y. Health Science Center, Syracuse, NY, has an extensive population of patients requiring surgery for ovarian cancer. At least 30 tumor samples per year are readily obtained, tissue from large benign tumors is available, and sections of normal human ovary from patients of various ages are accessible from our own patient population. Modern culture techniques, described by other participants in this workshop, have made feasible *in vitro* study of interactions between various cell types included in a particular tissue. Our laboratory has successfully cultured the ovarian epithelial tumor for over 6 years, and we are certain of our ability to perform this type of analysis.

One aspect of our investigation will be to identify a likely source of androgen substrate for tumor aromatase. It is probable that at least some other steroidogenic enzymes in addition to aromatase are expressed by ovarian cancer cells[15,16]. Experiments will include incubation of cells *in vitro* in the presence of labeled steroids which are commonly found in the enzymatic pathway between cholesterol and progesterone, followed by HPLC separation of products extracted from culture medium. Also, because an abundance of data has been recently published regarding DNA sequences for many of these enzymes, we are confident that we could identify mRNA for these enzymes in our cells with the polymerase chain reaction if it is present.

Our hypothesis for the mechanism by which androgen inhibits ovarian cancer cell proliferation *in vitro* is: High turnover of androgen substrate by aromatase, a cytochrome P-450 enzyme, produces an oxidative stress which accumulates to toxic level over a time course of several days. The rationale for this hypothesis includes several concepts. The first is that the dose-response range for inhibition of cellular proliferation by androgen is in the high μMolar range, concentration at which enzymes rather than receptors would be expected to function. Also the effect of androgen on cell proliferation was not correlated with the presence or absence of steroid receptors in the various cell lines studied. It is also significant that toxic steroids were androgens, compounds normally synthesized in ovary, while the adrenal steroid cortisol was without effect. There is an extensive literature describing free radical intermediates in the hydoxlylation of compounds by cytochrome P-450 enzymes. The high Km and Vmax of tumor aromatase, which adds three hydoxyls to the steroid during conversion of androgen to estrogen[23], would be consistent with possible release of free radicals at elevated substrate and rapid turnover. The long time required to observe toxic effects of androgen, several days, would also be consistent with accumulation of free radical damage to the cells which ultimately led to their death. Cells, which survived high dose androgen insult, were able to recover and resume division if androgen was removed from culture medium. This would be in agreement with the concept that sublethal doses of free radical damage can be repaired by cellular housekeeping mechanisms.

CONCLUSIONS

In conclusion, we propose that development of ovarian cancer at menopause is influenced by the steroid hormone profile of the patient. We hypothesize that postmenopausal androgen secretion by ovarian stromal cells suppresses ovarian carcinoma. Our data show that suppression of ovarian tumor cell proliferation *in vitro* can be accomplished with micromolar doses of androgen, and this suppression is independent of steroid receptors. We plan to test if the molecular mechanism for this proposed stromalepithelial interaction is defined by the cytochrome P-450 steroidogenic enzymes present in the two cell types, and whether production of free radical damage is involved.

REFERENCES

1. Zaloudek, C. The Ovary. *In*: Gompel, C. and S. G. Silverberg, S. G. (eds.) Pathology In Gynecology And Obstetrics. J. B. Lippincott Company, Philadelphia (1985).

2. Young, J. L., Jr., Percy, C. L. and Asire, A. J. "Surveillance, epidemiology and end results: incidence and mortality data, 1973-1977. National Cancer Institute Monograph 57, DHHS no. (NIH) 81-2330. U. S. Government Printing Office, Washington, DC. pp 50-51 (1981).

3. Day, T. G. Jr. and Smith, J. P. Diagnosis and staging of ovarian cancer. *Semin. Oncol.* 2:217 (1975).

4. Smith, E. M. and Anderson, B. The effects of symptom and delay in seeking diagnosis on stage of disease at diagnosis among women with cancers of the ovary. *Cancer* 56:2727 (1985).

5. Hacker, N. F., Berek, J. S., Laguasse, L. D., Nieberg, R. K. and Elashoff, R. M. Primary cytoreductive surgery for epithelial ovarian cancer. *Obstet. Gynecol.* 61:413 (1983).

6. Adelson, M. D., Baggish, M. S., Seifer, D. B., Cassell, S. L. and Thompson, M. A. Cytoreduction of ovarian cancer with the Cavitron Ultrasonic Surgical Aspirator, *Obstet. Gynecol.* 72:140 (1988).

7. Brenner, D. E. and Greco, F. A. Multiagent chemotherapy in advanced ovarian carcinoma. *In*: Alberts, D. S. and Surwit, E. A. (eds.) Ovarian Cancer. Martinus Nijhoff, Boston, pp 147 (1985).

8. Louie, K., Ozols, R., Myers, C., Ostechega, Y., Jenkins, J. and Howser, D. Long-term results of a cisplatin containing combination chemotherapy regimen for the treatment of advanced ovarian carcinoma. *J. Clin. Oncol.* 4:1579 (1986).

9. Bourhis, J., Goldstein, L. J., Riou, G., Pastan, I., Gottesman, M. M. and Benard, J. Expression of a human multidrug reisistance gene in ovarian carcinomas. *Cancer Res.* 49:5062 (1989).

10. Slotman, B. J. Rationale For The Use Of Endocrine Therapy In Ovarian Cancer. Thesis Publishers, Amsterdam (1990).

11. Kuhnel, R.. de Graaff, J., Rao, B. R. and Stolk, J. G. Androgen receptor predominance in human ovarian carcinoma. *J. Steroid Biochem.* 26:393 (1987).

12. Kuhnel, R., Rao, B. R., Poels, L. G., Delemarre, J. F. M., Kenemans, P. and Stolk, J. G. Multiple parameter analysis of ovarian cancer: Morphology, immunohistochemistry, steroid hormone receptors and aromatase. *Anticancer Res.* 8:281 (1988).

13. Thompson, M. A., Adelson, M. D., Kaufman, L. M., Marshall, L. D. and Coble, D. A. Aromatization of testosterone by epithelial tumor cells cultured from patients with ovarian carcinoma. *Cancer Res.* 48:6491 (1988).

14. Kuhnel, R., Delemarre, J. F. M., Rao, B. R. and Stolk, J. G. Correlation of aromatase activity and steroid receptors in human ovarian carcinoma. *Anticancer Res.* 6:889 (1986).

15. Plotz, E. J., Wiener, M. and Stein, A. A. Steroid synthesis in cystadenocarcinoma of the ovaries. *Am. J. Obstet. Gynecol.* 94:189 (1966).

16. Plotz, E. J., Wiener, M., Stein, A. A. and Hahn, B. D. Enzymatic activities related to steroid synthesis in common ovarian cancer. *Am. J. Obstet. Gynecol.* 97:1050 (1967).

17. Hughesdon, P. E. Thecal and allied reactions in epithelial ovarian tumors. *J. Obstet. Gynecol. Br. Emo.* 63:702 (1958).

18. McNatty, K. P., Smith, D. M., Makris, A., DeGrazia, D. Tulchinsky, C., Osathanondh, R., Schiff, I. and Ryan, K. J. The intraovarian sites of androgen and estrogen formation in women with normal and hyperadrogenic ovaries as judged by *in vitro* experiments. *J. Clin. Endocrinol. Metab.* 50:755 (1980).

19. Longcope, C., Hunter, R. and Franz, C. Steroid secretion by the postmenopausal ovary. *Am. J. Obstet. Gynecol.* 138:564 (1980).

20. Judd, H. Hormonal dynamics associated with the menopause. *Clin. Obstet. Gynecol.* 19:775 (1976).

21. Freedman, R. S., Pihl, E., Kusyk, C., Gallager, H. S. and Rutledge, F. Characterization of an ovarian carcinoma cell line. *Cancer* 42:2352 (1978).

22. Tseng, L., Mazella, J., Mann, W. J. and Chumas, J. Estrogen synthesis in normal and malignant human endometrium. *J. Clin. Endocrinol. Metab.* 55:1029 (1982).

23. Cole, P. A. and Robinson, C. H. A peroxide model reaction for placental aromatase, *J. Am. Chem. Soc.* 110:1284 (1988).

PROSTATIC CANCER: AN AGE-OLD PROBLEM

John T. Isaacs

Johns Hopkins Oncology Center and the Department of
Urology, The Johns Hopkins School of Medicine
Baltimore, Maryland 21231

MAGNITUDE AND AGE RELATED NATURE OF PROSTATIC CANCER

During this year there will be approximately 30 thousand deaths due to prostatic cancer in the United States (1). This mortality rate makes prostatic cancer the second commonest fatal tumor in males of all ages in America (1). Besides a high annual mortality rate, prostatic cancer is now the most commonly diagnosed malignancy in males of all ages in the United States (1). These high annual incidence rates translate into the human reality that one of every 11 American white male will eventually develop clinical prostatic cancer during their lifetime (2). Rates for American black males are even higher such that the lifetime risk for cancer is one out of every 10 (3). In addition, the annual incidence rate of clinical prostatic cancer has increased steadily since 1930's to the present time (4).

Prostatic cancer incidence increases with age more rapidly than any other form of cancer; less than one percent of prostatic cancers are diagnosed in men under 50 years of age (5). This suggests that as the life expectancy of the general male population increases over time, the incidence of clinical prostatic cancer will also increase. This may explain why the annual incidence rate of clinical prostatic cancer has increased steadily since 1930 to the present time (4). Due to its age-related nature, prostatic cancer is often considered a disease of the very elderly. Of the 132,000 newly diagnosed prostatic cancers in the United States in 1992 (1), twenty-six thousand cases will occur in men under the age of 65 (5). These 26,000 cases under 65 years of age represents more than all the renal cancers and leukemias in men of all ages, more than all brain and central nervous system tumors of men and women of all ages, and will almost equal the number of buccal cavity/pharynx and rectal cancers in men of all ages (1).

The Underlying Molecular, Cellular, and Immunological Factors in Cancer and Aging, Edited by S.S. Yang and H.R.Warner, Plenum Press, New York, 1993

Although 106,000 cases occur each year in men over the age of 65, the impact of this disease in these later years is still significant. This is because even though the average life expectancy of U.S. men at birth is approximately 72 years, once a man has reached the ages of peak prostate cancer incidence, 70-74 years old, his life expectancy is another 9-11.5 years if he does not have prostate cancer (6). Horm and Sondik have calculated that the average man who dies of metastatic prostate cancer experiences a 9 year reduction in the length of his life (7).

RELATIONSHIP BETWEEN AGE AND THE MULTIPLE STEP NATURE OF PROSTATIC CANCER

Based on autopsy studies, 10% of men in the age range of 50-60 years and 50% in the 70-80 years range have histological deposits of cancer within their prostates (8,9). There are thus approximately 11 million men older than 45 to 50 years in the United States with histological prostate cancer (8). Despite the remarkable number of these cancers in the United States male population, it is well known that the majority of histological prostate cancers remain clinically silent and relatively few become clinically manifest during the lifetime of the host (8). These histological cancers found at autopsy have been referred to as latent, microscopic, incidental, dormant and so forth, and there are problems with all of these various labels. For example, latent implies that the biological potential of these histologically detectable cancers is known. However, presently it is not possible to predict with accuracy in an individual patient which of these cancers will produce clinical disease. The term microscopic is misleading because the lesions found at autopsy are by no means always microscopic. For example, data from the German Prostate Cancer Registry reveal that a third of these autopsy cancers are greater than 1 cm in diameter (10). In addition, these tumors are not always well differentiated histologically and in one study only 58% of the prostate cancers found at autopsy were well differentiated (11). Therefore, we used the term histological cancer, which implies nothing about the biological potential of the tumor, to describe the prostate cancers that exist in most older men based on autopsy data.

Although the factors involved in prostatic carcinogenesis are not known, it is well recognized based on a large body of experimental and clinical data that the development of a fully malignant cancer cell from a normal cell requires multiple malignant events. A fundamental issue with regard to prostatic carcinogenesis is the question of whether all histological prostate cancers already have completed all the steps necessary to become clinically manifest. In other words, what is the temporal relationship between the appearance of histologically recognizable prostatic cancer and the malignant events needed for such a lesion to produce a clinical disease. One possibility is that by the time prostate cancers are histologically recognizable they already have undergone all of the malignant events necessary to produce an aggressive clinical tumor. Thus, the only additional requirement for histological cancer to produce clinical symptoms would be the time required for the growth of the tumor to a clinically detectable size. Alternatively, it is possible that not all histologically recognizable prostate cancers have undergone all of the essential events necessary to produce a clinically relevant cancer. Thus, not only would further time be necessary for clinical manifestation but the occurrence of additional malignant events also would be necessary for these histological tumor to become clinical prostate cancer.

The resolution of whether histological prostate cancer requires further malignant events to produce a clinical tumor in addition to time, is possible based upon available clinical data. If further time (i.e. tumor growth) is the only requirement for a histologically recognizable prostate cancer to produce clinical disease, then the age specific prevalence of clinically manifest prostate cancers should be similar worldwide if two conditions are met: (1) that the age specific prevalence of histological prostate cancers is similar among male population worldwide, and (2) that the life expectancy of the populations being compared is the same.

Carter *et. al* have demonstrated that the age-specific prevalence of histological prostate cancer and the life expectancy is similar between Japanese and American males while there is a more than 10-fold difference in the age-specific prevalence of clinical prostatic cancer between these two populations (9). It should be noted that the marked difference in the age specific prevalence of clinical prostate cancer between Oriental and United States men is not simply due to better detection of prostate cancer in the United States. Prostate screening studies in Oriental men older than 55 years using transrectal ultrasound suggest that there exist marked differences in prostate cancer prevalence between United States and Oriental men (12, 13). In addition, Oriental pathologist use the same histological criteria to diagnose prostate cancer (14). This data is thus inconsistent with histological prostate cancer having undergone all of the steps necessary in order for it to produce a clinically detectable disease.

Using a mathematical model relating the prevalence of histological and clinical prostatic cancer to host age, Carter *et. al* demonstrated that more than one malignant event is required even for the development of histological prostate cancer, and that the probability of undergoing these multiple transformation events is similar in Japanese and United States men (8). This model also demonstrates that the progression from histological to clinical prostate cancer requires additional steps and that the number of additional malignant steps is similar in Japanese and United States men (9). The difference in the prevalence of clinical prostate cancer between Japanese and American men suggests that the probability of occurrence of the additional events necessary for progression of histological to clinical prostate cancer is lower in Japanese than the United States man. The probability of undergoing these further malignant changes appears to be determined predominately by environmental factors since when Japanese men migrate to California or Hawaii, the age-adjusted incidence for prostatic cancer dramatically increases in the first and second generations, and becomes more similar to the high rates of United States men than to the low rates of native Japanese (15, 16). This increase in the incidence of clinical prostate cancer among Japanese men migrating to a high prevalence area for prostate cancer does not support an inherent resistance to the development of clinical prostate cancer in the Japanese man. In contrast to the increase in clinical prostate cancer cases, the prevalence of histological lesions remains unchanged when Japanese men migrate to the United States (i.e. Japanese men in Japan or the United States, or American men in the United States all have a similarly high age specific prevalence of histological prostate cancer) (17).

IMPORTANCE OF DISTINGUISHING BETWEEN HISTOLOGICAL AND CLINICALLY MANIFEST PROSTATIC CANCER

Distinguishing the relationship between histological and clinical prostatic cancer has clinical importance with respect to diagnosis and therapy. If all histologically recognizable prostate cancers have undergone the malignant events necessary to produce a clinically aggressive cancer, it would seem prudent to detect and treat all of these histological prostate cancers, since the malignant potential of these tumors is similar and dependent only upon time (i.e. the natural history is predictable). In contrast, as described above, histological prostate cancers are heterogeneous with only a small subset having undergone all the required malignant changes while the vast majority of such lesion have not completed the process required to produce a clinically aggressive tumor. In addition, the majority of these histological prostate tumors, never undergo the further events required despite host longevity and ample time for tumor growth. Thus, the majority of the histological prostate disease will remain clinically silent and will not ever require treatment (8). Presently it is not possible to predict which histological cancers have undergone all of the steps needed for progression to clinical cancer and which have not (i.e. the nature history is unpredictable). Thus, the ability to predict which tumors have the capacity to manifest aggressive behavior requiring therapy becomes a critical issue as greater emphasis is placed upon screening for earlier detection of prostatic cancer.

This issue is critical since if such a patient with histologically detectable prostatic cancer is left untreated until definitive clinical evidence of metastatic disease outside of the prostate become apparent, then the ability to cure such a metastatic patient with presently available therapy is lost (18). However, it is impractical, unwarranted and unnecessary to definitively treat (e.g. surgical resection) all men with histological prostatic cancer since the majority of these men will never progress to a clinical disease during their lifetime. What is urgently needed is some type of diagnostic method to identify which histological prostate cancers have, and which have not, completed the progression to a stage which will produce a clinical disease and thus require therapeutic intervention.

THERAPY FOR METASTATIC PROSTATIC CANCER

Besides advances in the ability to correctly diagnose which histological prostatic cancer require therapy, the development of more effective therapy for metastatic prostate cancer also is urgently required. Since the pioneering work of Charles Huggins in the 1940's it has been known that like the normal prostate which requires a continuous supply of androgen to maintain its normal cell number and secretory activity, most metastatic prostate cancers retain an androgen responsiveness for stimulation of their growth. Metastatic prostatic cancer is thus often highly responsive to androgen ablation therapy. Nearly all men with metastatic prostatic cancer treated with androgen ablation therapy have an initial, often dramatic, beneficial response to such androgen withdrawal therapy (19). While this initial response is of substantial palliative value, essentially all treated patients eventually relapse to an androgen-insensitive state in which additional forms of antiandrogen therapy are ineffective no matter how aggressively given (20-22). Because of this nearly universal relapse phenomenon, the annual death rate from prostatic cancer has not decreased at all over the subsequent 50 years since androgen withdrawal has become standard therapy (1). Over the last 50 years, the superficially benign nature of androgen withdrawal therapy has tended to disguise the fact that metastatic prostatic cancer is still a fatal disease for which no therapy is available which effectively increases survival (23).

THERAPEUTIC IMPORTANCE OF ANDROGEN-INDEPENDENT PROSTATIC CANCER CELLS

Studies by a series of laboratories have demonstrated that a major reason for this universal relapse of metastatic prostatic cancer to androgen ablation is that prostatic cancer within an individual patient is heterogeneously composed of clones of both androgen-dependent and -independent cancer cells even before hormone therapy is begun (24-26). Development of such tumor cell heterogeneity can occur by a variety of mechanisms [e.g. multifocal origin of the tumor, adaptation, or genetic instability (27)]. Regardless of the mechanism of development of such cellular heterogeneity, once androgen-independent cancer cells are present with individual prostatic cancer patients, the patient is no longer curable by androgen withdrawal therapy alone, no matter how complete, since this therapy kills only the androgen-dependent cells without eliminating pre-existing androgen-independent prostatic cancer cells. To effect all the heterogenous prostatic cancer cell populations within an individual cancer, effective chemotherapy, specifically targeting against the pre-existing androgen-independent cancer cell must be simultaneously combined with androgen ablation to effect the androgen-dependent cells. The validity of each of these points has been demonstrated by a series of animal (28-32) and human studies (33). The animal studies demonstrated that only by giving such a combined chemo-hormonal treatment, that it is possible to produce any reproducible level of cures in animals bearing prostatic cancers (32). In order to produce cures however, treatment must be started early in the course of the disease, the chemotherapy must have definitive efficiency against androgen-independent cells, it must be given for a critical period, and it must be begun simultaneously with, and not sequential to androgen ablation. The cure rate however, even under these ideal conditions in animals, is not high, i.e. 25% (32). While the concept of early combinational chemohormonal therapy for prostatic cancer is valid, for such an approach to be therapeutically effective in humans, a chemotherapeutic agent which can effectively control the growth of the preexisting androgen-independent prostatic caner cells must also be available. There are presently no highly effective chemotherapeutic agents which can control the growth of androgen-independent prostatic cancer cells (18).

NEW APPROACHES TO CONTROL THE GROWTH OF ANDROGEN-INDEPENDENT PROSTATIC CANCER CELLS

The inability to control androgen-independent prostate cancer cells in human and rodent tumors by standard chemotherapeutic methods, has led to a search for new approaches. Growth of a cancer is determined by the relationship between the rate of cell proliferation and the rate of cell death. Only when the rate of cell proliferation is greater than cell death does tumor growth continue. If the rate of cell proliferation is lower than the rate of cell death, then involution of the cancer occurs. Therefore a successful treatment of a cancer can be obtained by either lowering the rate of proliferation and/or by raising the rate of cell death so that the rate of cell proliferation is lower than the rate of cell death.

While the exact magnitude of either the cell proliferation rate or cell death rate has not been precisely determined for many human prostatic cancers, available data on the thymidine labelling index, suggest that it has both a low cell proliferation rate and a low cell death rate (34, 35). Successful treatment of slow growing prostatic cancers will probably require simultaneous anti-proliferative chemotherapy targeted at the small number of dividing cancer cells and some type of additional therapy targeted at increasing the low cell death rate of the majority of androgen-dependent cancer cells not proliferating within the prostatic cancer.

There are a large variety of effective anti-proliferative chemotherapy presently available which can lower the rate of cell proliferation without increasing the rate of cell death (i.e. cytostatic agents) or agents which lower the rate of cell proliferation and also increase the rate of cell death (i.e. cytotoxic agents). Unfortunately, the cytotoxic agent presently available only lead to death of cancer cells if they subsequently undergoes cell proliferation. Therefore cancer cells not in cycle (i.e. cell in the G_0 phase of the cell cycle) at the time of exposure or not undergoing cell division soon enough after exposure to the cytotoxic chemotherapeutic agent can repair the damage induced by cytotoxic agent and are thus not killed by the therapy. Therefore what is needed is some type of cytotoxic therapy which lead to the death of cancer cells not requiring the cell to undergo proliferation in order to be killed.

It is possible to induce the death of cells without requiring them to attempt to divide? The answer to this question is yes, as demonstrated by the rapid involution of the normal prostate following androgen ablation. Only 2% of the cells in the normal adult prostate of intact male rats are undergoing cell proliferation on any day (36). Androgen ablation (i.e. castration) of the male rat leads to a decrease in cell proliferation and to an increase in the rate of cell death such that 20% of the cells present per day die within the prostate between 2-7 days following castration (36). By 7 days following castration >70% of the total number of cells in the rat prostate have died (36, 37). Thus the vast majority of prostatic cells which die following castration did not undergo cell proliferation (i.e. the cells are in the G_0 phase when they die).

PROGRAMMED CELL DEATH IN PROSTATE FOLLOWING ANDROGEN ABLATION

Studies from a variety of investigators have demonstrated that the death of a cell occur via one of two major pathways (38). The first type of cell death is termed necrotic cell death. Necrotic death is a response to pathological changes initiated outside of the cell and can be elicited by any of a large series of rather non specific factors which produce a hostile microenvironment for the cells (i.e. freezing and thawing, osmotic stock, ischemia, solubilizing agents, membranes ATPase inhibition, etc). In necrotic cell death, the cell has a passive role in initiating the process of cell death (i.e. the cell is "murdered" by its hostile microenvironment). In addition to this necrotic type of cell death, there is a second type of cell death termed programmed cell death. In contrast to necrotic cell death which is a pathological process, programmed cell death is a physiological process whereby a cell is activated by specific signals to undergo an energy-dependent process of cell death (i.e. the cell is induced to commit "suicide" by specific signals in an otherwise normal microenvironment) (38, 39). Programmed cell death is a widespread phenomenon occurring normally at different stages of morphogenesis, growth and development of metazoans (40). It also occurs in adult tissues (40). Programmed cell death is initiated in specific cell types by tissue specific extra cellular agents generally hormones or locally diffusing chemicals. The activation of this programmed cell death can occur either due to the positive presence of a tissue specific inducer [e.g. glucocorticoid induce death of small thymocytes (41, 42)] or due to the negative lack of a tissue specific repressor [e.g. decrease in serum ACTH results in cell death in the zona reticularis of the adrenal (43)]. Once initiated, either by the positive presence of inducer or the negative lack of a repressor, programmed cell death leads to a cascade of biochemical and morphological events which result in the irreversible degradation of the genomic DNA and fragmentation of the cell (41, 42, 44-46). The morphological pathway for programmed cell death is rather stereotypic and has been given the name apoptosis to distinguish this process from necrotic cell death.

Apoptosis was originally defined by Kerr *et. al* (39) as the orderly and characteristic sequence of structured changes resulting in the programmed death of the cell. The temporal sequences of events of apoptosis comprise chromatin aggregation, the nuclear and cytoplasmic condensation, and the eventual fragmentation of the dying cell into a cluster of membrane-bound segment (apoptotic bodies), which often contain morphological intact organelles. For example, in apoptosis (as opposed to necrotic death), mitochondria do not swell and lose their function as an early event in the process. Instead, functionally active mitochondria are often contained in apoptotic bodies. These apoptotic bodies are rapidly recognized, phagocytosed and digested by either macrophages or adjacent epithelial cells.

In an intact adult male, the supply of androgen is normally sufficient to maintain a balance between prostatic cell death and proliferation such that neither involution nor overgrowth of the gland occurs (36). Biochemical and morphological studies have demonstrated that the involution of the normal prostate following castration is not due to necrotic cell death but is an active process brought about by the initiation of a series of specific biochemical steps which led to the program death (apoptosis) of the androgen-dependent glandular epithelial cells within the prostate (36, 37, 47-53). In the androgen maintained ventral prostate of an intact adult male rat, the rate of cell death is very low, approximately 2% per day and this low rate is balanced by an equally low rate of cell proliferation, also 2% per day (36). If animals are castrated, the serum testosterone levels drop to less than 10% of the intact control value within two hours (37). By 6 hour post-castration the serum testosterone level is only 1.2% of intact control (37). By 12-24 hour following castration the prostatic dihydrotestosterone (DHT) levels (i.e. the active intracellular androgen in prostatic cells) are only 5% of intact control values) (37). This lowering of prostatic DHT leads to changes in nuclear androgen receptor function (i.e. by 12 hour after castration, and androgen receptors are no longer retained by biochemically isolated ventral prostatic nuclei) (37). These nuclear receptor changes results in the synthesis of a series of proteins normally not present in the intact prostate (54, 55), due to the novel expression of genes normally repressed in the intact prostate. The most notable of these are the TRPM-2 gene [i.e. testosterone repressed prostate message-2] (56), the Ca^{+2} responsive *c-fos* gene (57), the heat shock (70 kilodalton protein) gene (57) and the TGF_{B_1} gene (58).

Based upon *in vivo* data using calcium channel blockers (47, 59), these changes and/or others in gene expression probably result in an increase in the intracellular free Ca^{+2} levels. This increase in intracellular free Ca^{+2} would explain what activates the Ca^{+2} Mg^{+2} dependent endonuclease activity within the nucleus to begin to fragment the genomic DNA into low molecular weight [<1000 base pairs (bp)] nucleosomal oligomers which lack intranucleosomal break points and which contain non-degraded histones (37). This genomic DNA fragmentation process begins in some cells within the first day post-castration. Once the genomic DNA fragmentation process is initiated within an individual androgen-dependent prostatic cell, the cell fragments all of its genome into low molecular weight (i.e. <1000 BP) pieces (37).

While the process of DNA fragmentation is completed in a portion of the androgen-dependent glandular epithelial cells in the prostate as early as one day following castration, the first morphological signs of apototic bodies formation occurs during the second day following castration (48, 49, 52). This demonstrates that the fragmentation of the genomic DNA does not occur after the cells are dead but instead occurs as an irreversible commitment step for viable cells to die. During the next several days (i.e. day 2-7 following castration), the level of the $Ca^{+2}Mg^{+2}$ dependent endonuclease (37, 47, 48), TRPM-2 gene expression (56), TGF_B (58), and a series of other proteins (54) continues to increase with the maximal levels[1] obtained on day 4 post castration. The fragmentation of the genomic DNA of the androgen-dependent glandular epithelial cells likewise continues, as does the production of apoptotic bodies (37, 47, 48) and the decrease in mRNA for the secretory proteins (60). By day 10 following castration, the androgen-dependent glandular epithelial cells have all died and there is no longer any indication of either DNA fragmentation, TRPM-2 expression, or apoptotic bodies. These temporal studies demonstrate that DNA fragmentation is an important irreversible commitment step in the process of the programmed cell death of the androgen-dependent glandular epithelial cells in the prostate following castration.

Additional studies have demonstrated that it is possible to use prostatic organ culture to study the effects of increased Ca^{+2} levels on prostatic cell death *in vitro* under conditions in which neither drug toxicity to the host nor lymphocytic infiltration into the gland is a problem (61). Using this organ culture system, it has been demonstrated that rate of programmed death of the glandular epithelial cells can be shifted from 5% to ~12% of the cells dying per day when testosterone plus 10 μM of the Ca^{+2} ionophore, A23187 are both in the media (62). Thus, in the presence of the ionophore, the rate of cell death in the presence of testosterone is identical to that induced when testosterone is not present. Additional studies have demonstrated that if the organ cultures are maintained in media lacking testosterone, but containing 10 μM of the Ca^{+2} channel blocks, nifedipine, the rise in the rate of cell death from 5% to 12% of the cells dying per day usually induced can be totally prevented (i.e. in the presence of nifedipine the rate is also 5%) (62). These results suggest that increases in intracellular free Ca^{+2} probably derived from extracellular Ca^{+2} pools, are a critical early event involved in triggering the subsequent process of programmed cell death (i.e., specifically DNA fragmentation) in the rat ventral prostate following androgen ablation. Regardless of the specific mechanism, once a prostate cell fragments its genomic DNA into such small pieces, the DNA is no longer functional for cell replication or gene expression, as evidenced by the fact that the mRNA levels for the major secretory proteins decrease abruptly (60) and thus the cell is terminally committed to death.

PROGRAMMED CELL DEATH OF HUMAN PROSTATIC CANCER CELL FOLLOWING ANDROGEN ABLATION

Recent completed studies have demonstrated that not only normal rat prostatic cells but also human androgen-responsive prostatic cancer cells activate the pathway of programmed cell death following androgen ablation (63). The PC-82 human prostatic cancer is highly androgen-responsive when grown as a xenograft in nude mice (64). If intact male nude mice are inoculated with human PC-82 prostatic cancer, continuously growing tumors are produced. If the host mice is castrated when the PC-82 tumor is ~0.5 cc in size, the rate of cell proliferation decreases ~7-fold from 3.5% of the cells proliferating per day to 0.5% of the cells proliferating per day and the rate of cell death increases ~11-fold from 0.5% of the cells dying per day to 4.7% of the cells dying per day. Due to these changes the tumor involutes rapidly following castration reaching ~1/2 of its starting size within three weeks of castration. Biochemical analysis during this involution period has demonstrated that TRPM-2 mRNA levels and DNA fragmentation into nucleosomal size pieces are detectably increased within the first day following castration. The levels of both of these parameter increase to a maximum on day three following castration. In addition, if exogenous androgen is given back to the castrated host, DNA fragmentation ceases, TRPM-2 levels drop, involution stops and growth of the tumor resumes.

PROGRAMMED CELL DEATH IN ANDROGEN-INDEPENDENT PROSTATIC CANCER CELLS

While androgen-independent prostatic cancer cells do not activate the program of cell death following androgen ablation, these cells still retain the major portion of the program cell death pathway. This has been demonstrated using a series of Dunning R-3327 androgen-independent prostatic cancers established as continuously growing *in vitro* cell lines. For example, the Dunning AT-3 androgen-independent, highly metastatic, anaplastic prostatic cancer cells have been treated *in vitro* with a variety of non-androgen ablative agents which induce "thymine-less death" of the cells [e.g. cells treated with 5-fluoro-deoxyuridine (5-FdUR) or trifluorothymidine (TFT)]. Analysis has revealed that "thymine-less death" results in an increase in the expression of the TRPM-2 gene and an increase in the nuclear Ca^{+2} Mg^{+2} dependent endonuclease with the resultant fragmentation of the genomic DNA of the AT-3 cells into a similar nucleosomal ladder, as seen in the death of androgen-dependent prostate cells following castration (65). This cascade of events requires 6-12 hrs before fragmentation of the DNA is complete. The AT-3 cells are not "dead," as defined by their ability to metabolize a mitochondrial vital dye, however until 24 hrs of treatment. This demonstrates that the fragmentation of the genomic DNA is an early, irreversible, commitment step in that of programmed cell death of even androgen-independent prostatic cancer cells (65). If the AT-3 cells are treated with osmotic shock induced by exposure to distilled water or agents which inhibit the plasma membrane ATPase Activity (i.e. ouabain or iodoacetate), the cells rapidly lyse in less than 3 hours after treatment and do not metabolize the vital dyes (i.e. they are dead) even though they do not fragment their DNA into nucleosomal size pieces nor do they elevate TRPM-2 mRNA levels (65). This data demonstrates that agents which induce necrotic death of the AT-3 cells (i.e. osmotic effects) do not lead to the activation o f the programmed cell death of these cells. Programmed cell death can be activated, however, even in androgen-independent prostatic cancer by specific agents (e.g. those able to induce a "thymine-less" state).

The problem with agents of this latter type, however, is that cell proliferation is required for the "thymine-less" state to activate the program of cell death in these AT-3 cells. Therefore some type of agent which can likewise activate this death program in androgen-independent prostatic cancer cells not in the cell cycle and not requiring the cell to attempt to proliferate, still must be identified.

If AT-3 cells are treated *in vitro* with 10μM of either the calcium ionophores, A23187 or ionomycin, cell death can be induced. Using microfluorescence image analysis (66) on AT-3 cells loaded with the fluorescent dye "fura-2" to measure intracellular free Ca^{+2} level such ionomycin treatment has been demonstrated to elevate the intracellular free Ca^{+2} levels from < 80 nM to > 200 nM within the first minute of treatment. After the first few minutes, the intracellular free Ca^{+2} returned to ~100-150 nM. Such sustained elevations in intracellular free Ca^{+2} results in cell proliferation stopped within hours of treatment (i.e., cells go into G_0) and then the cells begin to die after ~24-36 hours (67). Biochemical analysis during this time course demonstrated that DNA fragmentation into nucleosomal oligomers begins as early as 6 hours after Ca^{+2} ionophores treatment. Interesting, there is no elevation of the TRPM-2 mRNA levels during the chronic elevation of intracellular free Ca^{+2} induced by ionophore (67). This may be significant since such chronic elevation in free Ca^{+2} levels does activate the DNA fragmentation suggesting that TRPM-2 elevation is not required for this step in the process of cell death. These results suggest that TRPM-2's site of action in the cell death may be involved in inducing an increase in intracellular free Ca^{+2} , which the ionophores are fully capable to doing without any TRPM-2 involvement. This possibility is further strengthened by the recent clarification that TRPM-2 is highly related if not identical to the previously identified sulfated glycoprotein 2 (SGP-2) normally secreted by rat sertoli cells (68). This SGP2 protein has been demonstrated to be secreted by sertoli cells and to bind to the acrosomal membrane of sperm (69). This may be significant since sperm in order to under the capitation reaction must proceed through an acrosomal reaction step which involves the breakdown of the acrosomal membrane, a process which is known to involve Ca^{+2}.

CONCLUSIONS - FUTURE NEEDS

Prostatic cancer is a major disease whose incidence is unfortunately rising.

Coupling this fact with the realization that presently it is impossible to cure the disease when it reaches the metastatic stage, has led to increasing attempts to diagnose the disease when in a localized form. Due to its age-related multi-step nature, such attempts at early detection will uncover large numbers of histological prostatic cancers which do not require therapy. What is urgently needed is some type of diagnostic method to identify which histological prostatic cancer have and which have not completed the progression to a stage which will produce a clinical disease requiring therapeutic intervention.

Besides advances in correctly diagnosing which histological prostatic cancer require therapy, the development of more effective therapy for metastatic prostatic cancer is also urgently need. This is because even with more aggressive screening procedures, a substantial number of men will already be metastatic at the time of initial diagnoses of the disease. To increase survival for men with metastatic prostatic cancer what is desperately needed is a modality which can effectively eliminate the clones of androgen-independent cancer cells already present even before therapy is begun within individual heterogeneous prostate cancers. By combining such an effective modality with any of the various types of androgen ablation presently available, all of the populations of tumor cells within individual heterogeneous prostatic cancer can be affected thus optimize the possibility for cure. Unfortunately, such an effective form of therapy for the androgen-independent prostatic cancer cell is not presently available. Effective chemotherapy for the androgen-independent prostatic cancer cell will probably require two types of agent; one having anti-proliferative activity affecting the small number of dividing androgen-independent cells, and the other able to increase the low rate of cell death among the majority of non-proliferating androgen-independent prostatic cancer cells present. Androgen-dependent prostatic epithelial cells can be made to undergo programmed death, even if the cells are not in the cell cycle (i.e. G_0 cells), simply by means of androgen ablation. Androgen-independent prostatic cancer cells retain the major portion of this programmed cell death pathway, only there is a defect in the pathway such that it is no longer activated by androgen ablation. The long term goal, therefore, is to develop some type of non-androgen ablative methods to activate this programmed cell death cascade in androgen-independent prostatic cancer cells distal to the point of the defect.

REFERENCES

1. Boring, C., Squires, T. and Tong, T. *Cancer Statistics - Cancer Journal for Clinicians* 42:19-38, 1992.

2. Seidman, H., Mushinski, M. H., Gelb, S. K. and Silverberg, E. Probabilities of eventually developing or dying of cancer: United States. *Cancer Journal for Clinicians* 35:36-56, 1985.

3. Mettlin, G. Epidemiology of prostate cancer in different population groups. *Clinics in Oncology* 2:287-300, 1983.

4. Devesa, S. S. and Silverman, D. T. Cancer incidence and morbidity trends in the United States: 1935-1947. *J. Natl. Cancer Inst.* 60:545-571, 1978.

5. Carter, H. B. and Isaacs, J. T. Experimental and theoretical basic for hormonal treatment of prostatic cancer. *Seminars in Urology* 4:262-268, 1988.

6. U.S. Bureau of the Census, Statistical Abstract of the United States 1989 (109th edition) Washington, DC, 1989.

7. Horm, J. and Sondik, E. Person-Years of life lost due to cancer in the United States 1970 and 1984. *Am. J. Public Health* 79:1490-1493, 1989.

8. Carter, H. and Coffey, D. Prostate cancer: The magnitude of the problem in the United States. In Coffey, D., Resnick, M., Dorr, F. *et. al* (eds): A Multidisciplinary Analysis of Controversies in the Management of Prostate Cancer. Plenum Press, New York, Pp. 1-9, 1988.

9. Carter, H. B., Piantadosi, S. and Isaacs, J. T. Clinical evidence for and implications of the multistep development of prostate cancer. *J. Urol.* 143:742-746, 1990.

10. Dhom, G. Classification and grading of prostatic carcinoma. *Recent Results Cancer Res* 60:14-26, 1977.

11. Hohbach, C. and Dhom, G. Pathology of prostatic cancer. *Scand. J. Urol. Nephrol.* 55:37, 1980.

12. Watanabe, H., Ohe, H., Inaba, T., Itakura, Y., Saitoh, M. and Nakao, M. A mobile mass screening unit for prostatic disease. *Prostate* 5:559, 1984.

13. Zhang, P., Cheng, S., Zhou, Y., He, A., Hu, J., Huang, S. General survey to detect prostatic disease in 1,165 aged males over 60. *Chinese J. Geriat.* 3:99, 1984.

14. Miller, G. J. Diagnosis of stage A prostate cancer in the People's Republic of China. In: A Multidisciplinary Analysis of Controversies in the Management of Prostate Cancer. Edited by D. S. Coffey, M. I. Resnick, F. A. Door, and J. P. Karr. Plenum Press, New York. Pp. 17-24, 1988.

15. Dunn, J. E. Cancer epidemiology in populations of the United States - with emphasis on Hawaii and California - and Japan. *Cancer Res* 35:3240, 1975.

16. Haenszel, W. and Kurihara, M. Studies on Japanese migrants. I. Mortality for cancer and other diseases among Japanese in the United States. *J. Natl Cancer Inst*. 40;43, 1968.

17. Akazaki, K. and Stemmerman, G. N. Comparative study of latent carcinoma of the prostate among Japanese in Japan and Hawaii. *J. Natl Cancer Inst.* 50:1137, 1973.

18. Raghavan, D. Non-hormone chemotherapy for prostate cancer: principles of treatment and application to the testing of new drugs. *Seminars in Oncology* 15:371-389, 1988.

19. Scott, W.W., Menon, M. and Walsh, P.C. Hormonal therapy of prostatic cancer. *Cancer* 45:1929-1936, 1980.

20. Schulze, H., Isaacs J.T. and Coffey, D. S. A critical review of the concept of total androgen ablation in the treatment of prostatic cancer. IN Murphy GP, Khoury S, Kuss R, Chatelain C, Denis L (eds). Prostate Cancer Part A: Research Endocrine Treatment, and Histopathology. *Progress in Clinical and Biological Research* Vol. 243A: pp. 1-19. Alan R. Liss, Inc., New York, 1987.

21. Smith, J. A., Eyse, H.J., Roberts, T. S. and Middleton, R. G. Transphenoidal hypophysectomy in the management of carcinoma of the prostate. *Cancer* 53:2385-2387, 1984.

22. Menon, M. and Walsh, P. C. Hormonal therapy for prostatic cancer. In Murphy GP (ed). Prostatic Cancer. Littleton, Mass, PSG Publ. Co., pp 175-200, 1979.

23. Lepor, H., Ross, A. and Walsh, P. C. The influence of hormonal therapy on survival of men with advanced prostatic cancer. *J. Urol.* 128:335-340, 1982.

24. Prout, G. R., Leiman, B., Daly, J.J., Macloughlin, R. A., Griffin, P. P., Young, H. H. Endocrine changes after diethylstilbestrol therapy. *Urology* 7:148-155, 1976.

25. Sinha, A. A., Blackhard, C. E., Seal, U. S. A critical analysis of tumor morphology and hormone treatment in the untreated and estrogen treated responsive and refractory human prostatic carcinoma. *Cancer* 40:2836-2850, 1977.

26. Isaacs, J. T. and Coffey, D. S. Adaptation vs selection as the mechanism responsible for the relapse of prostatic cancer to androgen ablation as studied in the Dunning R-3327 H adenocarcinoma. *Cancer Res* 41:5070-5075, 1981.

27. Isaacs, J. T. Cellular factors in the development of resistance to hormonal therapy. In Bruchovsky, N. and Goldie, J. (eds). Drug and Hormone Resistance in Neoplasia. Vol. 1. CRC Press, Boca Raton, Inc. Pp 139-156, 1982.

28. Ellis, W. J. and Isaacs, J. T. Effectiveness of complete vs partial androgen withdrawal therapy for the treatment of prostatic cancer as studied in the Dunning R-3327 system of rat prostatic carcinoma. *Cancer Res* 45:6041-6050, 1985.

29. Redding, T. W. and Schally, A. V. Investigation of the combination of the agonist D-Trp-6-LHRH and the antiandrogen flutamide on the treatment of Dunning R-3327 H prostatic cancer model. *The Prostate* 6:219-232, 1985.

30. Kung, T.T., Mingo, G. G., Siegel, M. I., Watnick, A. S. Effect of adrenalectomy, flutamide and leuprolide on the growth of the Dunning R-3327 prostatic carcinomas. *The Prostate* 12:357-364, 1988.

31. Isaacs, J. T. The timing of androgen ablation therapy and/or chemotherapy in the treatment of prostatic cancer. *The Prostate* 5:1-18, 1984.

32. Isaacs, J. T. Relationship between tumor size and curability of prostate cancer by combined chemohormonal therapy. *Cancer Res* 49:6290-6294, 1989.

33. Schulze, H., Isaacs, J. and Senge, T. Inability of complete androgen blockage to increase survival of patients with advanced prostatic cancer as compared to standard hormone therapy. *J. Urol.* 137:909-914, 1987.

34. Helpap, B., Steins, R. and Bruhl, P. Autoradiographic in vitro investigations of prostatic tissue with C-14 and H-3 thymidine double labelling method. Beitr *Pathol. Anat. Allgem. Path.* 151:65-72, 1974.

35. Meyer, J. S., Sufrin, G. and Martin, S. A. S. Proliferative activity of benign human prostate, prostatic adenocarcinoma and seminal vesicle evaluated by thymidine labeling. *J. Urol.* 128:1353-1356, 1982.

36. Isaacs, J. T. Antagonistic effect of androgen on prostatic cell death. *Prostate* 5:545-558, 1984.

37. Kyprianou, N. and Isaacs, J. T. Activation of programmed cell death in the rat ventral prostate after castration. *Endocrinology* 122:552-562, 1988.

38. Wyllie, A. H., Kerr, J. F.R. and Currie. A. R. Cell death: the significance of apoptosis. *Int. Rev. Cytol.* 68:251-306, 1986.

39. Kerr, J. F. R., Wyllie, A. H. and Currie, A. R. Apoptosis: a basic biological phenomenon with wide ranging implications in tissue kinetics. *Brit. J. Cancer* 26:239-257, 1972.

40. Bowen, I. D. and Lockshin, R. A. Cell Death in Biology and Pathology. London: Chapman and Hill, 1981.

41. Wyllie, A. H. Glucocorticoid induces in thymocytes a nuclease-like activity associated with the chromatin condensation of apoptosis. *Nature* 284:555-556, 1980.

42. Umansky, S. R., Korol, B. A. and Nelipovich, P. A. *In vivo* DNA degradation in thymocytes of -irradiated or hydrocortisone-treated rats. *Biochim. Biophys. Acta* 655:9-17, 1981.

43. Wyllie, A. H., Kerr, J. F. R, Macaskill, I. A. M. and Currie, A. R. Adrenocortical cell deletion: the role of ACTH. *J. Pathol.* 111:85-94, 1973.

44. Cohen, J. J. and Duke, R. C. Glucocorticoid activation of a calcium-dependent endonuclease in thymocyte nuclei leads to cell death. *J. Immunol.* 132:38-42, 1984.

45. Wyllie, A. H., Morris, R. G., Smith, A. L., Dunlop, D. Chromatin cleavage in apoptosis: association with condensed chromatin morphology and dependence on macromolecular synthesis. *J. Pathol.* 142:67-77, 1984.

46. Compton, M. M. and Cidlowski, J. A. Rapid *in vivo* effects of glucocorticoids on the integrity of rat lymphocyte genomic deoxyribonucleic acid. *Endocrinology* 118:38-45, 1986.

47. Kyprianou, N., English, H. F. and Isaacs, J. T. Activation of a Ca^{+2}-Mg^{+2}-dependent endonuclease as an early event in castration-induced prostatic cell death. *The Prostate* 13:103-118, 1988.

48. English, H. F., Kyprianou, N. and Isaacs, J. T. Relationship between DNA fragmentation and apoptosis in the programmed cell death in the rat prostate following castration. *The Prostate* 15:233-250, 1989.

49. Kerr, J. F.R. and Searle, J. Deletion of cells by apoptosis during castration-induced involution of the rat prostate. *Virchow Archiv B* 13:87-102, 1973.

50. Lesser, B. and Bruchovsky, N. The effects of testosterone, 5 -dihydrotestosterone and adenosine 3',5'-monophosphate on cell proliferation and differentiation in rat prostate. *Biochim. Biophys. Acta* 308:426-437, 1973.

51. Lee, C. Physiology of castration-induced regression of the rat prostate. *Prog. Clin. Biol. Res.* 75A:145-159, 1982.

52. Sanford, M. L., Searle, J. W. and Kerr, J. F. R. Successive waves of apoptosis in the rat prostate after repeated withdrawal of testosterone stimulation. *Pathology* 16:406-410, 1984.

53. Stanisic, T., Sadlowski, R., Lee, C., Grayhack, J. T. Partial inhibition of castration-induced ventral prostate regression with actinomycin D and cycloheximide. *Invest. Urol.* 16:19-22, 1978.

54. Lee, C. and Sensibar, J. A. Protein of the rat prostate: synthesis of new proteins in the ventral lobe during castration-induced regression. *J. Urol.* 138:903-908, 1985.

55. Salzman, A. G., Hiipakka, R. A., Chang, C., Liao, S. Androgen repression of the production of a 29 kilodalton protein and its mRNA in the rat ventral prostate. *J. Biol. Chem.* 262:432-437, 1987.

56. Montpetit, M. L., Lawless, K. R. and Tenniswood, M. Androgen repressed messages in the rat ventral prostate. *The Prostate* 8:25-36, 1986.

57. Buttyan, R., Zaker, Z., Lockshin, R. and Wolgemuth, D. Cascade induction of *c-fos*, *c-myc* and heat shock 70K transcripts during regression of the rat ventral prostate gland. *Mol. Endocrinol.* 2:650-657, 1988.

58. Kyprianou, N. and Isaacs, J. T. Expression of transforming growth factor-*B* in the rat ventral prostate during castration-induced programmed cell death. *Mol. Endocrinol.* 3:1515-1522, 1989.

59. Connor, J., Sawdzuk, I. S., Benson, M. C., Tomashersky, P., O'Tool, K. M., Olsson, C. A. and Buttyan, R. Calcium channel antagonists delay regression of androgen-dependent tissues and suppress gene activity associated with cell death. *The Prostate* 13:119-130, 1988.

60. Viskochil, D. H., Perry, S. T., Lea, D. A., Stafford, D. W., Wilson, E. M., French, F. S. Isolation of two genomic sequences encoding the mr ~ 1400 subunit of rat prostatein. *J. Biol. Chem.* 258:8861-8866, 1983.

61. Martikainen, P. and Isaacs, J. T. An organ culture system for the study of programed cell death in the rat ventral prostate. *Endocrinology* 127:1258-1267, 1990.

62. Martikainen, P. and Isaacs, J. T. Role of calcium in the programmed death of rat prostatic glandular cells. *The Prostate* 17:175-187, 1991.

63. Kyprianou, N., English, H., and Isaacs., J. T. Programmed cell death during regression of PC-82 human prostatic cancer. *Cancer Res.* 50:3748-3753, 1990.

64. van Steenbrugge, G. J., Groen, M., Romijn, J. C. and Schroder. F. Biological effects of hormonal treatment regimens on the transplantable human prostate tumor line (PC-82). *J. Urol.* 131:812-817, 1984.

65. Kyprianou, N. and Isaacs, J. T. Thymine-less death in androgen-independent prostatic cancer cells. *Biochem. Biophys. Res. Comm.* 165:73-81, 1989.

66. Tucker, R. W., Meade-Cobun, K., Loats, H. Measurement of free intracellular calcium (Ca) in fibroblasts. Digital image analysis of Fura 2 fluorescence. In Fiskum, G. (ed), Plenum Publ. Corp. Pp 239-248, 1989.

67. Martikainen, P., Kyprianou, N., Tucker, R. W. and Isaacs, J. R. Programmed death of nonproliferating androgen-independent prostatic cancer cells. *Cancer Research* 51:4693-4700, 1991.

68. Bettuzzi, S., HYiipakka, R. A., Gilna, P., Liao, S. Identification of an androgen-repressed mRNA in rat ventral prostate as coding for sulphated glycoprotein 2 by cDNA cloning and sequence analysis. *Biochem. J.* 257:293-296, 1989.

69. Sylvester, S. R., Skinner, M. K. and Griswold, M. D. A sulfated glycoprotein synthesized by Sertoli cell and by epididymal cells is a component of the sperm membrane. *Biol. Reproduc.* 31:1087-1101, 1984.

STROMAL - EPITHELIAL PARACRINE INTERACTIONS IN THE NEOPLASTIC RAT AND HUMAN PROSTATE

Daniel Djakiew[1], Beth Pflug and Makoto Onoda

Department of Anatomy and Cell Biology
Georgetown University Medical School
3900 Reservoir Road N.W., Washington D.C. 20007

ABSTRACT

Homotypic paracrine interactions in the rat and human prostate have been investigated using prostatic stromal cells and neoplastic epithelial cells (PA-III, rat; TSU-pr1, human). Secretory proteins prepared from each cell type were used to determine the dose dependent regulation of growth (DNA synthesis) of the corresponding homotypic responder cell, as determined by ^{3}H-thymidine incorporation. PA-III secretory protein stimulated rat stromal cell proliferation by 1.8-fold. This stimulatory activity of PA-III protein on stromal cell proliferation was partially reduced (approximately 35%) by treatment with nerve growth factor (NGF) antibody, whereas neither acidic fibroblast growth factor (aFGF) antibody nor basic fibroblast growth factor (bFGF) antibody immunoneutralized the stimulatory activity of PA-III cell protein. In the corresponding opposite interaction, rat stromal cell protein modulated PA-III growth in a biphasic manner. At lower concentrations of stromal cell protein (1.25 ug/ml) PA-III cell growth was stimulated by 1.6-fold, whereas at higher concentrations of protein (100 ug/ml) PA-III cell growth was inhibited to 60%. Treatment of the stromal cell protein (1.25 ug/ml and 100 ug/ml) with NGF antibody reduced PA-III cell relative

[1]We thank Dr. C. Freeman, Dr. S. S. Yang and the National Institutes of Health for the invitation to present our research. This work was funded by N.I.H. grant CA50229 (D.D.).

growth to approximately 30% and 5%, respectively. bFGF antibody treatment of stromal cell protein at 1.25 ug/ml did not influence relative growth, whereas bFGF antibody treatment of 100 ug/ml stromal cell protein reduced relative growth by an additional 40%. Treatment of the stromal cell protein (1.25 ug/ml and 100 ug/ml) with aFGF antibodies reduced relative growth from that observed at these two protein concentrations by approximately 50% in both cases. Human epithelial TSU-pr1 protein stimulated human stromal cell proliferation approximately 1.7-fold. Treatment of TSU-pr1 protein with NGF antibody resulted in stimulation of human stromal cell proliferation (4-fold). In the corresponding opposite interaction, human stromal cell secretory protein stimulated TSU-pr1 epithelial cell proliferation in a dose-dependent manner up to a maximum of 2.6-fold. This stimulation of TSU-pr1 proliferation by stromal cell secretory protein was reduced to 20% of maximal levels by treatment with antibody against NGF, whereas antibodies against bFGF and aFGF did not significantly influence the stimulatory effect of stromal cell secretory protein mediated proliferation of TSU-pr1 cells. These results suggest that prostatic stromal cells and neoplastic epithelial cells secrete several paracrine factors. One of these factors is nerve growth factor-like, and appears to have a major non-neurotrophic influence on the paracrine regulation of prostatic growth.

INTRODUCTION

Prostate cancer has surpassed lung cancer as the leading incidence of cancer in men (Reis et al., 1990). The major risk factor associated with prostate cancer is age. The first manifestations of prostate cancer typically occur after the age of 40 with 80% of cases diagnosed in men over the age of 65 (Reis et al., 1990). Indeed, men over the age of 65 that do not present with the symptoms of prostate cancer during life almost universally are found to contain microscopic lesions of prostatic neoplasms upon autopsy (Carter et al., 1990). Hence, a better understanding of the mechanisms which regulate prostatic growth and protein secretion in the normal and neoplastic prostate may facilitate the eventual clinical manipulation of aberrant prostatic growth. Prostatic growth and protein secretion has been shown to be regulated through 1) endocrine factors, 2) extracellular matrix effects, 3) autocrine growth factors, and 4) paracrine growth factors, all of which may be interdependent to various degrees. With respect to endocrine regulation the dependence of stromal cells (Shannon & Cunha, 1984) and epithelial cells (Brandes, 1974) on dihydrotestosterone for their growth and development has been elegantly evaluated (Coffey, 1988). Moreover, in an animal model Pollard and Luckert (1986) showed that the spontaneous formation of prostatic adenocarcinomas was increased by testosterone administration. In regard to the extracellular matrix, there is considerable support for the concept of structural links, formed from components of the extracellular matrix, mediating and transducing signals between the stroma and epithelia (Isaacs et al., 1981; Coffey, 1988), thereby controlling prostatic growth and development. In addition, the recent observations that basic fibroblast growth factor (bFGF) binds with a strong affinity to components of the extracellular matrix such as heparan sulfate proteoglycans and glycosaminoglycans, and that these bound forms of the bFGF can be mobilized in a stable form by proteolytic cleavage of the extracellular matrix (Rifkin and Moscatelli, 1989), suggest another mechanism whereby the extracellular matrix may regulate prostatic growth and development. Autocrine regulation of prostatic growth appears to involve a variety of growth factor polypeptides. In this context, epidermal growth factor (EGF)-like and bFGF-like molecules account for a considerable amount of the growth factor activity in the prostate (Jacobs et al., 1988). In addition, acidic FGF (aFGF) (Mansson et al., 1989), transforming growth factor-beta (TGF-b) (McKeehan and Adams, 1988; Matuo et al., 1990), and nerve growth factor (NGF) (Harper et al., 1979; Schwarz et al., 1989) have been identified in the prostate or prostatic tumor cell lines. Some of these growth factors are presumed to have a paracrine role in prostatic growth and development. Paracrine regulation of prostatic growth was first suggested by Franks et al., (1970) after observing a lack of growth capacity of epithelia which had been separated from their stroma. Subsequently, Cunha (1973) and Cunha et al., (1980) demonstrated that fetal mesenchyme (stroma) induced prostatic epithelial morphogenesis from urothelium, with increased amounts of mesenchyme relative to epithelium increasing the total prostatic growth (Chung and Cunha, 1983). Furthermore, the proliferation of epithelial cells within the prostatic acini exhibit a regional heterogeneity, indicating that local control mechanisms, such as paracrine interactions with stroma, regulate differentiation and development (Sugimura et al., 1985; 1986). Indeed, recent studies by Djakiew et al., (1990) have shown that such a paracrine factor(s) secreted by stromal cells stimulates total protein secretion from a neoplastic prostatic epithelial cell line, and induces the secretion of a novel peptide (SE-1) from these cells consistent with the inductive action of stroma on epithelial morphogenesis. Moreover, the recent work of Swinnen et al., (1989) has identified one of these stromal cell paracrine secretagogues as P-Mod-S. Curiously, even though several growth factors have been identified in the prostate from whole tissue homogenates (Jacobs et al., 1988; Kyprianou and Isaacs, 1989) and various cell lines (Story et al., 1989; Matuo et al., 1990), the specific growth factor interactions between epithelial cells and stromal cells, and therefor their identity as paracrine growth factors, remains to be investigated. In this communication homotypic paracrine interactions between prostatic stromal cells from the rat and human, and neoplastic epithelial cells from the prostate of the rat (PA-III) and human (TSU-pr1) were investigated.

METHODS

Culture of Prostatic Epithelial Tumor Cells

A variety of rat and human prostatic epithelial tumor cell lines were grown *in vitro*. The rat cell lines were PA-III (Chang and Pollard, 1977) and RVP-47 3G (Terracio and Nachtigal, 1988). The human cell lines were TSU-pr1 (Iizumi et al., 1987), DU-145 (Mickey et al., 1977) and PC-3 (Kaighn et al., 1979). These cells were maintained in RPMI-1640 medium supplemented with 10% fetal calf serum (FCS), 10^{-7}M testosterone (T) and antibiotics and antimycotics (100 U/ml penicillin, 100 ug/ml streptomycin and 0.25 ug/ml fungizone), in 5% CO2/95% air at 37° C.

Isolation and Culture of Prostatic Stromal Cells

Rat prostatic stromal cells were isolated from 45 day-old Sprague-Dawley rats by sequential collagenase digestion followed by isopyknic Percoll gradient centrifugation, as previously described (Djakiew et al., 1990). Human prostatic stromal cells were obtained from an adult male undergoing transurethral prostatic resection for benign prostatic hyperplasia (BPH). The BPH tissue was minced into small blocks (1-3 mm^3) and sequentially digested in a collagenase enzyme solution as previously described (Djakiew et al., 1990). The resulting single cells and small fragments of digested tissue were rinsed in RPMI-1640 medium and resuspended in RPMI-1640 medium supplemented with 10% FCS/T, and plated into 75 mm flasks. After three days unattached cells were removed and the remaining adherent cells allowed to proliferate to confluence. Medium was replaced every second day.

In some cases, the rat and human stromal cells were detached from the flasks by trypsinization, and resuspended in aliquots of 25% FCS/10% dimethylsulfoxide and frozen at -130° C. These cells were periodically thawed and used as a seed stock to initiate new cultures of stromal cells.

In order to confirm the purity of the seed stock, human stromal cells seeded on glass coverslips were screened for vimentin intermediate filament immunofluorescence as previously described for the rat stromal cells (Djakiew et al., 1990).

Ploidy Analysis of Prostatic Epithelial and Stromal Cells

The ploidy of the epithelial and stromal cells was kindly analyzed by Dr. Owen Blair (Lombardi Cancer Research Center, Georgetown University Medical Center, Washington, D.C.) by the method of Vindelov (1983) using propidium iodide as the nuclear stain for the flow cytometry. Chicken erythrocytes and human lymphocytes were used as the internal standard cell types.

Preparation of Epithelial and Stromal Cell Secretory Protein

Stromal cells from the rat and human prostate and the neoplastic epithelial cell line (TSU-pr1) were grown to confluence in RPMI-1640 medium supplemented with 10% FCS/T. The rat epithelial PA-III cells were grown in a serum free defined medium (SFDM) as previously described (Djakiew et al., 1990). At confluence all cell lines were washed three times in F12/DME medium and cultured in F12/DME containing 10-7M testosterone for 24 hours. These conditioned media were collected and the cells incubated in fresh F12/DME/T for a second 24 hour period. Conditioned media were centrifuged at 1,000 x g to remove particulates and pooled over several collection periods by freezing at -20° C. Conditioned media were concentrated/dialyzed on ice with a hollow-fiber filter cartridge of 10 kD molecular weight exclusion limit (Cole-Parmer Instruments Co., Chicago IL) using ice cold distilled water for dialysis. The concentrated filtrates were lyophilized and stored at -20° C until use. At that time epithelial cell and stromal cell secretory protein were reconstituted separately in F12/DME/T.

Growth Assays and Immunoneutralization Studies

Preliminary studies determined the appropriate cell density for each cell type to be plated in 24-multiwell tissue culture plates (Falcon, Becton Dickinson & Company, Oxnard, CA). The rat and human stromal cells, and the TSU-pr1 epithelial cells were plated at 50 x 10^3 cells per well, whereas the rat PA-III epithelial cells were plated at 100 x 10^3 cells per well. The following day the cells were washed three times in F12/DME medium. Subsequently, the stromal cells were incubated in various concentrations of reconstituted epithelial cell secretory protein, and the epithelial cells were incubated in various concentrations of reconstituted stromal cell secretory protein for 24 hours at 37° C in 5% CO_2/95% air. Some of the reconstituted epithelial and stromal secretory protein (1.5 ml) were mixed with 15 ul of polyclonal antibody against either bovine bFGF (R & D Systems Inc., Minneapolis, MN), bovine aFGF (U.B.I., Inc., Lake Placid, N.Y.) or murine NGF (Collaborative Research Inc., Bedford, MA). All of the antibodies are known to cross react with their homologous human and rat growth factors. A non-immune rabbit IgG was used as a control. Subsequently, the antibody/secretory protein mixture was allowed to complex for 1 hour at room temperature, followed by centrifugation at 10,000 x g. The supernatant was subsequently incubated with the epithelial or stromal cells as above. Additional control treatments included cultures in F12/DME media alone, F12/DME/T, 10% FCS in F12/DME/T and 1% FCS in F12/DME/T. After a 24 hour incubation with the secretory protein or the control treatments, the cells were further incubated with 1 uCi of ^{3}H-thymidine per well for 6 hours. Each well was washed with 1 ml of ice cold phosphate buffered saline (3X) and the cells fixed with 5% trichloracetic acid (4° C) for 20 minutes. The cells were further washed (3X) in 1 ml of 5% trichloracetic acid (4° C) and dissolved in 0.5N NaOH (0.3 ml) for 10 minutes at room temperature. This solution was neutralized with 0.5N HCl (0.3 ml) and incorporation of radioactivity was determined by liquid scintillation spectrometry using a Beckmann Scintillation counter.

RESULTS

Ploidy Analysis of Cell Lines

Various epithelial and stromal cell lines were analysed for their ploidy as shown in Table 1. Cells with a DNA index (D.I.) of 1.0 (range of 0.9 to 1.1) were considered diploid (D). Cells with a D.I. below 0.9 or above 1.1 were considered aneuploid (A).

Characterization of Human Stromal Cells

Figures 1A and 1B show a phase contrast image and the corresponding indirect immunofluorescence of vimentin intermediate filaments in human prostatic stromal cells grown *in vitro*. The phase contrast image of the stromal cells (Fig. 1A) shows an attenuated, squamous morphology with numerous stress fibers and a few particulate inclusions in the cytoplasm. The corresponding immunofluorescence image of these cells (Fig. 1B) shows prominent vimentin intermediate filaments in the cytoplasm. This is consistent with a previous report showing vimentin localization in rat prostatic stromal cells (Djakiew et al., 1990). These human stromal cells have been subcultured up to 15 population doublings and then stored at -130° C. The stromal cells were seeded *ad libitum* from the stock vials for growth assays. Based on the immunofluorescence images the purity of the human prostatic stromal cell line is 100%.

Table 1. The DNA Index (D.I.) of Epithelial and Stromal Cell Lines.

Epithelial Cell D.I.		Stromal Cell D.I.	
TSU-pr1	1.63 (A)*	Rat stromal cells	1.02 (D)*
RVP-47 3G	1.74 (A)	Human stromal cells	0.98 (D)
DU-145	1.34 (A)	Murine 3T3s	1.69 (A)
PC-3	1.47 (A)		
PA-III	0.98 (D)		

*Aneuploid (A), Diploid (D).

Paracrine Influence of Neoplastic Epithelial and Stromal Cell Secretory Proteins on Cell Growth

Figure 2 shows the dose dependent stimulation of rat stromal cell proliferation as indicated by ^{3}H-thymidine incorporation in response to increasing concentrations of rat PA-III cell secretory protein. Cell growth is expressed relative to cultures incubated in F12/DME/T. Stromal cell proliferation was stimulated in a dose-dependent manner up to a concentration of 25 ug/ml PA-III cell protein at which there was a

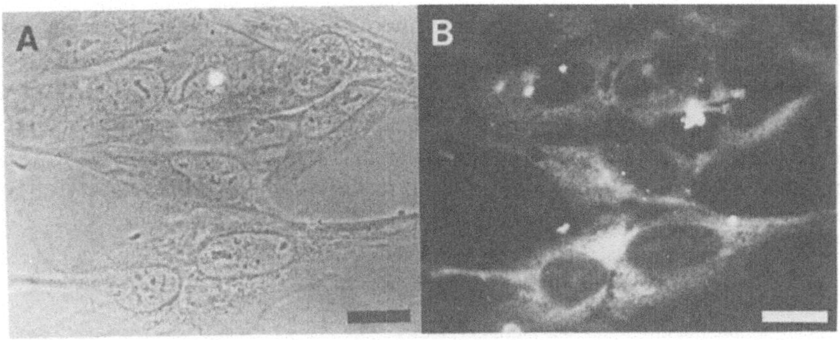

Figure 1. *Human prostatic stromal cells.*
Phase contrast image of stromal cells is presented in A and the corresponding indirect immunofluorescence of vimentin intermediate filaments in the same stromal cells is presented in B. Bar = 5 um.

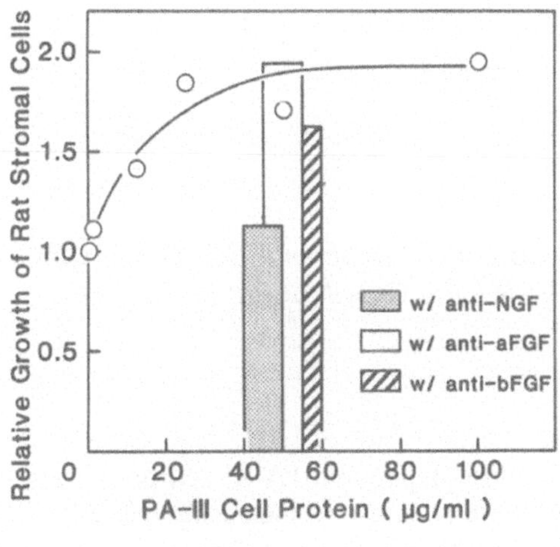

Figure 2. *Influence of Rat PA-III Cell Secretory Protein on The Relative Growth of Rat Stromal Cells.*

1.8-fold enhancement of relative growth. Stromal cells grown in 10% FCS/DME/T were stimulated in relative growth 2.6-fold compared to stromal cells grown in 1% FCS/DME/T which were stimulated in relative growth 1.8-fold. At a saturated stimulatory concentration of PA-III cell protein (50 ug/ml), prior immunoprecipitation of the PA-III cell protein with polyclonal antibodies directed against aFGF and bFGF did not significantly modify the stimulatory effect of the PA-III protein on stromal cell proliferation. In contrast, prior immunoprecipitation of the PA-III cell protein with a polyclonal antibody directed against NGF reduced the stimulatory effect of the PA-III protein to 65% from maximal stromal cell proliferation. Non-specific, control IgG treatment of the PA-III cell protein did not eliminate the stimulatory effect of the PA-III cell protein on stromal cell proliferation (data not shown).

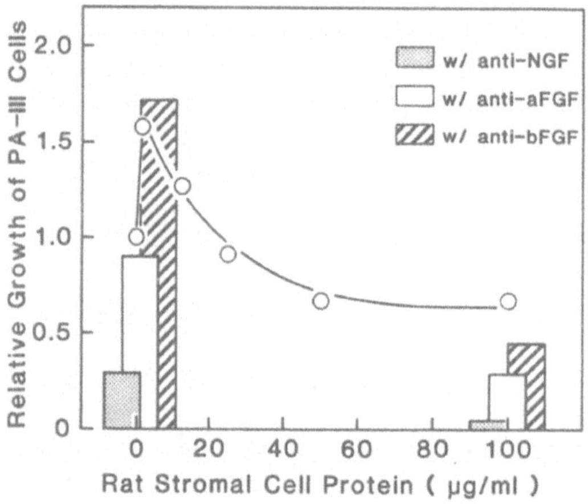

Figure 3. *Influence of Rat Stromal Cell Secretory Protein on The Relative Growth of Rat PA-III Cells.*

Figure 3 shows the dose dependent PA-III cell proliferation, as indicated by ^{3}H-thymidine incorporation, in response to increasing concentrations of rat stromal cell secretory protein. Cell growth is expressed relative to cultures incubated in F12/DME/T. PA-III cell proliferation was stimulated in a biphasic manner by stromal cell secretory proteins. PA-III cell relative growth was maximally stimulated 1.6-fold with 1.25 ug/ml of stromal cell secretory protein, whereas at a higher concentration of stromal cell secretory protein (25 ug/ml) no change in relative growth was observed. Even higher concentrations of stromal cell protein up to 100 ug/ml reduced relative PA-III cell growth by 40%. Treatment of the stromal cell secretory protein (1.25 ug/ml and 100 ug/ml) with NGF antibody reduced to 30% and 5% the PA-III cell relative growth at these protein concentrations, respectively. bFGF antibody treatment of stromal cell protein (1.25 ug/ml) did not influence relative growth, whereas bFGF antibody treatment with 100 ug/ml stromal cell protein reduced relative growth by an additional 40%. Treatment of the stromal cell protein (1.25 ug/ml and 100 ug/ml) with aFGF antibody reduced relative growth by approximately 50% at both protein concentrations. The non-specific IgG treated control cell culture resulted in relative growth of PA-III cells similar to that treated with 100 ug/ml of stromal cell protein (data not shown).

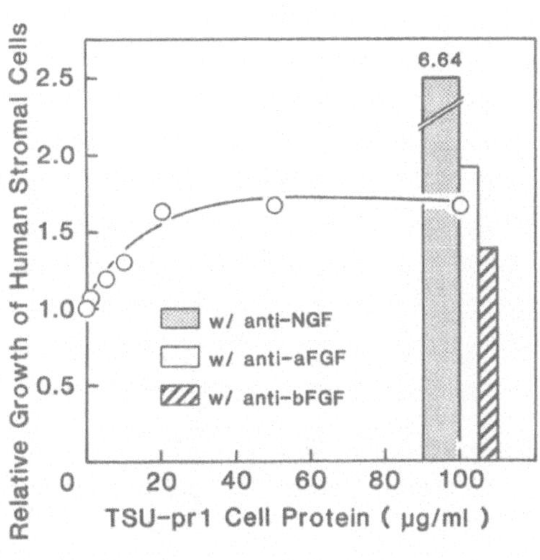

Figure 4. *Influence of Human TSU-pr1 Secreted Protein on The Relative Growth of Human Prostatic Stromal Cells.*

Figure 4 shows the dose dependent effect of human TSU-pr1 epithelial cell protein on the relative proliferation of human prostatic stromal cells. Stromal cell proliferation was maximally stimulated 1.7-fold by TSU-pr1 protein at a concentration of 25 ug/ml. Prior immunoprecipitation of this TSU-pr1 protein with NGF antibody further facilitated stromal cell proliferation 4-fold above this maximal level. Prior immunoprecipitation of the TSU-pr1 proteins with antibodies against aFGF and bFGF did not significantly modify the relative growth of the human stromal cells.

Figure 5 shows the dose dependent effect of human stromal cell secretory protein on the proliferation of human TSU-pr1 relative growth. Human epithelial proliferation, as indicated by ^{3}H-thymidine incorporation, was stimulated in a dose dependent manner; maximal growth stimulation was observed at a stromal cell protein concentration of

20 ug/ml, at which relative growth enhancement was 2.6-fold. Prior immunoprecipitation of human stromal cell protein (20 ug/ml) with antibody against NGF reduced relative growth of TSU-pr1 cells to 20% of maximal growth response. Antibodies against aFGF and bFGF did not significantly modify the ability of the stromal cell protein to maximally stimulate TSU-pr1 relative growth.

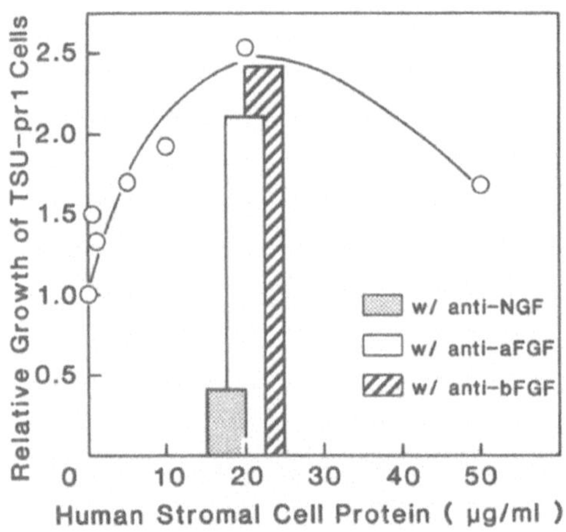

Figure 5. *Influence of Human Stromal Cell Secretory Protein on The Relative Growth of Human TSU-pr1 Neoplastic Epithelial Cells.*

DISCUSSION

The immunocytochemical localization of vimentin intermediate filaments in the human stromal cells (Fig. 1B) and rat stromal cells (Djakiew et al., 1990), in addition to the diploid characterization of the rat and human prostatic stromal cell lines is consistent with these cells maintaining at least some characteristics of their *in vivo* counterparts. The aneuploid nature of the human TSU-pr1 epithelial cells seems to be consistent with their derivation from a prostatic carcinoma (Iizumi et al., 1987). Interestingly, the rat PA-III epithelial cell line, which was derived from a prostatic adenocarcinoma (Chang and Pollard, 1977), and can form metastatic tumors in aged germ-free Wistar rats (Pollard & Luckert, 1979), was found to be diploid. Since there appears to be a general associate between the degree of malignancy and the degree of aneuploidy (Ruddon, 1987), the TSU-pr1 cells may be more malignant than the PA-III epithelial cells used in these studies.

At least four experimental approaches to the study of paracrine interactions between epithelial and stromal cells have been utilized by various investigators. These experimental approaches include 1) the addition of known growth factors to specific cell types, 2) Northern blot analysis of cell lines to determine potential expression of growth factors and other proteins, 3) co-culture of epithelial and stromal cells, and 4) immunoprecipitation and immunoneutralization of paracrine growth factors from secretory protein prior to the addition of that protein to the responding cell type. With respect to the modulation of growth by the addition of growth factors to cultured cells, the observations that numerous growth factors will bind to receptors of other growth factors illustrates a lack of specificity of this approach. In this respect, transforming growth factor-alpha (TGF-a) will bind to the receptor of epidermal growth factor (EGF) (Roberts and Sporn, 1988). Insulin-like growth factor-II (IGF-II) and mannose-6-phosphate share a common receptor (MacDonald et al., 1988). Indeed, both TGF-beta1 precursor (Purchio et al., 1988) and proliferin (Lee and Nathans, 1988) also bind to the IGF-II/mannose-6-phosphate receptor which in turn activates inositol triphosphate production (Rogers et al., 1990). Furthermore, IGF-I, IGF-II and insulin will all bind to each others' receptors with differing affinities (Rodeck et al., 1987; Dickson and Lippman, 1988). In addition, aFGF and bFGF will com-

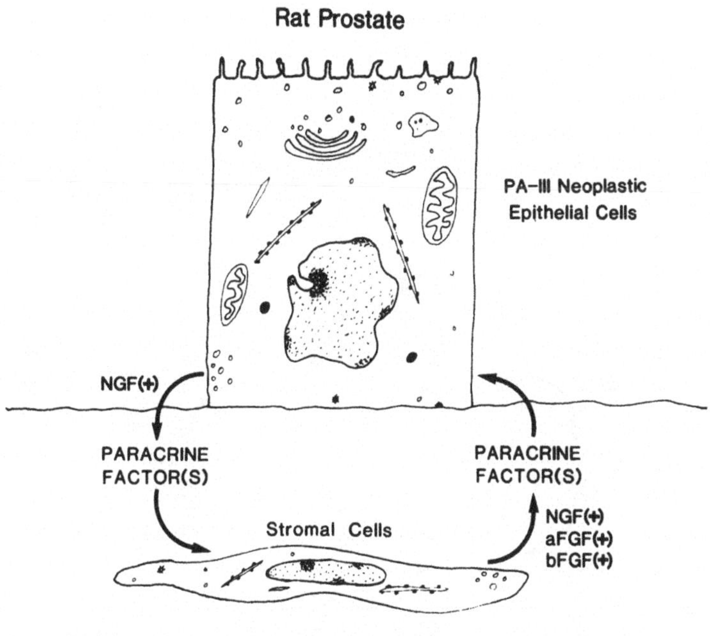

Figure 6. *A Schematic Representation of The Stimulatory (+) Actions of Growth Factors on Neoplastic Epithelial Cells And Stromal Cells of The Rat Prostate.*

pete for the same binding site on prostatic epithelial cells (McKeehan and Adams, 1988). The second experimental approach of determining growth factor mRNA in cells does not address whether the protein is secreted, or whether the target cell type has receptors capable of responding to that growth factor. Indeed, neither aFGF nor bFGF have classical hydrophobic leader sequences for their cellular secretion (Thomas, 1987). Since both these growth factors lack a standard signal peptide, the mechanism by which these proteins are released from cells remains an enigma (Thomas, 1987). The third approach, whereby epithelial and stromal cells are co-cultured is confounded by difficulty of determining which cell type elicits the biological effect. Even the use of a filter, such as in the bicameral chambers (Djakiew et al., 1990), to physically separate the two cell types does not address the issue of which cell type elicits the biological effect. Considering these caveats we have utilized the approach whereby specific growth factors were depleted from secretory protein of one cell type by immunoprecipitation prior to the addition of the secretory protein on the putative responder cell. Considering the specificity of antibodies this approach has the advantage of removing and concurrently identifying the specific paracrine growth factor while maintaining the presence of all the other secretory proteins which may be required for the full biological function and/or response of the intact cell.

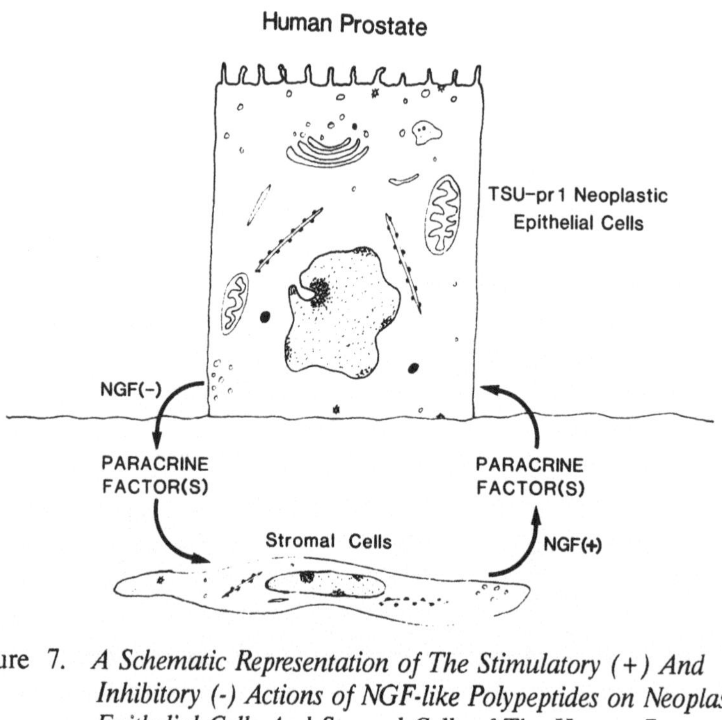

Figure 7. *A Schematic Representation of The Stimulatory (+) And Inhibitory (-) Actions of NGF-like Polypeptides on Neoplastic Epithelial Cells And Stromal Cells of The Human Prostate.*

In this report we examined the paracrine regulation of prostatic growth between neoplastic epithelial cells and stromal cells, and the role of aFGF, bFGF and NGF-like polypeptides in those cell-to-cell interactions. It is apparent that depending on the species and cell type, these growth factors can differentially modulate growth of stromal cells and neoplastic epithelial cells in a paracrine interactive manner. Following the demonstration of a prostatic osteoblastic factor (Jacobs et al., 1979) several laboratories characterized bFGF in the prostate gland (Story et al., 1987; Jacobs et al., 1988) and in neoplastic epithelial cells (Mansson et al., 1989). In addition, aFGF has been demonstrated in the epithelium of the normal prostate gland and in the epithelium and stroma of prostatic tumors (Mansson et al., 1989). Indeed, since aFGF and bFGF compete for the same binding site on prostatic epithelial cells, their actions in the paracrine regulation of prostatic growth may lack complete specificity. In any event, it is of interest that stromal cell secreted acidic and basic FGF modulated the rat neoplastic epithelial cell (PA-III) proliferation (Fig. 6) whereas human neoplastic epithelial cell (TSU-pr1) proliferation (Fig. 7) was not dependent on these growth factors. This latter observation does not necessarily indicate that the human stromal cells do not secrete acidic and basic FGF but that the TSU-pr1 neoplastic epithelial cells may lack functional FGF receptors and/or have escaped their growth regulation during malignant progression.

Subsequent to the early work of Harper et al. (1979) demonstrating the presence of NGF in the guinea pig prostate, it was found that NGF is widely distributed throughout the male sex organs of mammals (Harper and Thoenen, 1980). Nevertheless, our demonstration of the paracrine regulatory effect of a NGF-like polypeptide between stromal cells and neoplastic epithelial cells of the rat and human prostate is a novel, albeit surprising observation. The ability of antibody against murine NGF to completely inhibit the biological activity of prostate extracts in tissue culture (Harper et al., 1979) provides support for the identification of a major paracrine factor as NGF-like by the immunoneutralization technique. Moreover, malignant tumors of the prostate (Carstens, 1980) and benign epithelium of the prostate (Cramer, 1981) show a marked epithelial neurotropism. Indeed, since NGF has been suggested to induce invasive properties in nerves (DeSchryver-Kecskemeti et al., 1987) it is tempting to speculate that, in addition to its non-neurotrophic role as a mitogen, it may also facilitate the invasive process in the malignant prostate. In this respect, the ability of NGF-like polypeptides to inhibit human stromal cell proliferation while stimulating TSU-pr1 epithelial cell proliferation (Fig. 7) is consistent with tumor cells preventing the stromal cells from competing for space and nutrients during neoplastic growth and/or metastasis.

Based on the immunoneutralization studies, it appears that human and rat stromal cells secrete an NGF-like substance which can stimulate human and rat neoplastic epithelial cell growth. Since the NGF antibody eliminated the growth of the neoplastic epithelial cells, a potential strategy for the treatment of prostatic tumors could include the localized administration of NGF antibodies. Since, the human epithelial cells appear to secrete a NGF-like polypeptide which inhibits stromal cell growth a potentially confounding effect of treating prostate tumors with antibody to NGF may be the escape of stromal cells from NGF-like inhibition of growth. Indeed, since the initial lesion of benign prostatic hyperplasia involves a fibrostromal proliferation (Moore, 1943; Pradhan and Chandra, 1975), it would be of interest to determine whether these stromal cells exhibit an escape from NGF-like inhibited growth.

REFERENCES

Brandes, D Hormonal regulation of fine structure, in: Male Accessory Sex Organs, edited by D. Brandes, Academic Press, New York (1974).

Carstens, P. H. B. Perineural glands in normal and hyperplastic prostates. *J. Urol.*, 123: 686 (1980).

Carter, B., Pianpadosi, F. and Isaacs, J. T. Clinical evidence for the implications of the multistep development of prostate cancer. *J. Urol.*, 143: 742 (1990).

Chang, C. F. and Pollard, M. *In vitro* propagation of prostate adenocarcinoma cells from rats. *Invest. Urol.*, 14: 331 (1977).

Chung, L. W. K. and Cunha, G. R. Stromal-epithelial interatcions: II. Regulation of prostatic growth by embryonic urogenital sinus mesenchyme. *Prostate* 4: 503 (1983).

Coffey, D. S. Androgen action and the sex accessory tissues, in: The Physiology of Reproduction, edited by E. K. Knobil and J. D. Neill, Raven Press, New York (1988).

Cramer, S. F. Benign glandular inclusion in prostatic nerve. *Am. J. Clin. Pathol.*, 75: 854 (1981).

Cunha, G. R. The role of androgens in epithelio-mesenchymal interactions involved in prostatic morphogenesis in embryonic mice. *Anat. Rec.* 175: 87 (1973).

Cunha, G. R., Chung, L. W. K., Shannon, J. M., and Reese, R. A. Stromal-epithelial interactions in sex differentiation. *Biol. Reprod.* 22: 19 (1980).

DeSchryver-Kecskemeti, K., Balogh, K. and Neet, K. E. Nerve growth factor and the concept of neural-epithelial interactions. *Arch. Pathol. Lab. Med.* 111: 833 (1987).

Dickson, R. B. and Lippman, M. E. Control of human breast cancer by estrogen, growth factors, and oncogenes, in: Breast Cancer: Cellular and Molecular Biology, edited by M. E. Lippman and R. B. Dickson. Kluwer Academic Publishers, Boston (1988).

Djakiew, D., Tarkington, M. A. and Lynch, J. H. Paracrine stimulation of polarized secretion from monolayers of a neoplastic prostatic epithelial cell by prostatic stromal cell proteins. *Can. Res.* 50: 1966 (1990).

Franks, L. M., Riddle, P. N., Carbonell, A. W., and Gey, G. O. Comparative study of the ultrastructure and lack of growth capacity of adult human prostate epithelium mechanically separated from its stroma. *J. Pathol.* 100: 113 (1970).

Harper, G. P., Barde, Y. A., Burnstock, Y. A., Carstairs, J. R., Dennison, M. E., Suda, K. and Vernon, C. A. Guinea pig prostate is a rich source of nerve growth factor. *Nature* 279: 160 (1979).

Harper, G. P. and Thoenen, H. The distribution of nerve growth factor in the male sex organs of mammals. *J. Neurochem.* 34: 893 (1980).

Iizumi, T., Yazaki, T., Kanoh, S., Kondo, I. and Koiso, K. Establishment of a new prostatic carcinoma cell line (TSU-pr1). *J. Urol.* 137: 1304 (1987).

Isaacs, J. T., Barrack, E. R., Isaacs, W.B. and Coffey, D. S. The relationship of cellular structure and function: The matrix system , in : The Prostate Cell Structure and Function, Part A edited by G. P. Murphy, A. A. Sandberg, and J. P. Karr. Alan R. Liss, New York (1981).

Jacobs, S. C., Pikna, D. and Lawson, R. K. Prostatic osteoblastic factor. *Invest. Urol.* 17:195 (1979).

Jacobs, S. C., Story, M. T., Sasse, J. and Lawson, R. K. Characterization of growth factors derived from the rat ventral prostate. *Prostate* 15: 355 (1988).

Kaighn, M., Shakar Narayan, K., Ohnuki, Y., Lechner, J. and Jones, L. Establishment and characterization of a human prostatic carcinoma cell line (PC-3). *Invest. Urol.* 17: 16 (1979).

Kyprianou, N. and Isaacs, J. T. Expression of transforming growth factor-beta in the rat ventral prostate during castration-induced programmed cell death. *Mol. Endocrinol.* 3: 1515 (1989).

Lee, S.-J. and Nathans, D. Proliferin secreted by cultured cells binds to mannose 6-phosphate receptors. *J. Biol. Chem.* 263: 3521 (1988).

MacDonald, R. G., Pfeffer, S. R., Coussens, L., Tepper, M. A., Brocklebank, C. M., Mole, J. E., Anderson, J. K., Chen, E., Czech, M. P. and Ullich, A. A single receptor binds insulin-like growth factor II and mannose-6-phosphate. *Science* 239: 1134 (1988).

Mansson, P.-E., Adams, P., Kan, M. and McKeehan, W. L. Heparin-binding growth factor gene expression and receptor characteristics in normal rat prostate and two transplantable rat prostate tumors. *Can. Res.* 49: 2485 (1989).

Matuo, Y., Nishi, N., Takasuka, H., Masuda, Y., Nishikawa, K., Isaacs., Adams, P., McKeehan, W. L. and Sato, G. H. Production and significance of TGF-beta in AT-3 metastatic cell line established from the dunning rat prostatic adenocarcinoma. *Biochem. Biophys. Res. Commun.* 166: 840 (1990).

McKeehan, W. L. and Adams, P. Heparin-binding growth factor/prostatropin attenuates inhibition of rat prostate tumor epithelial cell growth by transforming growth factor type beta. *In Vitro Cell. Dev. Biol.* 24: 243 (1988).

Mickey, D., Stone, K., Wunderli, H., Mickey, G., Vollmer, R. and Paulson, D. Heterotransplantation of a human prostatic adenocarcinoma cell line in nude mice. *Can. Res.* 37: 4049 (1977).

Moore, R. A. Benign hypertrophy of the prostate: A morphological study. *J. Urol.* 50: 680 (1943).

Pollard, M. and Luckert, P. H. Patterns of spontaneous metastasis manifested by three rat prostate adenocarcinomas. *J. Surg. Oncol.* 12: 371 (1979).

Pollard, M. and Luckert, P. H. Production of autochthonous prostate cancer in Lobund-Wistar rats by treatment with N-Nitroso-N-methylurea and testosterone. *J. Nat. Cancer Inst.* 77: 583 (1986).

Pradhan, B. K. and Chandra, K. Morphogenesis of nodular hyperplasia-prostate. *J. Urol.* 113: 210 (1975).

Purchio, A. F., Cooper, J. A., Brunner, A. M., Lioubin, M. N., Gentry, L. E., Kovacina, K. S., Roth, R. A. and Marquardt, H. Identification of mannose 6-phosphate in two asparagine-linked sugar chains of recombinant transforming growth factor-beta1 precursor. *J. Biol. Chem.* 263: 14211 (1988).

Reis, L. A., Hankey, B. F. and Edwards, B. K. (ed.) Cancer Statistics Review, 1973-1987. The Surveillance program-DCPC, N.I.H., U. S. Department of Health and Human Services (1990).

Rifkin, D. B. and Moscatelli, D. Recent developments in the cell biology of basic fibroblast growth factor. *J. Cell Biol.* 109: 1 (1989).

Roberts, A. B. and Sporn, M. B. Transforming growth factor-beta. *Adv. Can. Res.* 51, 107 (1988).

Rodeck, U., Herlyn, M., Menssen, H. D., Furlanello, R. W. and Koprowski, H. Metastatic but not primary melanoma cell lines grow *in vitro* independently of exogenous growth factors. *Int. J. Cancer* 40: 687 (1987).

Rogers, S. A., Purchio, A. F. and Hammerman, M. R. Mannose 6-phosphate-containing peptides activate phospholipase C in proximal tubular basolateral membranes from canine kidney. *J. Biol. Chem.* 265: 9722 (1990).

Ruddon, R. W. Cancer Biology. Oxford University Press, New York (1987).

Schwarz, M. A., Fisher, D., Bradshaw, R. A. and Isackson, P. J. Isolation and sequence of a cDNA clone of beta-nerve growth factor from the guinea pig prostate gland. *J. Neurochem.* 52: 1203 (1989).

Shannon, J. M., and Cunha, G. R. Characterization of androgen binding and deoxyribonucleic acid synthesis in prostate-like structures induced in the urothelium of testicular feminized (Tfm/Y) mice. *Biol. Reprod.* 31: 175 (1984).

Story, M. T., Sasse, J., Jacobs, S. C. and Lawson, R. K. Prostatic growth factor: Purification and structural relationship to basic fibroblast growth factor. *Biochemistry* 26: 3843 (1987).

Story, M. T., Livingston, B., Baeten, L., Swartz, S. J., Jacobs, S. C., Begun, F. P. and Lawson, R. K. Cultured human prostate-derived fibroblasts produce a factor that stimulates their growth with properties indistinguishable from basic fibroblast growth factor. *Prostate* 15: 355 (1989).

Sugimura, Y., Norman, J. T., Cunha, G. R. and Shannon, J. M. Regional differences in the inductive activity of the mesenchyme of the embryonic mouse urogenital sinus. *Prostate* 7: 253 (1985).

Sugimura, Y., Cunha, G. R., Donjacour, A. A., Bigsby, R. M. and Brody, J. R. Whole autoradiography study of DNA synthetic activity during postnatal development and androgen activity during postnatal development and induced regeneration in the mouse prostate. *Biol. Reprod.* 34: 985 (1986).

Swinnen, K., Cailleau, J., Heyns, W. and Verhoeven, G. Stromal cells from the rat prostate secrete androgen-regulated factors which modulate Sertoli cell function. *Mol. Cell. Endocrinol.* 62: 147 (1989).

Terracio, F. and Nachtigal, M. Oncogenicity of rat prostate cells transformed *in vitro* with cadmium chloride. *Arch. Toxicol.* 61: 450 (1988).

Thomas, K. A. Fibroblast growth factor. *Fed. Amer. Soc. Exp. Biol. J.* 1: 434 (1987).

Vindelov, L. L. A detergent-trypsin method for the preparation of nuclei for flow cytometric DNA analysis. *Cytometry* 3: 223 (1983).

HEPARIN-BINDING FIBROBLAST GROWTH FACTORS AND PROSTATE CANCER

Wallace L. McKeehan, Jinzhao Hou, Pamela Adams, Fen Wang, Guo-Chen Yan and Mikio Kan

W. Alton Jones Cell Science Center, Inc.
10 Old Barn Road, Lake Placid, N.Y. 12946

ABSTRACT

Studies of model rat prostate tissue and derived cells indicate the insulin-like (IGF), epidermal growth factor (EGF), transforming growth factor beta (TGF-β) and heparin-binding fibroblast growth factor (HBGF) families and their receptors may play important roles in regulation of normal prostate cell growth. Tumor cells at different levels in the progression from slow-growing, hormone-dependence to fast-growing, hormone-independence exhibit distinct alterations in expression of specific growth factors and their receptor phenotype. Distinct IGF-I and HBGF mRNAs are constitutively expressed in the mesenchymal cells of slow-tumors, but alteration in HBGF receptor phenotype occurs in the epithelial cells. Fast-tumors exhibit even higher constitutive expression of multiple HBGFs. Splice variants in cDNA for the HBGF receptor in fast-tumors suggest constitutive expression of an intracellular receptor, that together with intracellular HBGFs, may constitute an intracellular autocrine system that is independent of exogenous hormones and growth factors.

INTRODUCTION

The incidence of prostatic carcinoma increases with age, and is characterized by progression from a slow-growing hormone (androgen)-sensitive tumor to a highly malignant, hormone-independent state (see Isaacs, this volume). A relatively unique feature of the disease which complicates diagnosis and treatment is "latency", that is a much larger number of individuals exhibit histologically abnormal prostate cells early in life than will suffer with clinical symptoms of the disease with advancing age (see also Isaacs). An understanding of the molecular cell biology underlying development and progression of prostatic carcinoma is especially important in order to develop diagnostic markers and eventually strategies for prevention and treatment. Intense study of the mechanism of action of androgen and its metabolism has failed to reveal the mechanism of progression of hormone-

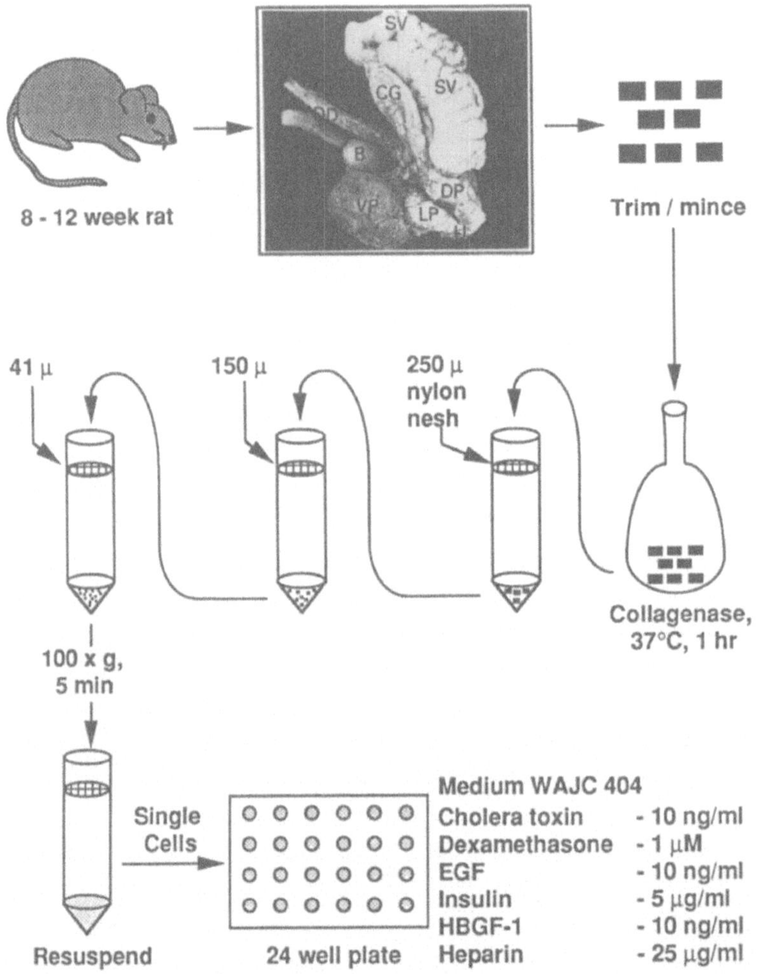

Fig. 1 Preparation of prostate epithelial and mesenchymal cells in defined cell cultures. The ventral or dorsal prostate (DP) lobes were removed, minced and dissociated with collagenase. Single cells were selected by progressive filtration to remove undissociated aggregates of cells. Cell cultures were initiated in 24-well plates in the indicated defined medium for epithelial cells. Addition of serum and omission of cholera toxin resulted in stromal cell cultures. The photo of formaldehyde-fixed rat sex accessory tissue was courtesy of Dr. F. French (12). SV = seminal vesicle, CG = coagulating gland; DD = ductus deferens; B = bladder; VP = ventral prostate; LP = lateral prostate; DP = dorsal prostate.

dependent tumors to hormone-independence and to suggest avenues of restoration of hormone-dependence in anaplastic tumors. Studies of the hormone-dependence of both isolated normal and slow-tumor prostate cells suggest that a significant fraction of both epithelial-like and mesenchymal-like cells with significant proliferation potential are not directly responsive to androgen. This has led to a study of the direct-acting hormones that support proliferation of both normal and abnormal prostate cells. The molecular cloning and biochemical characterization of numerous polypeptide growth factors and their receptors from various sources have generated the required tools to begin to dissect the role of such factors in the prostate.

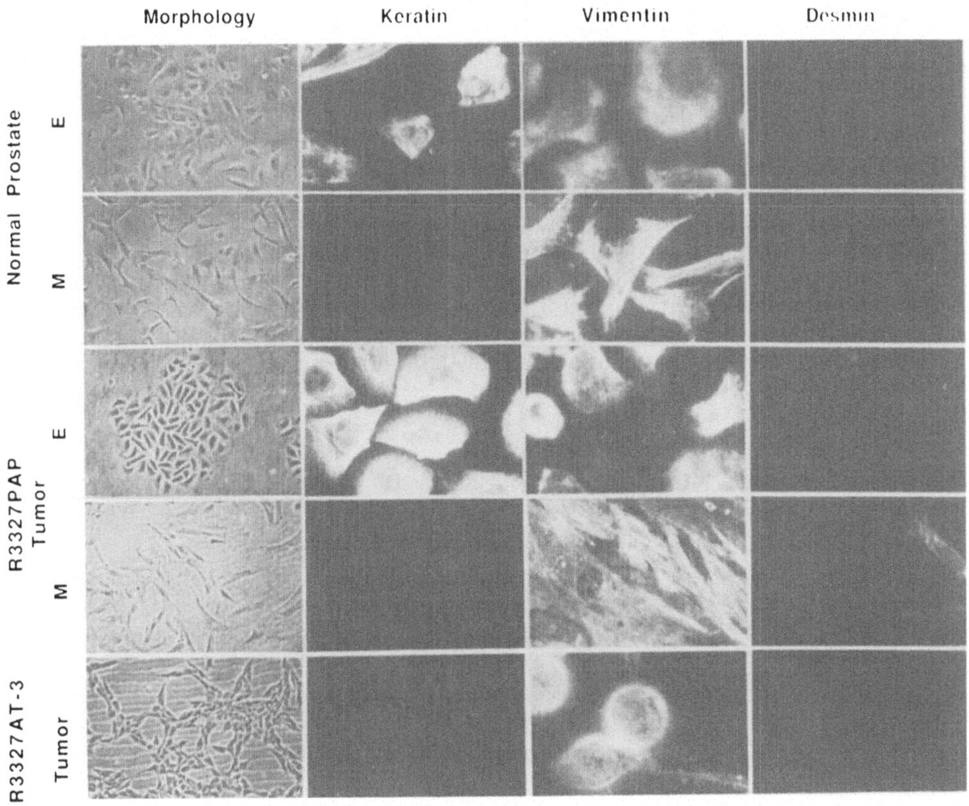

Fig. 2 Selection of epithelial and mesenchymal cells in defined medium. The indicated cell cultures were prepared as described in Fig. 1 and ref. 1. The R3327PAP tumor is an androgen-responsive, slow-growing tumor with well-developed epithelium and stroma. The AT-3 tumor is a completely androgen-independent, highly-malignant tumor derived from a similar tumor to the R3327PAP by passage in castrated males. Only a single cell type emerges from the AT-3 tumor. Reprinted by permission from ref. 8. See ref. 8 for experimental methods.

Polypeptide Growth Factors and Prostate Cells

Homogenous cell cultures of different prostate cell types provide a means to identify and characterize the factors that act directly on prostate cells. Cell cultures bear the caveat that certain phenomena evident in vitro may not always be expressed in vivo. However, cultured cell models reveal possibilities that can unfold in physiological situations that cannot be obtained by alternate methods. The history of discovery using cultured cell models has proven that observations made in vitro are rarely without an in vivo counterpart once adequate analytical tools are available to document the phenomena in vivo.

Analysis of growth responses of both isolated epithelial and mesenchymal cells (Figs. 1,2) from normal prostate have revealed that five major polypeptide growth factor families are active on prostate cells (1-4). These include one or more members of the insulin-like growth factor (IGF), epidermal growth factor (EGF), heparin-binding (fibroblast) growth factor (HBGF) and the transforming growth factor type beta (TGF-β) families (Table 1). Currently, there is no evidence for a "prostate-specific" polypeptide or steroid growth factor. Polypeptide growth factor families act on a variety of cell types and consists of multiple gene products that are not classical circulating endocrine hormones. Individual factors are expressed locally by tissue cells or are delivered to local sites by blood cells (platelets and monocytes). The key to regulation of proliferation of prostate cells by these factors probably lies in the control of expression of specific members of the families in prostate cells, their access to signal-generating receptor sites, and expression and activity of specific growth factor receptors in the prostate cell themselves. Conceivably, blood cells may contribute growth factors to the local prostate tissue during compensatory and pathological growth of the prostate.

Table 1

"Growth Factor" Families at Play in the Prostate

Insulin-like Growth Factors (IGF)
Insulin, IGF-I, IGF-II

Epidermal growth factor
EGF, TGF-α

Heparin-binding (fibroblast) growth factors
HBGF-1, HBGF-2

Transforming growth factor beta (TGF-β)

Polypeptide Growth Factor Expression in the Prostate

The pattern of expression and cell type of origin of each member of the four major families of growth factors that are active on prostate cells during compensatory or androgen-stimulated growth during prostatic hyperplasia and in various prostate tumors is incomplete. Analyses in our laboratory using rat prostate models and some human tissues show that normal prostate tissues express a major IGF-I mRNA transcript at 3.4 kB (Fig. 3). A second transcript at 8 kB is apparent in young rats (6-8 weeks) and is not detectable in 18 week old animals. Specifically the 8 kB signal increases during androgen-stimulated regeneration of the prostate in castrated rats (Fig. 3). The slow-growing, androgen-responsive Dunning R3327PAP tumor constitutive expresses the 8 kB transcript in addition to the 3.4 kB species (Fig. 3). Castration of slow-tumor-bearing males does not decrease expression of the 8 kB, however, androgen treatment of the castrates does cause a transient boost in expression which drops back to controls after 6 days (Fig. 3). An androgen-

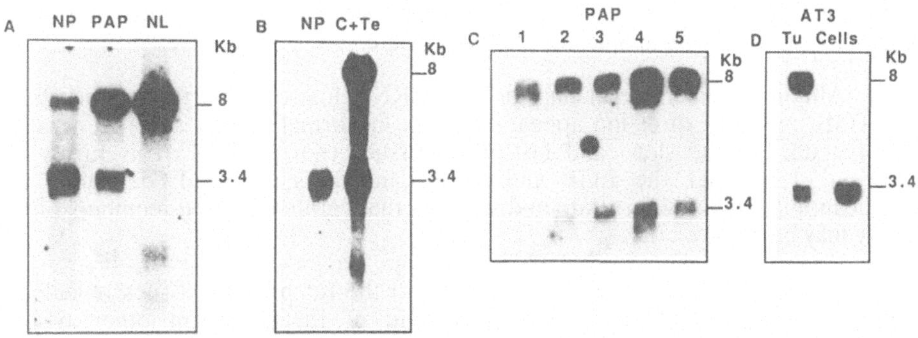

Fig. 3 Analysis of IGF-I gene expression. The rat IGF-I cDNA was obtained from Dr. L.J. Murphy (5). The cDNA was isolated, nick-translated and Northern analysis performed as described (8). A. Poly(A+)RNA (5 mg) from normal 6-8 week old rat prostate (NP), R3327PAP tumors (PAP) and normal rat liver (NL). B. Poly(A+)RNA from normal 18 week old rat prostate (NP) and the same aged animals two weeks after castration followed by 2 days of testosterone treatment (2 mg/day). C. R3327PAP tumors were implanted for 60 days in 7-8 week old hosts and poly(A+)RNA analyzed: 1, control tumor; 2, 7 days after castration; 3, 10 days after castration; 4, 14 days after castration followed by 2 days testosterone treatment; 5, same as 4, but after 4 days testosterone treatment. D. Poly(A+)RNA from AT3 tumors implanted for 7 days. Tu is the tumor tissue, Cells are from pooled primary through tertiary cultures.

independent, highly anaplastic variant tumor (R3327AT3) constitutively expresses both 8 and 3.4 kB transcripts and neither transcript is affected by sex of host nor castration of male hosts nor androgen treatments. Analysis of IGF-I expression in isolated cells from the normal-regenerating and slow tumor revealed that the mesenchymal (fibroblast-like) cell types are likely the source of IGF-I mRNA in the tissues (not shown). Noteworthy is the absence of expression of the 8 kB transcript in cultured fast-tumor cells (Fig. 3) despite the fact that tumor tissue from the subsequently transplanted tissues express the 8 kB species similar to the original tumor (not shown). In sum, these results suggest that expression of the 8 kB IGF-I mRNA is elevated in the stromal cells during normal prostate regeneration, and is constitutively expressed in slow-tumor stromal cells. Whether the transient stromal cell expression of 8 kB IGF-I mRNA in normal prostate is (i) directly induced by androgen; (ii) a consequence of stromal cell proliferation during androgen stimulation; or (iii) a causal factor driving normal prostate regeneration is an open question. The contribution of the 3.4 kB species of IGF-I-like mRNA to local IGF-I-like factor expression in the prostate is also unclear. The constitutive expression of the 8 kB transcript in the fast-tumor tissue, but not the derived cells in culture poses further questions. The 8 kB IGF-I mRNA expression apparent in tumors may be induced in host cells by the transplanted tumor cells, or expression in the tumor cells may require factors present in vivo that are absent in culture. The origin and character of the AT3 tumor cell population, whether epithelial mesenchymal or a transitional cell type is unknown. This is a key question and may be central to the understanding of the progression of prostate tumors from the slow, hormone-responsive to the highly anaplastic, malignant state.

Although detectable at high poly(A+)RNA loads on Northern blots, EGF and TGFα-mRNA expression appear very low in normal resting and regenerating rat prostate and the slow- and fast-tumor tissues (not shown). This raises the question of whether the EGF and TGF-α members of the EGF family are significant players in the prostate and suggests that yet unidentified members of the family may be at play.

Analysis of TGF-β mRNA expression in the rat prostate tissues revealed a pattern expected from reports of expression of the factor in other tissues. Significant expression was not detectable in normal tissues or normal cells derived in culture (Figs. 1,2), however, both slow- and fast-tumors expressed equal and constitutive levels of 2.5 kB TGF-β_1 mRNA (not shown). Whether TGF-β transcripts and the active factor are significantly induced during androgen-induced prostate regeneration and the cell type or origin remains to be tested. Level of expression of the TGF-β transcript in slow-tumors appears unaffected by castration and androgen-treatment of the host (not shown). TGF-β mRNA expression was reduced, but significant in cultured fast-tumor cells relative to intact tumor tissue. TGF-β clearly is composed of multiple genes and receptors are equally heterogeneous. A complete study of TGF-β subtypes and its receptor awaits molecular characterization in the prostate as well as other tissues.

Heparin-Binding Fibroblast Growth Factor Expression in the Prostate

The heparin-binding (fibroblast) growth factor family has been the most recent family of polypeptide growth factors to be implicated in prostate cell growth. Of all prostate growth factor families, the HBGF family is so far the most diverse and therefore, likely the most complicated. Currently, seven cloned genes constitute the family (6). The gene products exhibit sequence homology of 28 to 55%, are widely distributed in tissues and exhibit a broad spectrum of biological activities which include both stimulation and inhibition of cell growth and modification of specific gene expression. The HBGF family, as the name implies, has a unique affinity for heparin-like glycosaminoglycans (6). Heparin-like molecules stabilize and protect HBGF against proteolytic degradation and may be obligatory for activity of certain members of the family, HBGF type one (acidic fibroblast growth factor) in particular (6). Since heparin-like molecules are concentrated in the pericellular matrix of tissues, the stability, life-time and activity of HBGF in the local tissue environment is affected by the composition and metabolism of the extracellular matrix. HBGF activity is present in various prostate tissue extracts and the presence of HBGF type 2 (basic fibroblast growth factor) has been confirmed by sequence analysis (7). Our laboratory has rigorously examined the expression of HBGF-1 and HBGF-2 in rat normal and slow- and fast-tumors and their derived cells (8). An analysis of the other five members of the family is in progress. Expression was analyzed most extensively at the mRNA level by Northern blot. Although every condition described below was not analyzed at the activity and antigen level, whenever activity and antigen were measured the differences correlated with differences in level of mRNA transcript. HBGF-1 mRNA expression in normal rat prostate tissue is age-dependent. Significant levels appear in 6-8 week old rats. Expression declines at 14 weeks and is undetectable at 35 weeks. HBGF-1 appears to be expressed in specifically the epithelial cells of young animals. In the slow-growing, androgen-responsive R3327PAP tumor, which consists of a well-defined epithelium and stroma, HBGF-1 is expressed at constitutive levels equal to 6-8 week old normal tissue. In contrast to young normal tissue, HBGF-1 expression appears to originate in specifically the stromal cells of the tumor tissue (8). This is surprising since the PAP tumor is thought to be an adenocarcinoma whose properties are dominated by abnormalities in the epithelial cell compartment of the tumor. Constitutive and presumably abnormal expression of HBGF-1 in the stromal cells suggest that this tumor may consist of both abnormal epithelial and stromal cells and might more correctly be called an "adenocarcinosarcoma". Southern restriction fragmentation analysis of genomic DNA with HBGF-1 cDNA also indicated an abnormal band in specifically the cultured mesenchymal cells from the slow-tumor (8). Comparative studies on expression of HBGF-1 and HBGF-2 in both normal and slow tumor tissues and derived cells suggest that HBGF-1 exceeds that of HBGF-2 ten-fold in all conditions examined. In contrast to the slow-PAP tumor, the derived fast AT3 tumor expresses 5 times the HBGF-1 mRNA transcript than that expressed in the slow-tumor. In addition, the fast tumor expresses at least 30- to 50-fold more HBGF-1 transcript (7 kB) than the slow-tumor. The expression of HBGF-1 mRNA was significantly reduced in the single cell type that emerges from the fast-tumor tissue in culture (8). HBGF-2 mRNA was undetectable in the cultured fast-tumor cells. This differential expression of mRNA levels between intact tumor tissue and derived cultured cells was similar to that described earlier for the 8 kB IGF-I transcript. Either the tumor is inducing expression of HBGF-1 and HBGF-2 in host tissues or the in vivo environment supports a higher level of expression of both factors in the tumor cells relative to the in vitro conditions.

The HBGF Receptor in Prostate

Both normal and tumor-derived prostate epithelial and mesenchymal cells display specific HBGF receptor sites (8). Covalent affinity cross-linking of ligand to receptor sites reveal a broad band with a mean molecular mass of 144 kilodaltons (Kd) or 129 kDa minus the ligand. The most striking difference between the receptor properties of normal and tumor cells is the curvilinearity of Scatchard plots in normal cells relative to the linear plots in tumor cells. Whether the curvilinearity in normal cells reflects heterogeneity in receptor species or negative cooperative effects of ligand occupancy is unclear (8). Both slow-tumor-derived epithelial cells and fast-tumor cells exhibit a dramatic reduction in requirement of HBGF for proliferation relative to normal epithelial and mesenchymal cells and slow-tumor mesenchymal cells. The combined data on receptor properties and mitogenic response of normal and tumor prostate cells suggests an alteration in receptor properties of tumor epithelial cells in particular that relax the stringent requirement for HBGF to support cell proliferation.

Our laboratory has recently determined the structure and heterogeneity of the HBGF receptor family in human hepatoma cells by cDNA cloning, use of the polymerase chain reaction (PCR), and DNA-directed expression of receptor cDNA variants in host mammalian cells (9). Three variants in the aminoterminal (extracellular) domain, two variants in the juxtamembrane and two variants in tyrosine kinase concensus sequences in the intracellular domain suggest a minimum of six and potential maximum of twelve receptor species may be expressed in a single cell population (Fig. 4). Aminoterminal variants consist of a three (HBGF-Rα) and two (HBGF-Rβ) immunoglobulin-like disulfide loop structures and a third variant (HBGF-Rγ) which predicts an intracellular homologue of the HBGF-Rβ type molecule. Juxtamembrane variants consist of presence (a type) or absence (b type) of a 6 base pair (bp) sequence coding for a threonine-valine which is a potential threonine protein kinase phosphorylation site. Previous results from our lab show that phorbol ester, presumably through activation of protein kinase C activity, down-regulates high-affinity HBGF receptors (10). Intracellular variants consist of a conventional tyrosine kinase structure and numerous potential tyrosine phosphorylation sites and a truncated carboxyterminus which is unlikely a kinase and in which many of the potential tyrosine phosphorylation sites are deleted. The heterogeneity in predicted HBGF-R translation products in the hepatoma cell line appears to occur by alternate splicing that generates the diverse mRNA species detected in cDNA.

We have applied a similar analysis to analyze and determine structure of mRNA variants in the rat prostate AT3 tumor and to a limited extent normal rat prostate (11). Multiple clones of PCR-generated DNA fragments indicate that all three sources express mRNA encoding the extracellular motif characteristic of the mature two loop HBGF-Rβ transmembrane receptor (Fig. 5). Cloned DNA fragments from the AT3 tumor represent additional unique splice variants of the HBGF-Rα coding sequence with a 5 bp deletion at the putative splice insertion site of the 267 bp sequence coding for the unique IgG-like loop that characterizes HBGF-Rα. The 5 bp deletion causes appearance of multiple stop codons that truncates the predicted translation product initiated at the consensus site for HBGF-R isoforms. The alternate predicted translation products is the same one predicted from the HBGF-Rα variant cDNA from human hepatoma cells. In contrast to this rat prostate tumor cDNA, the human hepatoma cDNA (described above) exhibits a substitution of the 267 bp an IgG-like loop sequence with a 144 bp DNA fragment which also causes multiple stop codons in reading frames headed by the HBGF-R consensus initiation site. A second cloned prostate tumor cDNA containing the HBGF-R aminoterminal coding sequence also could code for an intracellular translation product. This cDNA variant also appears to be a splice variant that exhibits an insert downstream of the HBGF-R consensus translational initiation site and then a duplication of part of the 5'-non-coding sequence and the consensus initiation site and aminoterminal membrane translocation sequence. The insertion is in frame with the first initiation site, but the subsequent aminoterminal sequence is unlikely a membrane translocation signal and an intracellular isoform of the receptor is predicted. Alternate translational initiation at the second site would yield simply the two loop HBGF-Rβ isoform of the transmembrane receptor. A comprehensive analysis of expression and effect of various receptor isoforms on ligand-binding, tyrosine kinase activity, substrate-specificity, cellular location and metabolism in tumor and normal prostate tissues will be required to clarify the role of the HBGF family and its receptor in prostate tumor progression. Although it appears that coding sequences for structural variants may be heterogenous in different tumors, the diverse changes may have a common consequence. An intracellular autocrine loop between intracellular HBGF and its receptor is an attractive mechanism to explain autonomous prostate tumor growth. HBGF-1 and HBGF-2 have no apparent secretory signal sequences for translocation to the extracellular environment and are mostly associated with cells and pericellular matrix rather than present in extracellular fluids (6). If splice error at sites in the HBGF-R gene which generate normal HBGF-R variants is selected at the cellular level by the growth advantage conferred by a constitutive intracellular receptor, then this event together with constitutive intracellular HBGF-1 and HBGF-2 expression may contribute to prostate tumor progression.

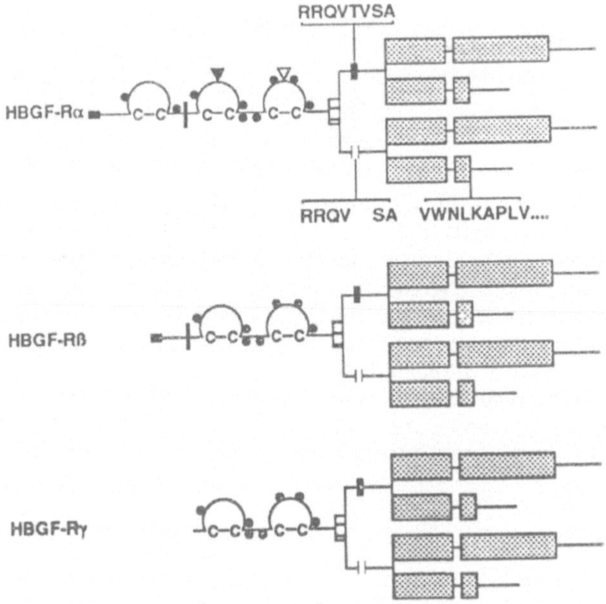

Fig. 4 Twelve possible variants of the HBGF receptor in HepG2 cells. The predicted α, β and γ NH_2-terminal motifs are shown fused to the **a** and **b** juxtamembrane sequence variants and the type **1** and **2** COOH-termini. The common initiation site and signal sequence for α and β motifs is indicated (■). Potential glycosylation sites are indicated by circles. The acidic-rich sequence (▌), the transmembrane domain (▤) and tyrosine kinase consensus sequences (◘) are indicated. The T/C:val/ala site (▽) and the EcoRI site (▼) are indicated in the α motif (top). See ref. 9 for sequence and methods.

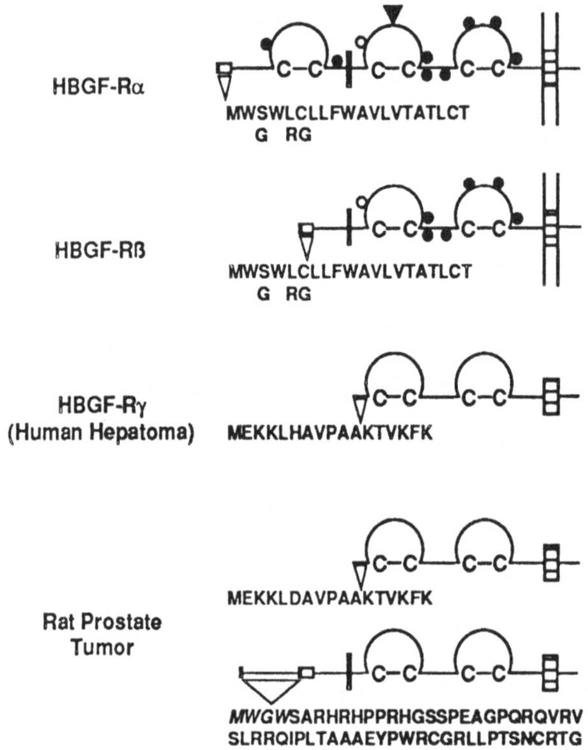

Fig. 5 Schematic diagram of aminoterminal HBGF-R variants predicted from cDNA. The concensus HBGF-R translational initiation site and the membrane translocation signal is indicated by the short black box and open box, respectively. Putative asparagine-linked glycosylation sites are indicated by circles. Rat HBGF-R exhibits a serine substituted for the third site in the human isoforms (open circle). The transmembrane domain sequence is hatched. The predicted aminoterminal sequences of variants are indicated. Rat differences are shown under the human sequence. The acidic residue-rich region is indicated by the vertical black bar. Only the aminoterminal variants are indicated. The full-length COOH-terminal structures of normal and tumor prostate have not been determined.

REFERENCES

1. McKeehan, W.L., Adams, P.S., and Rosser, M.P., 1984, Direct mitogenic effects of insulin, epidermal growth factor, glucocorticoid, cholera toxin, unknown pituitary factors and possibly prolactin, but not androgen, on normal rat prostate epithelial cells in serum-free, primary cell culture, Cancer Res., 44:1998.
2. Chaproniere, D.M., and McKeehan, W.L., 1986, Serial culture of single adult human prostatic epithelial cells in serum-free medium containing low-calcium and a new growth factor from bovine brain, Cancer Res., 46:819.

3. McKeehan, W.L., Adams, P.S., and Fast, D., 1987, Different hormonal requirements for androgen-independent growth of normal and tumor epithelial cells from rat prostate, In Vitro Cell. Devel. Biol., 23:147.
4. McKeehan, W.L., and Adams, P.S., 1988, Heparin-binding growth factor/prostatropin attenuates inhibition of rat prostate tumor epithelial cell growth by transforming growth factor beta, In Vitro Cell. Devel. Biol., 24:243.
5. Murphy, L.J., Bell, G.I., Duckworth, M.L., and Friesen, H.G., 1987, Identification, characterization, and regulation of a rat complementary deoxyribonucleic acid which encodes insulin-like growth factor-I., Endocrinol., 121:684.
6. Burgess, W.H., and Maciag, T., 1989, The heparin-binding (fibroblast) growth factor family of proteins., Ann. Rev. Biochem., 58:575.
7. Story, M.T., Sasse, J., Jacobs, S.C., and Lawson, R.K., 1987, Prostatic growth factor: purification and structural relationship to basic fibroblast growth factor, Biochemistry, 26:3843.
8. Mansson, P.E., Adams, P., Kan, M., and McKeehan, W.L., 1989, Heparin-binding growth factor gene expression and receptor characteristics in normal rat prostate and two transplantable rat prostate tumors, Cancer Res., 49:2485.
9. Hou, J., Kan, M., McKeehan, K., McBride, G., Adams, P., and McKeehan, W.L., 1990, Fibroblast growth factor receptors from liver vary in three structural domains, Science (in press).
10. Hoshi, H., Kan, M., Mioh, H., Chen, J-K., and McKeehan, W.L., 1988, Phorbol ester-dependent reduction in receptor number correlates with attenuation of heparin-binding growth factor-dependent DNA synthesis in human adult large vessel endothelial cells, FASEB J., 2:2797.
11. Hou, J., Wang, F., McBride, G., McKeehan, K., Kan, M., and McKeehan, W.L., 1991, Different splice variations encoded in complementary DNA from a human hepatoma and a rat prostate tumor predict similar intracellular isoforms of the heparin-binding fibroblast growth factor receptor, (in preparation).
12. Wilson, E.M., and French, F.S., 1980, Biochemical homology between rat dorsal prostate and coagulating gland., J. Biol. Chem., 255:10946.

AGE RELATED CHANGES IN ADULTS WITH ACUTE LEUKEMIA

Charles A. Schiffer and O. Ross McIntyre[*1]

Division of Hematologic Malignancies, University of Maryland
Cancer Center, School of Medicine, Baltimore, MD 21201
Norris Cotton Cancer Center, Dartmouth Medical School
Hanover, NH 03756[*]

INTRODUCTION

There are well known differences between children and adults in both the incidence of different types of acute leukemia and the response to treatment. Whereas acute lymphoblastic leukemia (ALL) constitutes 85-90% of cases of acute leukemia in children, the converse is true in adults, approximately 85% of whom have acute myeloid leukemia. There are no proven explanations for this discrepancy in incidence, although it has been postulated that the antigenic stimulation of new clones of lymphocytes during the maturation of the immune system in infants and children may be associated with an increased mutation rate and hence leukemias occurring in cells of lymphoid lineage (1). There are also major differences in responsiveness to therapy, particularly in ALL where there is a progressive age related decline in both initial complete response rate as well as long term disease free survival; adolescents fare more poorly than younger children with subsequent decreases in survival with advancing patient age in adults (Figure 1)(2-8).

This observation is somewhat less apparent in AML patients with deterioration in response occurring at a much higher age range. Table 1 summarizes the results of induction treatment of an ongoing Cancer and Leukemia Group B (CALGB) trial. There is a decline in response rate with increasing age which is most prominent in patients greater than 60 years of age. Of note is that in younger

[1]For the Cancer and Leukemia Group, Lebanon, NH 03766

patients, the major cause of initial treatment failure is drug resistance, a circumstance in which the patient survives initial therapy, but the bone marrow reveals persistent leukemia. In contrast, non-response in older adults occurs both because of persistent leukemia as well as failure to survive the initial treatment, in approximately equal frequency. Given the rigorous nature of current anti-leukemic therapy, this is not particularly surprising. Elderly patients with pre-existing cardiac or renal disease are more likely to succumb to side effects related to neutropenia and infection. They are less able to tolerate the nephrotoxic consequences of treatment with some antibiotics and amphotericin B. In addition, the administration of antibiotics, blood products, total parenteral nutrition and hydration for amphotericin B present substantial intravenous fluid loads which can be quite difficult to manage in older patients with cardiac dysfunction. These difficulties in supportive care affect not only the results of initial induction therapy, but also the ability to deliver even moderately intensive post remission treatment. Most AML and some ALL protocols currently emphasize intensive post-remission therapy as a means of maximizing disease free survival. Complications encountered during induction often become more chronic problems in elderly patients thereby making the delivery of post remission therapy unsafe.

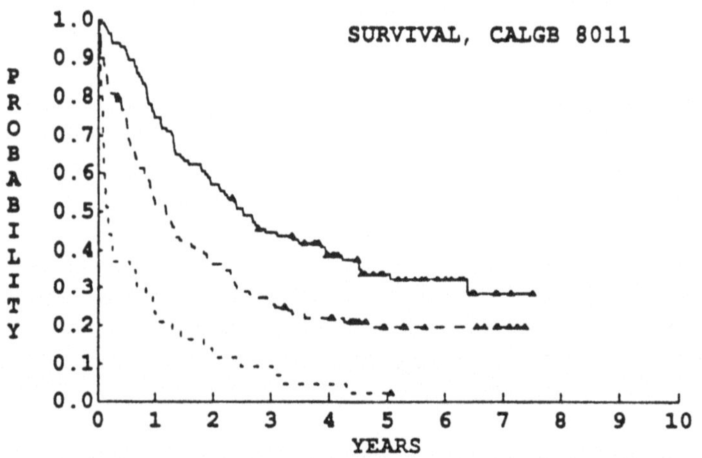

	AGE GPS	ALIVE	DEAD	TOTAL	MEDIAN
——	15-29	39	75	114	2.5
- - - -	30-59	26	94	120	1.2
· · · · ·	60+	1	42	43	0.2

Fig 1. *These age related differences in survival in adults with ALL treated by the CALGB are representative of results in other adult treatment programs (7).*

TABLE 1. Response Rate And Cause of Treatment Failure in Adult AML[2]

PATIENT AGE (YEARS)	<u><40</u>	<u>40-60</u>	<u>>60</u>
COMPLETE REPONSE	78%	71%	49%
RESISTANT DISEASE	13	12	20
DEATH DURING APLASIA/EARLY DEATH	9	17	31
NO. OF PATIENTS	281	321	342

[2]CALGY 8525 (10).

Until recently, it had been assumed that it was these difficulties with supportive care which accounted for the major decline in the short and long term outcome of more elderly patients with acute leukemia, despite major advances in both infectious disease and transfusion medicine supportive care (9). It has become apparent however, that there are additional, more fundamental "biologic" differences between adults and children and amongst adults themselves, which are age related and of critical importance. This review will briefly discuss some of these issues in patients with both AML and ALL.

ACUTE MYELOID LEUKEMIA

Multiple statistical analyses of CALGB treatment programs have defined increasing patient age as the major independent risk factor associated with poorer prognosis in patients with AML (10-13). Recently, a number of studies have demonstrated that cytogenetic findings also independently predict outcome and contribute a great deal to the effect associated with increased patient age (14-18). It is now apparent that there are a number of favorable karyotypes, usually characterized by balanced chromosomal translocations, which are associated with high complete response rate, low incidence of initial chemotherapy drug resistance, improved long-term disease free survival and younger median patient age. Conversely, other chromosomal changes such as deletions of all or part of chromosomes 5 and 7, trisomy 8 and abnormalities of chromosome 11q23, produce precisely opposite results with very few long term survivors and median patient ages of 60 years or greater. Younger patients with these latter chromosomal abnormalities have a similarly grim outlook suggesting the critical association of these chromosomal changes and resistance to treatment. Of interest is that these same chromosomal changes are frequently seen in patients with secondary leukemia following prior chemotherapy for another disorder as well as in patients with leukemia following prior myelodysplasia. Both of these entities are also refractory to current chemotherapeutic approaches (15-19). Furthermore, these cytogenetic changes have been seen in patients in whom there is a suspicion of occupational exposure in the etiology of the leukemia (20), suggesting that the increased frequency of these findings in elderly patients may represent cumulative exposure to as yet undefined environmental toxins.

Table 2. Common Cytogenetic Abnormalities in AML

	FAB MORPHOLOGY	MEDIAN AGE	APPROX. FREQUENCY IN DE NOVO AML
FAVORABLE			
t(8;21)	M2 (AML with maturation & Auer rods)	30 yrs	5-7%
t(15;17)	M3 (progranulocytic)	40 yrs	5-8%
abn 16q22	M4Eo (myelomonocytic with eosinophilia)	35-40 yrs	5%
UNFAVORABLE			
-5,-7 (alone or in combination)	variable	> 60 yrs	15-20%
+8	variable	> 60 yrs	5-10%
abn11q23	usually M5 (monocytic)	> 50 yrs	3%

As summarized in Table II, the favorable translocations are closely associated with distinct morphologic subtypes of AML. In contrast, more elderly patients with -7, -5, +8, can present with a variety of FAB histologies. Of interest is that FAB M6 (erythroleukemia) and FAB M7 (megakaryocytic) leukemias usually have these cytogenetic findings, sometimes in association with other complex abnormalities. Based on morphologic findings of trilineage dysplasia and recent molecular studies, there is a strong suggestion that the leukemia in such patients is likely to be a hematopoietic stem cell disorder (21). Other leukemias which primarily affect less differentiated cells, such as chronic myeloid leukemia in blast crisis and morphologically undifferentiated leukemias characterized immunologically by the presence of CD34, also are refractory to conventional therapy (22-24). This observation makes sense teleologically in that hematopoiesis must persist effectively for the life of the organism. It would therefore seem appropriate that stem cells have intrinsic protection against the host of environmental agents to which they are exposed during these many years. Further inferential support for this contention is provided by the observation that the hematopoietic stem cells can reconstitute otherwise lethally treated bone marrow transplant recipients despite *in vitro* incubation with extremely high concentrations of cytotoxic drugs. It is postulated that the multidrug resistance phenotype, expressed normally in high levels in the gastrointestinal tract, serves such a protective function for other organs (25). Further understanding of the mechanisms by which stem cells maintain resistance to cytotoxic agents may therefore provide clues which may permit improvements in treatment for a substantial fraction of older adults with AML.

ACUTE LYMPHOCYTIC LEUKEMIA

The systematic characterization of large cohorts of patients entered on clinical trials with newer immunologic, cytogenetic and molecular genetic techniques, has identified important differences in the leukemia cells from adults and children. These factors are related to the major difference in cure rate between adults (~ 20% disease free survival) and children (~ 60% DFS, > 80% in "good risk" categories). This section will review these findings as well as other variables affecting outcome.

Immunophenotype

The blasts from the majority of adults and children with ALL are of the pre-B cell phenotype as defined by reactivity with antibodies against CD10 (CALLA) and CD19 (using B4) and confirmed more recently by detection of immunoglobulin gene rearrangements (4, 26). About 15% of both adults and children have leukemia with a T cell phenotype. Although older studies suggested a poorer prognosis for patients with T-cell ALL, recent reports using more intensive regimens indicate a very high remission rate and overall survival similar to other immunologic subtypes (27). B-cell ALL (surface immunoglobulin positive, FAB- L3, increased incidence of CNS leukemia, +/- abdominal masses, t(8;14) karyotype) occurs as a small proportion of cases in all age groups, and has a uniformly poor outcome.

Adults and children do seem to differ however in the frequency with which their leukemia cells co-express antigens generally felt to be associated with a commitment to myeloid differentiation. Sobol et al, from the CALGB, reported that 33% of adults with ALL had either CD13 or CD33 detectable on greater than 20% of their blasts with the strong inference that these antigens were expressed on the same cells bearing lymphoid antigens (28). These individuals were older than patients without associated myeloid "positivity" (44 years vs 32 years) and had a statistically significantly inferior CR rate and survival. The incidence of myeloid antigen positivity may be lower in children. Mirro et al detected myeloid antigens in 19% of children (29); there was no effect on CR rate or event free survival. Further studies to quantitate the clinical impact of this apparent discrepancy are in order and considerable attention is now being focused on the multiple types of mixed or hybrid phenotypes which can be detected in both AML and ALL using combinations of immunologic, molecular biologic and enzymatic techniques (30,31).

Cytogenetics

Although cytogenetic analyses in ALL can be somewhat more difficult technically, experienced laboratories utilizing a direct technique can successfully study greater than 90% of patients with ALL (32). Cytogenetic findings differ markedly according to age in patients with ALL. In a series of 366 consecutive children with ALL reported by Williams, et al from St. Jude's Hospital, a bimodal distribution of chromosome number was noted (32,33). Forty-two percent of patients had normal chromosome numbers although most of these had detectable structural abnormalities or translocations. Approximately the same fraction of patients had hyperdiploid karyotypes, with 20% of specimens having between 47 and 50 chromosomes and 27% with greater than 50 chromosomes. Children with marked hyperdiploidy had the best prognosis with patients with 47-50 chromosomes having a somewhat poorer prognosis. Both groups however, had a markedly better failure free outcome than patients with translocations. Some translocations were specifically associated with B lineage ALL while others are associated with T lineage. As techniques improve, it is likely that more such non-random abnormalities will be described. At this time, it is unknown why patients with numerical additions of apparently intact chromosomes have a distinctly superior prognosis. The Philadelphia chromosome [t(9;22)(q34;q11)] is uncommon in childhood ALL and is found in only about 3% of cases (32, 34).

Although there are fewer large studies in adults, it is clear that hyperdiploidy is extremely unusual. Some translocations, such as t(4;11) and t(8;14) (associated with FAB-L3, B cell ALL) occur in approximately the same frequency in adults and children and confer a very poor prognosis (35). Most importantly, however, the Philadelphia chromosome can be detected in a much higher fraction of adults with ALL. Early studies utilizing cytogenetic analyses alone (35) indicated that 15-20% of adults with ALL had detectable t(9;22). Using Southern blotting techniques and probes for the bcr/abl region which is the hallmark of the (9;22) translocation in patients with chronic myelogenous leukemia, the frequency of the Philadelphia chromosome appears even higher. Recent data indicate that the abl oncogene from chromosome 9 can be translocated to two distinct regions of the bcr locus on chromosome 22 (36). One translocation is in the same area found in classic CML, while the other is considerably downstream in the bcr region, codes for the production of a protein of different molecular weight, and can only be detected using pulse field gel electrophoresis technology (37). Until recently, it was felt that approximately 50% of the translocations occurred within the bcr itself (similar to CML) with the other 50% occurring downstream. Utilizing samples from adults studied and treated by the CALGB, Hooberman *et. al*, have recently reported an overall frequency of 32% Philadelphia chromosome positivity utilizing both molecular techniques with most translocations detected outside of the bcr region (38). Molecular abnormalities were always present in patients in whom the

Philadelphia chromosome could be recognized cytogenetically. Importantly, however, the molecular techniques detected the translocations in some patients in whom cytogenetic analysis could not be done, suggesting that these techniques, including pulse field gel electrophoresis, will become a critical feature of the evaluation of adults with ALL in the future.

In both adults and children, the presence of the Philadelphia chromosome confers a poor prognosis. In adults, all Philadelphia positive patients have B cell precursor ALL and no patients with T cell phenotypes have been detected in the CALGB series as yet (39). Such patients have a decreased rate of complete remission (40-50%) and there are no long term disease free survivors using chemotherapeutic approaches. The median age of Philadelphia chromosome positive adults is higher (47 years) than other adults with ALL and it is very likely that this major difference in the frequency of t(9;22) accounts for much of the difference in response to therapy and long term survival between children and adults. The higher median age also suggests that bone marrow transplantation will not be a suitable option for many Philadelphia chromosome positive adults, although preliminary results in small numbers of patients indicate potential benefit from allogeneic BMT (40). Further studies in children using molecular technology are in progress but it is highly unlikely, even with the enhanced sensitivity of these techniques, that the incidence of t(9;22) will begin to approach that noted in adults.

Pharmacokinetics/Pharmacodynamics Of Chemotherapeutic Agents

Doses of chemotherapeutic agents are generally administered according to patient's weight or body surface area without regard for potential variability in drug disposition and clearance amongst different individuals. Recent studies have demonstrated wide interpatient variability in the steady state levels of different antineoplastic agents in patients given the same apparent "dose". Evans *et. al* demonstrated a three fold variability in serum concentration of methotrexate in children with ALL receiving high dose methotrexate therapy. Patients with lower methotrexate concentrations had a statistically significantly shorter duration of complete remission and the methotrexate clearance was found to be an independent prognostic factor for remission duration (41). Similar studies have not been conducted in adults with ALL, but there are obvious potential differences between adults and children with regard to the following: the incidence of obesity which could affect drug distribution; baseline renal and hepatic function; the frequency of cardiac dysfunction; compliance with the large number of oral medications used in ALL treatment. Indeed, a recent report has suggested that variable absorption and metabolism of 6-mercaptopurine may be correlated with differing treatment outcome in childhood ALL (42). Whether these variables can account for some of the differences in response are unknown, but such studies would be of interest in adults, particularly since there is growing interest in designing treatment programs in which certain drugs could be administered in differing individualized doses with the intent of achieving a predetermined serum level (43).

In addition to potential dissimilarities in drug disposition, there are also differences between children and adults in terms of tolerance of side effects of particular chemotherapeutic agents. One of the most successful chemotherapeutic programs described in children utilizes an intensive program of administration of high dose l-asparaginase for 20 weeks after complete remission is achieved (44). Although toxicity was noted in these children, more than 90% of the children were able to continue to receive these high doses. In contrast, most investigators treating adult ALL have found it extremely difficult to administer continuous high dose l-asparaginase because of gastrointestinal side effects, hepatic dysfunction, hyperglycemia, and sporadic episodes of pancreatitis. Other ALL programs in children have utilized sequences of high dose therapy with a variety of different drugs during both remission induction and post remission therapy (45). The CALGB is currently piloting such an approach in adults. Although it appears that most patients less than 50-60 years of age can receive most of the specified doses, the toxicity appears to be greater than that in children. Indeed, in adults greater than the age of 60, drug associated mortality was excessive and doses have had to be attenuated. In addition to intolerance of asparaginase, there is concern, particularly in adults, about the increased infectious risks associated with the prolonged course of corticosteroids which is administered during induction. Many adult centers now note an increasing rate of fungal infections, which although usually controllable with Amphotericin B, can preclude or delay the administration of subsequent therapy. It is of interest that there are no contemporary comparative studies determining the ideal duration of corticosteroid therapy; such an evaluation would be of interest.

FUTURE PROSPECTS

Until the mechanisms by which specific cytogenetic changes are associated with resistance to treatment, detection of these abnormalities does not provide specific insight into new therapeutic options. Presumably, these changes are associated with the over or under production of normal or mutated protein products resulting in biochemical or cytokinetic changes or both, which confer resistance to available therapies. It is hoped that identification and subsequent study of the functions of these gene products will permit the development of rationally designed rather than empiric treatment for both younger and older patients in the future. Characterization of the structure and function of the lineage specific cell membrane antigens, with possible pharmacologic or immunologic modification of their function would also be of interest (46). Although bone marrow transplantation is a logical, albeit empiric approach to adults with poor prognosis ALL, there is no evidence that BMT in first remission is of benefit to adults who are more "standard risk" (Philadelphia chromosome, t(4;11) negative, low WBC count). The overall results of BMT are poorer in adults than children with a much higher relapse rate in the former (47). Prospective trials in "poorer risk" adults are needed.

In the interim, other approaches may help improve therapy in more elderly individuals. Closer pharmacologic monitoring of cancer agents with potential individualization of dosing may help to optimize treatment benefit while reducing toxicity. Because of the intrinsic biologic resistance of the leukemias found most commonly in the elderly, however, it is likely that such manipulations will have the potential to reduce toxicity but not necessarily markedly enhance cure rate. Studies of agents such as verapamil, cyclosporine and progesterone which can partially or completely reverse the multidrug resistance phenotype in vitro, are being evaluated and have the theoretic potential of enhancing the activity of already available drugs, hopefully without increasing toxicities (25).

A number of studies have also demonstrated that administration of hematopoietic growth factors (granulocyte macrophage colony stimulating factor (GM-CSF)), (granulocyte colony stimulating factor (G-CSF)), can shorten the period of neutropenia following a variety of cytotoxic regimens and bone marrow transplantation (48). This is particularly relevant to elderly patients in whom problems with supportive care still represent a major cause of treatment failure. Although there is a concern that these hematopoietic growth factors may stimulate the proliferation of myeloid leukemia, preliminary studies have demonstrated that this is an infrequent occurrence when GM-CSF is administered after the completion of induction chemotherapy to patients with AML (49,50). There was also a suggestion that the period of neutropenia was shortened and the CALGB is currently conducting a randomized study in patients greater than 60 years of age in which patients are randomized to receive either GM-CSF or placebo to be begun on the day after completion of standard induction chemotherapy. The goal of this study is to determine whether neutropenia can be shortened with an accompanying decrease in infectious complications and death. Such an approach may also be of value in decreasing the complications of intensive post remission therapy. A conceptually similar study using G-CSF will be begun shortly in adults with ALL. In addition, the CALGB is initiating a study in patients with AML in relapse to determine whether *pre-treatment* with GM-CSF will stimulate proliferation of leukemic cells so as to enhance the cytotoxic effects of cell cycle specific agents such as cytarabine. A parallel approach to patients with ALL would be of interest when appropriate lymphokines are cloned and available for clinical trial.

In summary, there are a number of biologic differences between younger and older adults with both AML and ALL which, in addition to problems associated with tolerance of treatment, account for the major differences in outcome observed between these age groups. Combined clinical and laboratory investigations hold promise for more precise determinations of the mechanisms of refractoriness to treatment with the potential for new approaches to reverse this resistance.

REFERENCES

1. Greaves, M.F. Speculations on the causes of childhood acute lymphoblastic leukemia. *Leukemia* 2:120 (1988).

2. Gaynor, J., Chapman, D., Little, C., McKenzie, S., Miller, W., Andreeff, M., Arlin, Z., Berman, E., Kempin, S., Gee, T., Clarkson, B. A cause-specific hazard rate analysis of prognostic factors among 199 adults with acute lymphoblastic leukemia: the memorial hospital experience since 1969. *J. Clin. Oncol.* 6:1014 (1988).

3. Baccarani, M., Carbelli, G., Amadori, S., Drenthe-Schonk, A., Willemze, R., Meloni, G., Cardozo, P.L., Haanen, C., Mandelli, F., Tura, S. Adolescent and adult acute lymphoblastic leukemia: prognostic features and outcome of therapy. A study of 293 patients. *Blood* 60:677 (1982).

4. Crist, W., Pullen, J., Boyett, J., Falletta, J., van Eys, J., Borowitz, M., Jackson, J., Dowell, B., Russell, C., Quddus, F., Ragab, A., Vietti, T. Acute lymphoid leukemia in adolescents: clinical and biologic features predict a poor prognosis - a Pediatric Oncology Group study. *J. of Clin. Onc.* 6:34 (1987).

5. Linker, C.A., Levitt, L.J., O'Donnell, M., Reis, C.A., Link, M.P., Forman, S.J., Farbstein, M.J. Improved results of treatment of adult acute lymphoblastic leukemia. *Blood* 69:1242 (1987).

6. Gottlieb, A.J., Weinberg, V., Ellison, R.R., Henderson, E.S., Terebelo, H., Rafla, S., Cuttner, J., Silver, R.T., Carey, R.W., Levy, R.N., Hutchinson, J.L., Raich, P., Cooper, M.R., Wiernik, P,. Anderson, J.R., Holland, J.F. Efficacy of daunorubicin in the therapy of adult acute lymphocytic leukemia: a prospective randomized trial by Cancer and Leukemia Group B. *Blood* 64:267 (1984).

7. Ellison, P.R., Mick, R., Cuttner, J., Schiffer, C., Sobol, R. Prognostic factors affecting response and survival in adults with acute lymphocytic leukemia treated on CALGB 8011. *Proc. Am. Soc. Clin. Oncol.* 5:156 (1986).

8. Hoelzer, D., Thiel, E., Loffler, H., Buchner, T., Ganser, A., Heil, G., Koch, P., Freund, M., Diedrich, H., Ruhl, H., Maschmeyer, G., Lipp, T., Nowrousian, M.R., Burkert, M., Gerecke, D., Pralle, H., Muller, U., Lunscken, C.H., Fulle, H., Ho, A.D., Kuchler, R., Busch, F.W., Schneider, W., Gorg, C.H., Emmerich, B., Braumann, D., Vaupel, H.A., von Paleske, A., Bartels, H., Neiss, A., Messerer, D. Progostic factors in multicenter study for treatment of acute lymphoblastic leukemia in adults. *Blood* 71:123 (1988).

9. Schiffer, C.A., Wade, J.A. Supportive Care: Issues in the use of blood products and treatment of infection. *Semin. Oncol.* 14:454 (1987).

10. Mayer, R.J., Schiffer, C.A., Peterson, B.A., Silver, R.T., Cornwell, G.G., Rai, K.R., Ellison, R.R., Maguire, M., Berg, D., Davis, R.B., McIntyre, O.R., Frei, E. Intensive post-remission therapy in adults with acute nonlymphocytic

leukemia using various dose schedules of Ara-C: A progress report from the CALGB. *Semin. Oncol.* 14:25-31 (1987).

11. Preisler, H., Davis, R.B., Kirshner, J., Dupre, E., Richards, III F., Hoagland, H.C., Kopel, S., Levy, R.N., Carey, R., Schulman, P., Gottleib, A.J., McIntyre, O.R., and the Cancer and Leukemia Group B. Comparison of three remission induction regimens and two postinduction strategies for the treatment of acute nonlymphocytic leukemia: A Cancer and Leukemia Group B study. *Blood* 69:1441 (1987).

12. Rai, K.R., Holland, J.F., Glidewell, O.J., Weinberg, V., Brunner, K., Obrecht, J.P., Preisler, H.D., Nawabi, I.W., Prager, D., Carey, R.W., Cooper, M.R., Haurani, F., Hutchinson, J.L., Silver, R.T., Falkson, G., Wiernik, P., Hoagland, H.C., Bloomfield, C.D., James, G.W., Gottlieb, A., Ramanan, S.V., Blom, J., Nissen, N.I., Bank, A., Ellison, R.R., Kung, F., Henry, P., McIntyre, O.R., Kaan, S.K. Treatment of acute myelocytic leukemia: a study by Cancer and Leukemia Group B. *Blood* 58:1203 (1981).

13. Schiffer, C.A., Mayer, R.J. for CALGB, Cancer and Leukemia Group B (CALGB) Studies in Acute Myeloid Leukemia. In: Acute Myelogenous Leukemia. R.P. Gale (eds), Wiley/Liss (*in press*).

14. Berger, R., Bernheim, A., Ochoa-Noguera, M.E., Daniel, M.T., Valensi, F., Sigaux, F., Flandrin, G., Boiron, M. Prognostic significance of chromosomal abnormalities in acute nonlymphocytic leukemia: a study of 343 patients. *Can. Genet. Cytogenet.* 28:293 (1987).

15. Fourth International Workshop on Chromosomes in Leukemia, 1982. Clinical significance of chromosomal abnormalities in acute non-lymphoblastic leukemia. *Can. Genet. Cytogenet.* 11:332 (1984).

16. Keating, M.J., Cork, A., Broach, Y., Smith, T., Walters, R.S., McCredie, K.B., Trujillo, J., Freireich, E.J. Toward a clinically relevant cytogenetic classification of acute myelogenous leukemia. *Leukemia Res.* 11:119 (1987).

17. Samuels, B.L., Larson, R.A., Le Beau, M.M., Daly, K.M., Bitter, M.A., Vardiman, J.W., Barker, C.M., Rowley, J.D., Golomb, H.M. Specific chromosomal abnormalties in acute nonlymphocytic leukemia correlate with drug susceptibility *in vivo*. *Leukemia* 2:79 (1988).

18. Schiffer, C.A., Lee, E.J., Tomiyasu, T., Wiernik, P.H., Testa, J.R. Prognostic impact of cytogenetic abnormalities in patients with *de novo* acute nonlymphocytic leukemia *Blood* 73:263 (1989).

19. Rowley, J.D. Association of specific chromosome abnormalities with type of acute leukemia and with patient age. *Can. Res.* 41:3407 (1981).

20. Golomb, H.M., Alimena, G., Rowley, J.D. Correlation of occupation and karyotype in adults with acute nonlymphocytic leukemia. *Blood* 60:404 (1982).

21. Keinänen, M., Griffin, J.D., Bloomfield, C.D., Machnicki, J., de la Chapelle, A. Clonal chromosomal abnormalities showing multiple-cell-lineage involvement in acute myeloid leukemia. *New England J Medicine* 318:1153 (1988).

22. Lee, E.J., Pollak, A., Leavitt, R.D., Testa, J.R., Schiffer, C.A. Minimally differentiated acute nonlymphocytic leukemia: A distinct entity. *Blood* 70:1400 (1987).

23. Vaughan, W.P., Civin, C.I., Weisenburger, D.D., Karp, J.E., Graham, M.L., Sanger, W.G., Grierson, H.L., Joshi, S.S., Burke, P.J. Acute leukemia expressing the normal human hematopoietic stem cell membrane glycoprotein CD34 (MY10). *Leukemia* 2:661 (1988).

24. Borowitz, M.J., Gockerman, J.P., Moore, J.O., Civin, C.I., Page, S.O., Robertson, J., Bigner, S.H. Clinicopathologic and cytogenetic features of CD34 (My 10)-positive acute nonlymphocytic leukemia. *Am. J. Clin. Pathol.* 91:265 (1989).

25. Moscow, J.A., Cowan, K.H. Review: Multidrug resistance. *J. Natl. Cancer Inst.* 80:14 (1988).

26. Sobol, R.E., Royston, I., LeBien, T.W., Minowada, J., Anderson, K., Davey, F.R., Cuttner, J., Schiffer, C., Ellison, R.R., Bloomfield, C.D, Adult acute lymphoblastic leukemia phenotypes defined by monoclonal antibodies. *Blood* 64:730 (1985).

27. Hoelzer, D., Thiel, E., Loffler, H., Buchner, T., Freund, M., Ganser, A., Heil, G., Hiddemann, W., Maschmeyer, G., Aul, C., Wendt, F.C., Bross, K., Pralle, H., Kuchler, R., Dietrich, H., Mettnernich, M., Lindemann, A., Lipp, T., Kaboth, W., Nowrousian, M.R., Koch, P., Busch, F.W., Heimpel, H., Gotz, G., Weiss, A., Kolb, H., Messerer, D. Intensification chemotherapy and mediastinal irradiation in adult T-cell acute lymphoblastic leukemia. *In*: R.P. Gale & D. Hoelzer, eds. "Acute Lymphoblastic Leukemia", New York, p. 221-229 (1990).

28. Sobol, R.E., Rosemarie, M., Royston, I., Davey, F.R., Ellison, R.R., Newman, R., Cuttner, J., Griffin, J.D., Collins, H., Nelson, D.A., Bloomfield, C.D. Clinical importance of myeloid antigen expression in adult acute lymphoblastic leukemia. *New Eng. J. Med.* 316:1111 (1987).

29. Mirro, J., Zipf, T.F., Pui, C-H., Kitchingman, G., Williams, D., Melvin, S., Murphy, S.B., Stass, S. Acute Mixed Lineage Leukemia: clinicopathologic correlations and prognostic significance. *Blood* 66:1115 (1985).

30. Schiffer, C.A. Hybrid Leukemias. *In*: R.P. Gale & D. Hoelzer, eds. "Acute Lymphoblastic Leukemia", New York, p. 129-142 (1990).

31. Ball, E.D., Griffin, J.D., Davis, R., Davey, F.R., Arthur, D., Wurster-Hill, D., Schiffer, C., Bloomfield, C.D. Prognostic value of lymphocyte surface markers in acute myeloid leukemia (AML): A Cancer and Leukemia Group B (CALGB) Study. *Blood* 72:187 (1988).

32. Williams, D.L., Raimondi, S.C., Pui, C-H., Rivera, G.K. Evolving chromosome patterns and new cytogenetic concepts in childhood acute lymphoblastic leukemia. *In*: R.P. Gale & D. Hoelzer, eds. "Acute Lymphoblastic Leukemia", New York, p. 91-100 (1990).

33. Williams, D.L., Harber, J., Murphy, S.B., Look, T.A., Kalwinksy, D.K., Rivera, G., Melvin, S.L., Stass, S., Dahl, G.V. Chromosomal translocations play a unique role in influencing prognosis in childhood acute lymphoblastic leukemia. *Blood* 68:205 (1986).

34. Crist, W., Carroll, A., Shuster, J., Jackson, J., Head, D., Borowitz, M., Behm, F., Link, M., Steuber, P., Ragab, A., Hirt, A., Brock, B., Land, V., Pullen, J. Philadelphia chromosome positive childhood acute lymphoblastic leukemia: clinical and cytogenetic characteristics and treatment outcome. A pediatric oncology group study. *Blood* 76:489 (1990).

35. Bloomfield, C.D., Goldman, A.I., Alimena, G., Berger, R., Borgstrom, G.H., Brandt, L., Catovsky, D., de la Chapelle, A., Dewald, G.W., Garson, O.M., Garwicz, S., Golomb, H.M., Hossfeld, D.K., Lawler, S.D., Mitelman, F., Nilsson, P., Pierre, R.V., Philip, P., Prigogina, E., Rowley, J.D., Sakurai, M., Sandberg, A.A., Secker Walker, L.M., Tricot, G., Van Den Berghe, H., Van Orshoven, A., Vuopio, P., Whang-Peng, J. Chromosomal abnormalities identify high-risk and low-risk patients with acute lymphoblastic leukemia. *Blood* 67:415 (1986).

36. Kurzrock, R., Gutterman, J.U., Talpaz, M. The molecular genetics of philadelphia chromosome-positive leukemias. *New Eng. J. Med.*, 319:990 (1988).

37. Hooberman, A.L., Rubin, C.M., Barton, K.P., Westbrook, C.A. Detection of the Philadelphia chromosome in acute lymphoblastic leukemia by pulsed-field gel electorphoresis. *Blood* 74:1101 (1989).

38. Hooberman, A.L., Westbrook, C.A., Davey, F., Schiffer, C., Spino, C., Bloomfield, C.D. Molecular detection of the philadelphia chromosome (PH^1) chromosome in adult acute lymphoblastic leukemia (ALL): clinical cytogenetic, and immunophenotypic correlations in a CALGB study. *Blood* 74:183 (1989).

39. Bloomfield, C.D., Wurster-Hill, D., Peng, G., Le Beau, M., Tantravahi, R., Testa, J., Davey, F.R., Ellison, R.R., Cuttner, J., Schiffer, C., Sobol, R.E., Lunghofer, B., Carey, M., Mick, R., Arthur, D. Prognostic significance of the philadelphia chromosome in adult acute lymphoblastic leukemia. *In*: R.P. Gale & D. Hoelzer, eds. "Acute Lymphoblastic Leukemia", New York, p. 101-109 (1990).

40. Forman, S.J., O'Donnell, M.R., Nademanee, A.P. Bone marrow transplantation for patients with Philadelphia chromosome-positive acute lymphoblastic leukemia. *Blood* 70:587 (1987).

41. Evans, W.E., Crom, W.R., Abromowitch, M., Dodge, R., Look, A.T., Bowman, W.P., George, S.L., Pui, C.H. Clinical pharmacodynamics of high-dose methotrexate in acute lymphocytic leukemia. *New Eng. J. Med.* 314:471 (1986).

42. Lennard, L., Lilleyman, J.S. Variable mercaptopurine metabolism and treatment outcome in childhood lymphoblastic leukemia. *J. Clin. Oncol.* 7:1816 (1989).

43. Capizzi, R.L., Oliver, L., Friedman, J., Davis, R., Mayer R., Schiffer, C.A. Variations in Ara-C plasma concentrations at steady-state (C-ss) during remission induction and intensification therapy of AML. A population pharmacokinetics study by CALGB. *Proc. Amer. Soc. Clin. Onc.* 7:57 (1988).

44. Clavell, L.A., Gelber, R.D., Cohen, H.J., Hitchcock-Bryan, S., Cassady, J.R., Tarbell, N.J., Blattner, S.R., Tantravahi, R., Leavitt, P., Sallan, S.E. Four-agent induction and intensive asparaginase therapy for treatment of childhood acute lymphoblastic leukemia. *New Eng. J. Med.* 315:657 (1986).

45. Steinherz, P.G., Gaynon, P., Miller, D.R., Reaman, G., Bleyer, A., Finklestein, J., Evans, R.G., Meyers, P., Steinherz, L.J., Sather, H., Hammond, D. Improved disease-free survival of children with acute lymphoblastic leukemia at high risk for early relapse with the New York regimen - a new intensive therapy protocol: a report from the Children's Cancer Study Group. *J. of Clin. Onc.* 4:744 (1986).

46. LeBien, T.W., McCormack, T. The common acute lymphoblastic leukemia antigen (CD10): emancipation from a functional enigma. *Blood* 73:625 (1989).

47. Barrett, J.A., Horowitz, M.M., Gale, R.P., Biggs, J.C., Camitta, B.M., Dicke, K.A., Gluckman, E., Good, R.A., Herzig, H., Lee, M.B., Marmont, A.M., Masaoka, T., Ramsay, N.K.C, Rimm, A.A., Speck, B., Zwaan, F.E., Bortin, M.M. Marrow transplantation for acute lymphoblastic leukemia: factors affecting relapse and survival. *Blood* 74:862 (1989).

48. Groopman, J.E., Molina, J.M., Scadden, D.T. Hematopoietic growth factors: biology and clinical applications. *New Eng. J. Med.* 321:1449 (1989).

49. Büchner, T., Hiddemann, W., Koenigsmann, M., Zuhlsdorf, M., Wormann, B., Boeckmann, A., van de Loo, J., Maschmeyer, G., Wendt, F., Schulz, G. Human recombinant granulocyte macrophage colony stimulating factor (GM-CSF) for acute leukemias in aplasia and at high risk of early death. *Blood* 72:111a (1989).

50. Muhm, M., Andreeff, M., Geissler, K., Gorischek, C., Haas, O., Haimi, J., Hinterberger, W., Schulz, G., Speiser, W., Sunder-Plassmann, G., Valent, P., Lechner, K., Bettelheim, P. RhGM-CSF in combination with chemotherapy - a new strategy in the therapy of acute myeloid leukemia. *Blood* 74:117a (1989).

SIGNIFICANCE OF CHROMOSOMAL CHANGES IN PATIENTS OF DIFFERENT AGE GROUPS WITH ACUTE LEUKEMIA

Jacqueline Whang-Peng

Cytogenetic Oncology Section, Medicine Branch
Division of Cancer Treatment, National Cancer Institute
Bethesda, Maryland 20892

ABSTRACT

Chromosome abnormalities have been observed in about 50% of patients with acute leukemia. There have been several published reports which emphasized the chromosomal changes in relation to the age of the patient and the morphologic type of acute leukemia. All observations suggest that there are both age related similarities and differences. The karyotype is an important independent prognostic factor in acute leukemia; however, age alone (especially above age 70) is the single most important factor for a poor prognosis.

INTRODUCTION

There have been several published reports in which chromosomal changes have been examined to determine if any of these changes can be correlated with the age of the patient within different morphologic types of acute leukemia. All the observations suggest that there are both age related similarities and differences. In this lecture, I will present the published data on this subject, as well as some data from my laboratory.

MATERIALS AND METHODS

Cytogenetic studies of acute leukemia are usually confined to the bone marrow because it is the site of origin for leukemic cells, and usually contains ample mitotic activity. Several other tissues, such as peripheral blood, lymph nodes, chloromas, and spinal fluid are also good sources of mitotic leukemic cells. In the direct procedure, the cells are immediately transferred to a 0.1-0.2μg/ml Colcemid solution for 30-60 minutes; they are then harvested with sequential exposure to

The Underlying Molecular, Cellular, and Immunological Factors in Cancer and Aging, Edited by S.S. Yang and H.R.Warner, Plenum Press, New York, 1993

different solutions: a hypotonic solution (which swells the cells), 1% sodium citrate or 0.075 M KCl or mixture of these two for 20-30 minutes, followed by several changes of a fixation solution, a 3:1 mixture of absolute alcohol and glacial acetic acid for 10 minutes and 5 minutes. Slides are then made using any of a variety of techniques (e.g., air-dry, wet slide, dropping). Standard Giemsa stain and banding stains (Giemsa-trypsin, quinacrine, and-C-banding) are used to determine the exact chromosomal abnormality involved in the neoplastic cells. The whole procedure and a preliminary report can be completed within a few hours.

A standard Nomenclature for cytogenetic studies has been published in the ISCN (An International System for Human Cytogenetic Nomenclature, 1985). The upper short arm is termed the "p" arm and the lower part of the chromosome is the "q" arm. Each arm is divided into regions, bands, and subbands; plus (+) and minus (-) symbols in front of the chromosome indicate the gain or loss of the whole chromosome, whereas, if placed after the designated arm, indicate the gain or loss of part of the arm. Other common symbols include der(derived chromosome), ins(insertion), t(translocation), mar(marker), r(ring), and dic(dicentric).

Chromosomal abnormalities have been observed in about 50% of patients with acute leukemia. Both numerical and structural chromosomal abnormalities are seen in the leukemic cells. Structural abnormalities include deletions, translocations, inversions, and isochromosome formation.

ACUTE LYMPHOCYTIC LEUKEMIA

According to the FAB classification (1, 2), acute lymphocytic leukemia (ALL) can be divided into three morphological categories, Ll, L2, and L3.

Ll ALL: The predominant cell is small with small or not visible nucleoli and scanty cytoplasm.
L2 ALL: The cells have large nuclei and the amount of cytoplasm is often abundant.
L3 ALL: The cells are of the Burkitt's variety with a B-cell phenotype.

The cells can be further categorized according to their immunologic surface markets as T-, B-, common ALL and Pre-B ALL. Most data have indicated that Ll and L2 ALL show similar chromosomal abnormalities; however, at the Sixth International Workshop on Chromosomes in Leukemia (IWCL) in Lund, Sweden, (3) in 1987, data gathered from laboratories of several different countries, enabled the participants to subdivide Ll and L2 into several subgroups on the basis of cytogenetic abnormalities, and to correlate the chromosome abnormalities with morphology, immunological markers, and clinical behavior. The patients were divided into ten groups according to their pretreatment karyotypes. Those with no chromosomal abnormality (normal) and those with chromosomal abnormality (aneuploidy). Patients with aneuploidy were further divided into 8 subcategories: Ph^1 chromosome, t(4;11), 14q+, 6q-, <46, 46 (abnormal), 47-50, and >50.

In all types of ALL, the best survival was seen in patients with >50 chromosomes (58 months) and the lowest survivals were in the groups with t(4;11) and 14q+ (7-8 months). Further division of the patient population into children and adults revealed a median survival for children with >50 to be 96+ months, while the t(4;11) group has a survival of 9 months. In general, adults do more poorly regardless of the chromosome type; for example, the survival was 21 months for the group with >50 chromosomes and 7 months for the t(4;11) group.

The t(4;11)(q21;q23) translocation has been observed in only a specific subtype of acute leukemia which sometimes presents in newborns as a form of congenital leukemia. Leukemic blasts vary from lymphoid to monocytic myeloid in nature. These findings are rarely seen in older patients.

The presence of the Ph^1 chromosome in ALL is a poor prognostic sign, one which occurs three times more frequently in adults than it does in children: 29 adult patients verses 9 children were reported at the Sixth International Workshop. Using DNA Probe Assay it is now possible to differentiate the true typical Ph^1 positive CML, which is bcr+ and p210+, from Ph^1 positive *de novo* ALL, which is bcr- and p190+; the cells seen during a blast crisis of CML, which arise in multipotent stem cells and resemble those of acute leukemia, are bcr+ and p210+. Ph^1 positive T-ALL has been reported. The existence of T-ALL and t-cell lymphoid blast crisis in CML supports the theory that there is a common stem cell for the hematopoietic and lymphoid system. It is important to identify the molecular characteristics of the Ph^1 chromosome in patients because of the difference in survival in Ph^1 positive ALL and CML: 12 months versus 44 months, respectively.

A rearrangement involving chromosome band 8q24 is commonly observed in the t(8;14) translocation of L3 ALL. The median survival is 5 months, regardless of age. Figure 1 shows a patient with L3 ALL with both t(8;22) and t(14;18).

ACUTE NON-LYMPHOCYTIC LEUKEMIA (ANLL)

According to the French-American-British (FAB) classification system, ANLL can be divided into 9 categories as listed below:

MO:	*ANLL but diagnosis of ALL cannot be excluded*
Ml:	*Acute myeloblastic leukemia maturation*
M2:	*Acute myeloblastic leukemia with maturation*
M3(M3V):	*Acute promyelocytic leukemia and hypogranular variant*
M4:	*Acute myelomonocytic leukemia*
M5:.	*Acute monocytic leukemia*
M6:	*Acute erythrocytic leukemia*
M7:	*Acute megakaryocytic leukemia*
M8:	*Definitely ANLL but not otherwise classifiable*

Several chromosomal abnormalities are commonly seen in the different categories of ANLL (4, 5, 6).

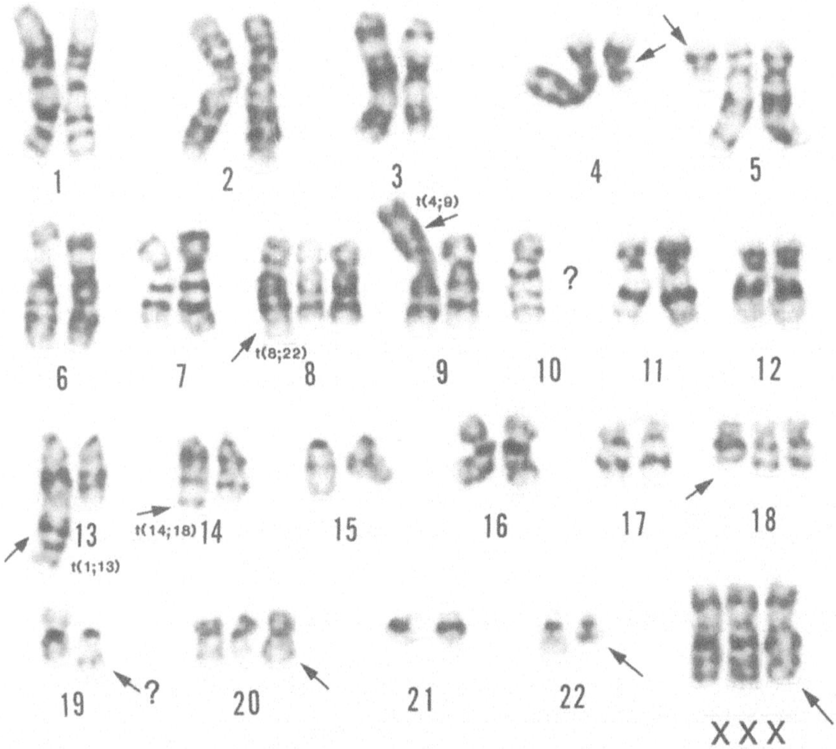

Fig. 1. *A karyotype from a patient with L3; 50,XXX,-10,+18,+20,+del(5)(q12), t(8;22)(q24;q11),t(4;9)(q21;p11),t(1;3)(q21;q34),t(14;18)(q32;q21),19q+.*

Ph[1] *chromosome*: This Ph[1] chromosome is indistinguishable from the one observed in CML (bcr). The incidence of the Ph[1] chromosome is lower in ANLL than in ALL; the percentage of affected patients varied from <1% (3 of 660 *de novo* cases) reported at the Fourth IWCL in 1982 (6) to 9.9% in Japanese patients reported by Sasaki, Kondo, and Tomiyasu (7). It has been noted that the age distribution of the Ph[1] varies in ANLL: the Ph[1] positive patients are evenly distributed throughout the various age groups under 80 years of age.

t(8;21)(q22;q22): Nearly all patients with this translocation have ANLL of the M2 variety, which is characterized by myeloid maturation and a low neutrophil alkaline phosphatase level. This chromosome abnormality occurs with greatest frequency in young patients under 45 years of age. Group Francais de Cytogeneticque Hematologique reported a total of 148 patients (33 children) with a mean age of 30.8 years. These patients had a remission rate of 90.7%, which was similar for both sexes regardless of age; however, the median survival was 24 months in children and only 16 months in adults.

+8: Trisomy 8 is seen in all FAB subgroups. According to the Fourth IWCL report (6), 92% of the cases ranged in age from 20 to >60 years (median 58 years). A complete remission was seen in 43% of the patients and the median survival was 6 months. (Patients with a normal karyotype had a median survival of 10 months).

-5, del(5q), -7, del(7q): These abnormalities of chromosomes 5 and 7 are often seen in secondary leukemia. Twenty nine of the 128 secondary leukemia patients reported at the Fourth IWCL (6) with these abnormalities, 17 (or 60%) of them were in the 50 to 85 year age group. In their study of chromosome 5 deletion, Wisniewski and Hirschhorn (8) reported that 21 of the 29 patients with refractory anemia, polycythemia vera, or ANLL, were aged 50 or more. It can thus be concluded that -5 and del (5q) are not seen in children, and both increase in frequency with progression in age. A substantial amount of evidence indicates that a greater proportion of patients exposed to chemotherapy or radiotherapy have an abnormal karyotype compared to nonexposed patients, and -5 and -7 are the most common chromosomal abnormalities seen in the exposed groups.

Chromosome 1: The age peak for abnormalities of chromosome 1 in the Fourth IWCL study was 60 and 70 years. The sex ratio in these patients showed a predominance of males (5:1). The most frequent type of ANLL was M5 (25%), followed by M2 (16%) and Ml (14%). Breakpoints were predominantly located on the short arm, near the centromere at pll in cases of trisomy lq, and in the terminal area at p36(33->36) in cases with reciprocal translocation. Survival in patients with these abnormalities was short, and death occurred during induction and early relapse in 80% of the cases.

Chromosome 3: Structural rearrangements involving chromosome bands 3q21 and 3q26 are associated with unusually high platelet counts, accompanied by morphological abnormalities of thrombopoiesis in ANLL. The most common 3q abnormalities noted in these patients were inv(3q), t(3q-; 3q+), ins(3;3), and ins (3;5) (4).

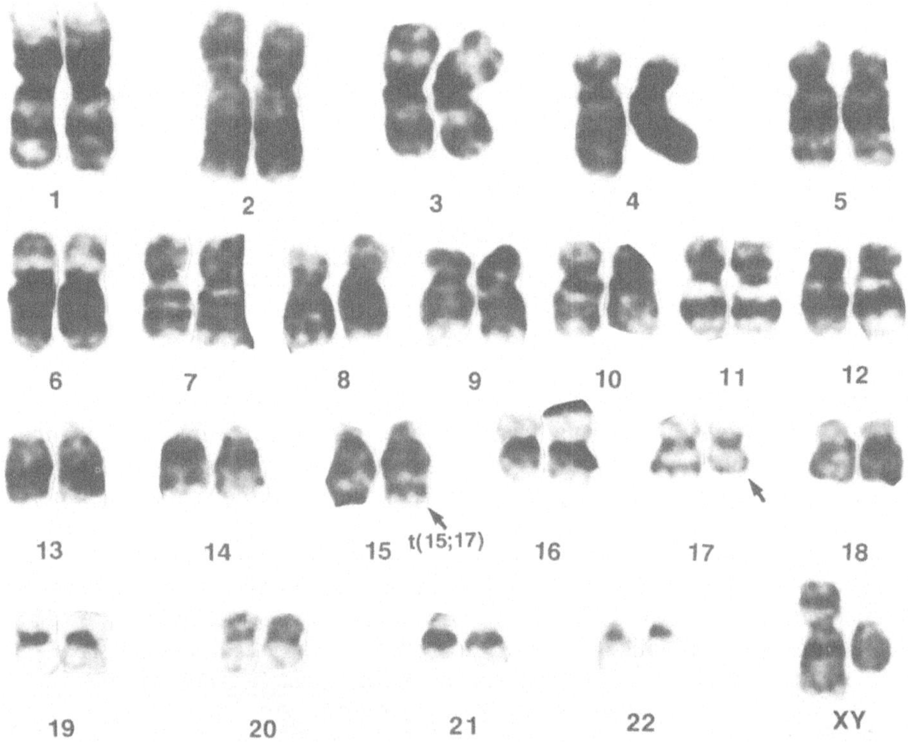

Fig. 2. *A karyotype from a patient with M3: 46,XX,t(15;17)(q24,q21).*

t(6;9) (p23;q34) and del(6)(q23): Patients with t(6;9) appeared to be in the younger age groups, and ranged from 5 to 51 years of age (average 40 years); the median survival was 5 months (4).

t(15;17) (q24;q21): This abnormality is seen exclusively in M3 ANLL (Figure 2).

Abnormalities of 12p, trisomy 13: Both abnormalities are associated with short survival (4).

Inversion 16 and del(16) (q22): No significant morphologic differences were noted between these two. Abnormal eosinophilia, ranging from 8% to 54%, was noted with inversion of chromosome 16, and these patients have a favorable prognosis with standard antileukemic therapy.

Figure 3 demonstrates chromosomal abnormalities (ring chromosome and other markers) in a patient with M4 ANLL.

Correlation of survival with age

Bernard et al (9) studied 78 adult patients with AML and found that increasing age was highly correlated with a shortened survival time. The greatest difference in heterogeneity was between patients under 59 years of age and those over 59. Of the 33 patients under age 59, clinical remission (CR) was obtained in 25 cases (75.8%). Of the 45 patients over 59, CR was obtained in only 13 cases (28.9%). This difference is highly significant. Further classification of patients with AA (aneuploid), AN (mixed normal and aneuploid) and NN (normal) karyotype correlated with age and showed that patients under 59 showed a significant difference between the AA group (CR rate of 20%) and the AN and NN groups (CR rate of 85.7%); in patients over 59, all groups showed significantly poorer remission rates (AA 11%, AN 30%, NN 34.6%).

Survival analysis of 711 patients, including 656 patients with de novo AML were done at the Sixth International Workshop in 1987. The findings were essentially identical to those reported earlier. Survival of older patients, particularly those over age 60, was much shorter than that of younger patients. In evaluating the 51 patients surviving more than 4 years, none of the patients was above 70 years of age at the time of diagnosis; 40 patients under age 50 and 11 patients between ages 50 and 69.

In conclusion, the karyotype is an important independent prognostic factor in acute leukemia; however, age alone, especially above 70 years, is the single most important factor for a poor prognosis.

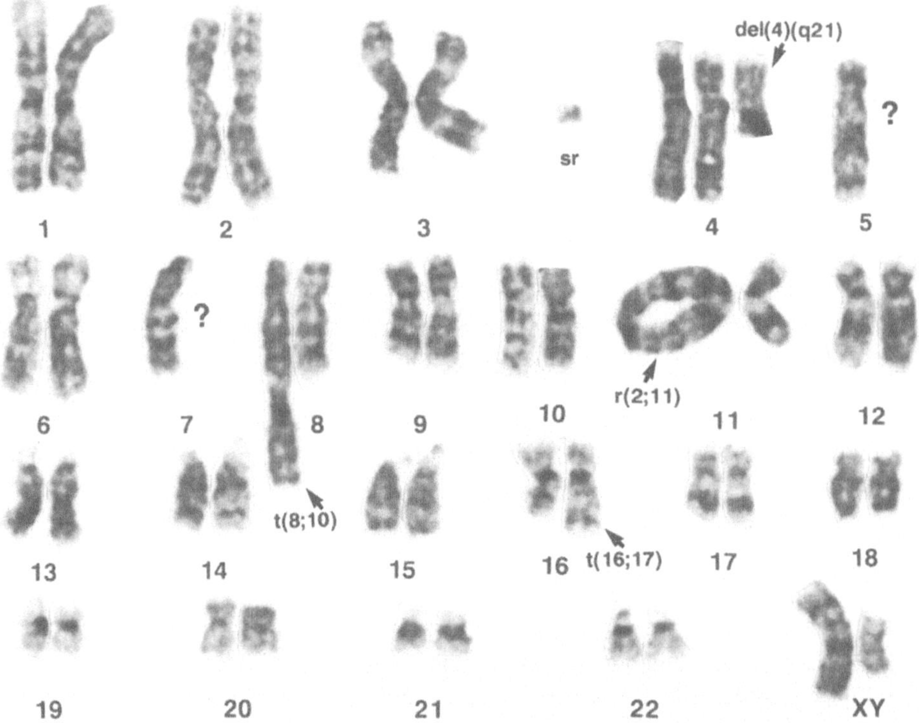

Fig. 3. *A karyotype from a patient with M4; 46,XY,-5,-7,-11,+del(4)(q21),t(8;10)(q24;q11),+r(2;11)(2p25;11p15q23;2q37),t(16;17)(q24;q22),+small ring.*

REFERENCES

1. Gralnick, H., Galton, D.A.G., Catoversusky, D., Sultan, C. and Bennett, J.M. Classification of acute leukemia. *Ann. Int. Med.* 87:740-753 (1977).

2. Bennett, J.M., Catovsky, D., Daniel, M., Flandrin, G., Galton, D.A.G., Gralnick, H.R., Sultan, C. Criteria for the diagnosis of acute leukemia of megakaryocyte lineage (M7). *Ann. Int. Med.* 103:460 (1985).

3. Bloomfield, C.D., Secker-Walker, L.M., Goldman, A.I., Van Den Berghe, H., De la Chapelle, A., Ruutu, T., Alimena, G. Garson, O.M., Golomb, H.M., Rowley, J.D., Kaneko Y., Whang-Peng, J., Prigogina, E., Philip, P., Sandberg, A.A., Lawler, S.D. and Mitelman, F. Six-year follow-up of the clinical significance of karyotype in acute lymphoblastic leukemia. *Cancer Genet. Cytogenet.* 40:171-185 (1989).

4. Whang-Peng, J. and Knutsen, T. The role of cytogenetics in the characterization of acute leukemia, acute lymphoblastic leukemia and acute myeloblastic leukemia. In The acute leukemias, S.A. Stass (ed), Mercel Dekker, Inc., New York (1987).

5. Whang-Peng, J. and Knutsen, T. Cytogenetic studies in neoplasia (human and animal): Implications, prognosis, and treatment. In Influence of tumor development on the host, L.A. Liotta (ed), Kluwer Academic Publisher, Dordrecht, Netherlands, pp. 133-175 (1989).

6. Fourth International Workshop on chromosomes in leukemia: A prospective study of acute non-lymphocytic leukemia. *Cancer Genet. Cytogenet.* 11:249 (1984).

7. Sasaki, M., Kondo, K. and Tomiyasu, T. Cytogenetic characterization of ten cases of Ph^1 positive acute myelogenous leukemia. *Cancer Genet. Cytogenet.* 9:119-128 (1983).

8. Wisniewski, L.P. and Hirschhorn K. Acquired partial deletions of the long arm of chromosome 5 in hematologic disorders. *Am. J. Hematol.* 15:295-310 (1983).

9. Bernard, P., Reiffers, J., Lacombe, F., Dachary, D., David, B., Boisseau, M.R. and Bronstet, A. Prognostic value of age and bone marrow karyotype in 78 adults with acute myelogeous leukemia. *Cancer Genet. Cytogenet.* 7:153-163 (1982).

GLUCOCORTICOID RECEPTORS IN LEUKEMIAS, LYMPHOMAS AND MYELOMAS OF YOUNG AND OLD

Javed Ashraf and E. Brad Thompson

Department of Human Biological Genetics and Chemistry
University of Texas Medical Branch
Galveston, Texas 77550

Glucocorticoids are well-known for their strong suppressive influence on certain cells of the immune system. These pharmacologic effects have long been taken advantage of to suppress immune responses and to treat leukemia and lymphomas. In recent years, a great deal has been learned of the mechanisms by which glucocorticoids affect lymphoid and related cells, and this information now provides a basis for studying the varying susceptibility to glucocorticoid therapy of the leukemias, lymphomas and myelomas in young and older patients. Expression of glucocorticoid receptors themselves is sometimes used as one predictive variable (Bloomfield, 1984; Thompson *et al.*, 1985; Iacobelli *et al.*, 1987). In this brief overview, we will outline the general pattern of expression with age of these groups of malignancies, discuss the recently established principles of glucocorticoid action, and describe some of our own experience with glucocorticoid effects on certain malignant lymphoid cell lines *in vitro*.

In considering steroid effects on malignancies of the hematopoietic system in the young and the old, one must first confront the fact that these are a diverse group of diseases. While leukemia can be classified broadly into four major classes: acute lymphocytic leukemia (ALL), chronic lymphocytic leukemia (CLL), acute myelocytic leukemia (AML) and chronic myelocyte leukemia (CML), each of these has many subdivisions based on cell type, expression of surface markers, and state of cell differentiation (Foon *et al.*, 1986, Soler *et al.*, 1988). There are in addition many rarer forms. The biological behavior and response to therapy of these various leukemias varies dramatically, and so do their behavior and responses to glucocorticoids, depending on the specific characteristics of the transformed cell

The Underlying Molecular, Cellular, and Immunological Factors in Cancer and Aging, Edited by S.S. Yang and H.R.Warner, Plenum Press, New York, 1993

involved. Malignant lymphomas represent cohesive tumorous lesions, primarily of lymphocytes, and are classified broadly into Non-Hodgkins' and Hodgkins' lymphomas, the latter characterized by the presence of unique Reed-Sternberg giant cells. As with the leukemias, the specific transformed cells involved result in many biologically important subclassifications. Myelomas are neoplasms of plasma or closely related cells which synthesize complete or incomplete immunoglobulins. All schemes of classification of these diseases are attempts to categorize so as to provide clean-cut information about origins, prognosis and response to therapy. That all these schemes remain suboptimal is attested by their continuing evolution and subdivision. The second point to consider is that the occurrence of different types of these malignancies tends to cluster at various ages: ALL and AML in young to mid-age adults; CLL, CML and myelomas in older adults. While these statements somewhat oversimplify the situation, they point up the basic truth that in considering the relation of aging to the morbidity and mortality caused by these diseases, one cannot easily follow the behavior of a single disease occurring in young to elderly patients. One old, basic question for which an answer would be very important is: Why do these differing types of hematologic malignancies cluster in certain age ranges? A third issue of importance is that among normal hematologic cells, glucocorticoid sensitivity varies widely. Immature T cells are inhibited, even lysed by glucocorticoids (Review: Homo-Delarche, 1984; Berczi, 1986), while mature T cells are much less sensitive. Subtypes of T cells appear to have variable sensitivity (Distelhorst and Benitto, 1981). B cells are generally found to be rather insensitive to inhibition by glucocorticoids, though there are exceptions. Fourth, and finally, the effects of glucocorticoids on normal cells of hematologic origin are both direct and indirect. These steroids are strong regulators of the genes for several lymphokines upon which the normal growth and function of hematologic cells depend. Thus for example, Interleukins 1 and 2 and Interferon γ are all down-regulated by glucocorticoids (Reviews: Munck *et al.*, 1984; Gessani *et al.*, 1988; Vacca *et al.*, 1990). Since T cell growth and function depend on such lymphokines, the steroid hormone's inhibition of the normal cells may be to a significant extent secondary to inhibition of lymphokine expression. Indeed, it has been proposed that this is the normal way which an immune response is damped (Munck *et al.*, 1984).

These four issues, then, must be kept in mind while attempting to evaluate the effect of glucocorticoids on leukemic diseases in elderly versus younger patients: the diversity of the diseases, the predominance of certain of these diseases in various age ranges, the natural categories of corticoid sensitivity or resistance among classes of normal lymphoid cells, and the potential of secondary control through regulation of some lympho/cytokines by corticoids. The last two factors will obviously affect the patient's own immune system, and the effect of aging on the immune system response to glucocorticoids must also be evaluated. Some exploration of this question in normals has been carried out (Review: Makinodan and Hirayama, 1985). Many malignant hematologic cells have lost or modified their dependence on lymphokines; so this level of control will vary greatly depending on the specific malignancy studied.

STRUCTURE OF GLUCOCORTICOID RECEPTOR

Most physiologic and pharmacologic glucocorticoid actions are mediated through specific intracellular receptors (GR), found in almost all mammalian cells. The human GR (hGR) is a protein of 87,000 Daltons as predicted from its DNA sequence (Hollenberg *et al.*, 1985) but which shows an apparent Mr of - 94,000 on denaturing polyacrylamide gel electrophoresis, presumably due to artifacts resulting from protein phosphorylation. It is coded by a single gene located on chromosome 5q32 (Francke and Foellner, 1989). After binding its specific class of ligand, the GR is activated, in which form it elicits specific cellular responses by regulating the expression of various responsive genes (Reviews: Yamamoto, 1985; Ringold, 1985; Evans, 1988; Beato, 1989; Burnstein and Cidlowski, 1989). The GR and other steroid hormone, thyroid, retinoic acid and vitamin D receptors are therefore ligand-dependent transcription factors, forming a large family, all members of which share certain features. A fragment of the rat GR cDNA was the first of these genes to be cloned (Miesfeld *et al.*, 1984), quickly followed by the hGR and its complete cDNA coding sequence (Hollenberg *et al.*, 1985). Other members of the steroid hormone receptor family followed. By mutagenesis followed by expression of the mutated receptor genes in transfected cells, three fundamental domains in the GR have been defined. In sequence from the amino-terminal end of the protein, these are the highly immunogenic/transactivation domain, the DNA binding domain, and the ligand binding domain (Weinberger *et al.*, 1985). They have been found in closely similar locations in rat and mouse GRs (Miesfeld *et al.*, 1986; Danielsen *et al.*, 1986). As other steroid receptors have been cloned, sequenced and examined, these same features have been evident (Reviews: Evans, 1988; Miesfeld, 1989; Carson-Jurica *et al.*, 1990). Homologies between the GR and the v-*erb*A protein led to the discovery of the thyroid hormone receptor(s) (Weinberger *et al.*, 1986; Sap *et al.*, 1986), and gene library searches with the sequences for the DNA binding regions of the GR and other related receptors resulted in the cloning of the vit D receptor (McDonnell *et al.*, 1987), the retinoic acid receptor (Petkovich *et al.*, 1987; Giguere *et al.*, 1987) and a score or more of related genes with as yet unknown ligands and function (Ryseck *et al.*, 1989, Watson and Milbrandt, 1989). All these genes together comprise what has come to be known as the steroid receptor gene superfamily. Figure 1 is a simple line diagram of some of the members of the family. Vertical marks show the limits of the DNA binding and steroid binding regions, where known. One can see that the size of the DNA binding region is rather constant through the array. The ligand binding region is less so, and the amino-ends are least similar in size. The constant size of the DNA binding region is a reflection of structural constancy also. The DNA binding regions of these proteins contain the sequences with the greatest degree of homology, and certain amino acids are invariant. The homologies are greatest among subsets of these proteins that bind identical ligands, even across species. For example, rat, mouse and human GRs' DNA binding regions are nearly identical. Between GRs and progesterone receptors, slightly greater differences in DNA binding regions exist. The extent of

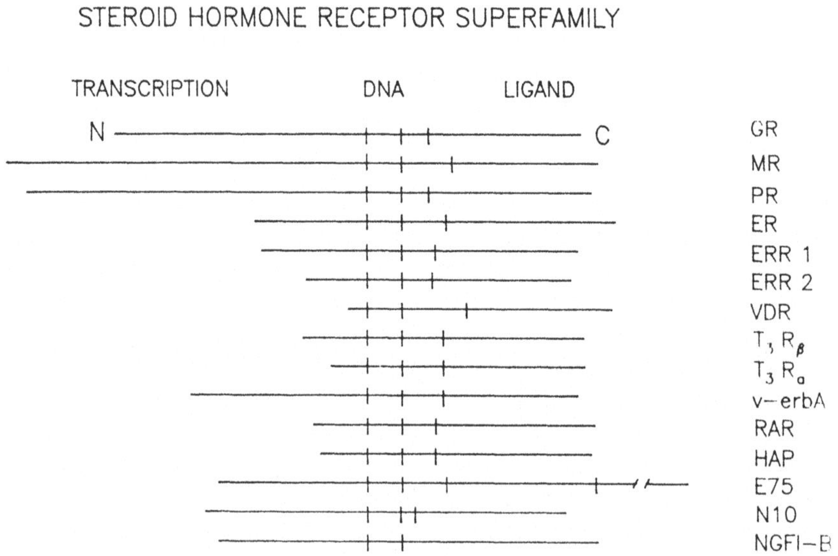

Figure 1. *Proteins of The Steroid Receptor Super Family.* The diagram shows a partial list of the members of this family of structurally related proteins. Each protein is shown as a horizontal line whose length is proportional to the length of the protein's amino acid sequence, amino terminal at the left (N) and carboxy terminal the right (C). The proteins are aligned at their nearly constant-sized DNA-binding regions, bounded by a pair of vertical lines under the heading DNA. The ligand-binding region lies to the carboxy-terminal end (LIGAND), with its amino-terminal limit, where known, indicated by a third vertical stroke. In those examples studied, the portion of the molecule towards the amino terminal relative to the DNA binding region is important for transcription activation; hence this region is under the heading TRANSCRIPTION. (It is well-known that other portions of these molecules also play important roles in regulation of transcription). The initials at the right signify the name of the particular family member, i.e. GR, glucocorticoid receptor; MR, mineralocorticoid receptor, T_3R, thyroid hormone receptor, etc. Several proteins shown indicate "orphan" members of the superfamily, proteins whose function and ligand (if any) are unknown, e.g. NGFIB, nerve growth factor induced gene B.

differences increase as one compares estrogen, thyroid, and other family members to the GR. There are lesser, but considerable homologies between ligand binding regions, and least between amino-terminal regions. One might predict the necessity for ligand class-specific distinctiveness in the ligand binding domains, to provide specific, high affinity fit between ligand and receptor. The variability of the proteins in the region amino-terminal to the DNA binding portion suggests that it may confer functions unique to each receptor. These three domains are functionally independent entities, as demonstrated by experiments involving interchanging ligand binding and DNA-binding domains of two unrelated receptors (Green and Chambon, 1987; Petkovich *et al.*, 1987; Harbour *et al.*, 1990).

i) *Amino terminal, trans-activation domain*

This region, between the amino-terminal and the DNA binding region, constitutes about half of the human GR protein (Weinberger *et al.*, 1985). This region is rich in acidic amino acids, like aspartate and glutamate. Use of yeast GAL4/hGR chimeras, in which the hGR DNA binding region was replaced with that of the yeast GAL4 protein, suggested that autonomous trans-activation signals reside both in the amino and carboxy terminal segments of the human GR (Evans, 1989). A strong transcription regulatory region found in amino terminal region of hGR is known as tau 1 (Giguere *et al.*, 1986; Hollenberg *et al.*, 1987). Mutants of the hGR having duplications of the tau 1 region were "super" active in driving the transcription of MMTV-CAT constructs. Deletion of this region caused virtual elimination of the transcription activity (Evans, 1989). The amino terminal domain of the GR may have interaction signals for other transcription factors (Schule *et al.*, 1988). The GR from an n^{ti} mutant of mouse lacks much of its amino terminal region and is defective in the lymphocytolysis process (Miesfeld, 1989 and references therein). Although the evidence points to a significant role for tau 1 in stimulation of transcription by the GR, the region is not fully mapped in terms of its overall contributions to the GR functions. This domain, in coordination with other domains of the GR, determines the optimal functioning of this protein for transcription enhancement.

ii) *DNA binding Domain*

The DNA binding domain of the GR is a region of about 65 amino acids. It can be cleaved from the rest of the GR by proteolysis (Carlstedt-Duke *et al.*, 1982). Analysis of deletion mutants showed that the amino-terminal and carboxy-terminal regions of the GR are not needed for site-specific *in vitro* binding to DNA (Rusconi and Yamamoto, 1987; Giguere *et al.*, 1986). As noted above, it is the DNA binding domain of the GR that has maximum homology with the analogous regions of other steroid receptors. This region is rich in cysteines, and many of them are conserved among all the steroid receptors (Reviews: Evans 1988, Miesfeld 1989, Carson-Jurica *et al.*, 1990). Site-directed mutagenesis of the DNA binding region showed all the conserved cysteines to be essential for optimal transcription activity, as tested in transfection experiments. Activation of transcription and ability of the GR to bind specific DNA sequences *in vitro* are closely related. However, DNA binding capability of the GR is not sufficient for optimal transcription activation (Miesfeld *et al.*. 1987; Evans, 1989 and see above). As shown in Figure 2, the DNA binding domain of the GR can be divided into two "zinc fingers", similar to that of transcription factor III A (Miller *et al.*, 1985) and numerous other transcription factors. By analyzing X-ray absorption and visible spectra, it was shown that two zinc molecules are involved in forming coordinated cysteine units in the zinc fingers of the rat GR (Freedman *et al.*, 1988). Both the fingers are required for the optimal activity of the GR (Hollenberg and Evans, 1988). However, the first or amino-terminal zinc finger of the GR and estrogen receptors is critical in determining the specificity of binding to target gene DNA (Green *et al.*, 1988, Hard *et al.*, 1990). In addition, a few amino acids within the "knuckle" C-terminal to the first zinc finger were found to be strongly involved in the sequence-specific binding of the GR (Danielsen *et al.*, 1989).

In the absence of ligand, the glucocorticoid receptor appears to exist primarily in the cell's cytoplasmic compartment (Walters, 1985, Antakly *et al.*, 1989). One molecular/genetic analysis implicated an arginine/lysine rich region close to the DNA binding domain as the signal for nuclear translocation (Picard and Yamamoto, 1987; Rusconi and Yamamoto, 1987). When this region of the protein was intact, addition of ligand to tissue culture cells resulted in shift of the GR to the nuclear compartment. Similar sequences of amino acids located similarly in other steroid receptors also seem to be essential for nuclear localization (Review: Carson-Jurica *et al.*, 1990), although these receptors are found in nuclei even in the absence of their ligands (King and Greene, 1984; Perrot-Applanat *et al.*, 1985).

iii) *Steroid Binding Domain*

Succeeding a short stretch of amino acids, the remaining 220 amino acids from 557 through 777, the carboxy-terminal, comprise the steroid binding domain. It appears that this region forms a tight but fragile structural unit responsible for proper hormone binding. Many amino acids participate critically in its structure, since mutations throughout the sequence drastically reduce the steroid binding of the GR (Hollenberg *et al.*, 1987, 1988, Godwski *et al.*, 1987; Miesfeld *et al.*, 1987; Danielson *et al.*, 1986). Some amino acids that make close contact with bound glucocorticoid have been identified. The covalent glucocorticoid affinity ligand dexamethasone mesylate (Simons and Thompson, 1981) has been found to bind to cysteine 656 of the rat GR (Simons *et al.*, 1987), and photo-activated labelling with TA identified met 622 and cys 754 as binding sites (Carlsted-Duke *et al.*, 1988) of the rat GR. Similar experiments showed that dexamethasone mesylate binds to cys 644 of the mouse GR (Smith *et al.*, 1988). The extremely tight binding of the synthetic phenylpyrozolo steroid cortivazol, a very potent glucocorticoid

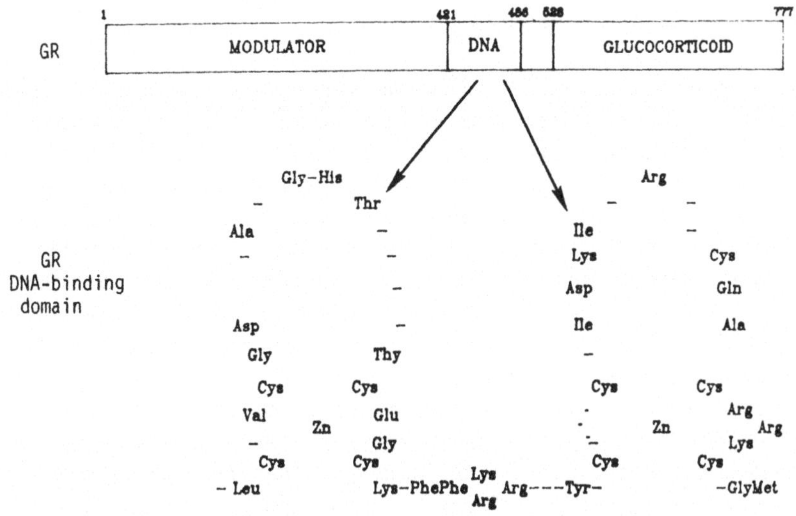

GRE consensus sequence GGTACAnnnTGTTCT

Figure 2. *Diagram of The hGR (Upper Horizontal Bar), Its DNA-binding Sequence Amino Acids 421-486, And The GRE Consensus Sequence to Which The DNA-binding Domain Binds.*

In GR, numbers at top indicate amino acid positions in the primary sequence. MODULATOR, DNA, and GLUCOCORTICOID refer to mapped regions of the protein. MODULATOR contains transcription-enhancing regions DNA is the core DNA-binding region. GLUCOCORTICOID refers to the steroid ligand binding region. The GR DNA-binding domain shows part of the amino acid sequence between 421 and 486 in the configuration of two "zinc fingers," with key amino acids named and variable ones shown by -. The model proposes that the invariant cys coordinate binding a Zn in each "finger" (from Danielsen *et al.*, 1986).

The GRE consensus sequence, compiled from several glucocorticoid- regulated genes, shows the DNA sequence critical for binding GR. Bases in the nucleic acid are given by the standard code in caps; lower case n's refer to three variable bases (from Beato, 1989).

(Harmon *et al.*, 1981; Schlecte *et al.*, 1985; Schlecte and Schmidt 1987; Thompson *et al.*, 1989) suggests that the ligand binding pocket must have a deep hydrophobic region to accept the phenyl group, which has been shown by X-ray crystallography to extend in planar arrangement from the pyrazolo-moiety fused to the A ring (Czerwinski and Thompson, unpublished results).

Aside from simply binding ligand, this region plays several critical roles in GR function. In the unliganded receptor, the steroid binding region appears to prevent the DNA binding region from interacting with its specific DNA binding site. This conclusion is based on experiments showing: that mutations destroying ligand binding block the ability of GR to activate genes carrying the appropriate binding site (Hollenberg *et al.*, 1988; Bronnegard *et al.*, 1988); that complete deletion of the steroid binding region results in a GR which is a weak but constitutive transcription activator (Hollenberg *et al.*, 1987, 1989; Miesfeld *et al.*, 1987) and that the unliganded GR in cell extracts is invariably found complexed to the protein HSP90. Ligand binding results in dissociation of HSP90 from GR concomitant with gain of site-specific DNA-binding and transcription stimulating activity (Review: Pratt, 1990). The amino acid sequence necessary for HSP90 binding is located in the steroid binding region (Denis *et al.*, 1988; Pratt *et al.*, 1989; Dalman *et al.*, 1989).The DNA and steroid binding regions interact to induce genes, but each can act as an independent unit. Thus chimeric receptors constructed with the DNA binding region of the GR replacing that of the estrogen receptor are activated by estradiol due to the ER-specific ligand binding domain, but activate GR-specific genes, determined by the GR's DNA binding domain interacting with its specific sites in those genes (Green and Chambon, 1987). These chimeric receptors also conveyed an estrogen-induced lethal response to leukemic cells normally killed only by glucocorticoids (Harbour *et al.*, 1990).

Finally, the steroid binding region has in its amino-terminal end a region, tau 2, that stimulates the transcriptional potency of the GR (Giguere *et al.*, 1986; Hollenberg *et al.*, 1988). Similar transactivation regions have been found in the carboxy terminal portions of estrogen receptors (Webster *et al.*, 1988) and are important for receptor dimerization (Fawell *et al.*, 1990). Binding of ligand not only frees the receptor to bind DNA, it also enhances that binding, at least in tests of estrogen, thyroid, retinoic acid receptors and chimeras of the DNA and ligand-binding regions between them (Wu and Pfahl, 1988). Receptor binds to specific DNA sequences as a dimer, in a cooperative fashion (Schmid *et al.*, 1989; Tsai *et al.*, 1989). It may be that the enhanced DNA binding by liganded receptor is due to enhanced dimerization (Eriksson and Wrange, 1990).

The GR not only stimulates gene transcription; it also down-regulates expression of certain genes (Reviews: Beato, 1989; Miesfeld, 1989; Carson-Jurica *et al.*, 1990). The trans activation domains of GR seem less important for this negative regulatory function, but detailed structure/function analysis of the negative regulation of genes by GR is still under investigation (Akerblom, *et al.*, 1988). It is intriguing that unliganded retinoic acid and thyroid receptors can act as negative transcription factors for certain genes normally stimulated by their ligands (Glass *et al.*, 1988; Graupner *et al.*, 1989). Analogous experiments have not as yet been carried out for GRs, but the cytoplasmic localization of unliganded GR makes such activity less likely.

Glucocorticoids and other steroids also regulate expression of some genes at post-transcriptional levels (Raghow *et al.*, 1986; Riegel *et al.*, 1987; Dong *et al.*, 1988; Rosewicz *et al.*, 1988). The role of receptor in this regulation is unknown.

GLUCOCORTICOID RESPONSE ELEMENTS

The *cis*-active, specific regulatory DNA sequences to which GRs bind when activated are referred to as glucocorticoid response elements (GREs). These were first identified in the mouse mammary tumor virus long terminal (MMTV LTR) (Buetti and Diggelmann, 1983; Scheidereit *et al.*, 1983; Payvar *et al.*, 1983) and have been located in several other glucocorticoid-induced genes, including tyrosine aminotransferase, glutamine synthetase, metallolthionein IIA, globulin, tryptophan oxygenase, thyrotropin-releasing hormone (Lee *et al.*, 1988), and others (Reviews: Yamamoto, 1985; Evans, 1988; Beato, 1989). The exact sequence of GREs varies slightly in various genes. However, a consensus GRE sequence, GGTACANNNTGT(T/C)CT has been defined (Beato *et al.*, 1987). The hexamer, TGTTCT, the partial dyad symmetry, and the spacing of the semi-symmetrical sequence are critical for the regulation of the transcription by the GR, and they have always been found in the GREs of glucocorticoid-induced genes studied, except that for phosphoenolpyruvate carboxy kinase (Review: Carson-Jurica *et al.*, 1990). Positive GREs are usually found in pairs or in multiples. They are usually present in the 5' flanking promoter region; however they can be found even 3' of the promoter, as in the first intron of the growth hormone gene (Slater *et al.*, 1985). Nuclease protection analysis of the promoter region of the tyrosine aminotransferase gene revealed the presence of two groups of GREs, which were present about 2.5 kb upstream from the transcription start site. The distal GRE in the gene was weakly active; however the proximal GRE could not function alone, probably because it is less **symmetrical.** Cooperative interaction between both GREs was needed for optimal transcriptional activity (Jantzen *et al.*, 1987). Two more physiologically important GREs have been identified farther upstream, about 5 kb upstream from the transcription start of the gene (Grange *et al.*, 1989). Cooperative interaction between pairs of GREs are also needed for the optimal transcriptional regulation of tryptophan oxygenase gene and mouse mammary tumor virus (Danesch *et al.*, 1987; Chalepakis *et al.*, 1988). GREs can also interact cooperatively with other enhancer elements (Review: Ptashne, 1988; Altschmied *et al.*, 1989).

GREs are also recognized with high affinity by progesterone and androgen receptors (Strahle *et al.*, 1987; Ham *et al.*, 1988; Danison *et al.*, 1989). The glucocorticoid and progesterone receptors can bind hormone response sequences in the lysozyme gene at sites that overlap but are not quite identical (von der Ahe *et al.*, 1985). A recent study compared the dual control of a hormonal response element by progestin and glucocorticoid in the same cell line (Nordeen *et al.*, 1989). Site directed mutagenesis experiments indicated that an estrogen response element (ERE) can be converted into a GRE by 1-2 base substitutions (Klock *et al.*, 1987). Two regions outside the loops were identified which were critical in differentiating between the glucocorticoid, estrogen or thyroid response elements (Umesono and Evans, 1989). In sum, gene induction by glucocorticoid usually requires GREs, but other receptors also can use these elements, and slight differences in sequence and interactions with other DNA elements and their binding factors probably have a lot to do with the specific response seen in each particular gene.

REPRESSION OF TRANSCRIPTION BY THE GR

A small number of genes have been studied so far that are negatively regulated by the glucocorticoid receptor. These include proopiomelancortin (POMC) (Eberwine and Roberts, 1984; Charron and Drouin, 1986; Beaulieu *et al.*, 1988), prolactin (Camper *et al.*, 1985; Sakai *et al.*, 1988), rRNA (Cavanaugh *et al.*, 1984), the α subunit of human glycoprotein hormones (Akerblom *et al.*, 1988) and the glucocorticoid receptor itself (Okret *et al.*, 1986; Kalinyak *et al.*, 1987; Dong *et al.*, 1988; Rosewicz *et al.*, 1988). Sequences which seem to mediate negative regulation by the GR have been identified in the prolactin and POMC genes. These sequences are dissimilar to the positive GRE sequences (Sakai *et al.*, 1988; Drouin *et al.*, 1989). It is believed that both transcriptional and post-transcriptional mechanisms are involved in the GR mediated down-regulation of its own mRNA (Dong *et al.*, 1988; Rosewicz *et al.*, 1988). One group has shown that GR interacts in the 3' untranslated sequences of its gene, and this might be involved in the negative regulation of its message (Okret *et al.*, 1986). About 3,000 bases of the promoter region of the GR gene from a human lymphocyte library have been sequenced in our laboratory. This region lacks any classical GRE, CAAT or TATA box and contains many binding sites for transcription factor Spl (Zong *et al.*, 1990). A 1.5kb fragment of this region containing the transcription start site was used to drive the expression of a reporter gene transfected into COS cells. Our preliminary results (Ashraf, Zong and Thompson, unpublished results) show that this promoter region of the GR gene may be involved in its negative regulation. In the case of the gene for the α-subunit of pituitary FSH and LH, interference between the GRE and an overlapping cyclic AMP response element seems to account for negative regulation (Akerblom *et al.*, 1988).

POSSIBLE MECHANISMS INVOLVED IN DETERMINING THE EFFICIENCY OF TRANSCRIPTIONAL REGULATION BY GLUCOCORTICOID RECEPTORS

The mechanisms involved in the transcriptional regulation by the GR are yet to be completely understood. On the basis of the studies to date, it can be concluded that there are involved: **1)** Cooperative interactions between GREs in responsive genes. In an *in vitro* transcription system, driven by GR, tandem GREs are considerably stronger than single ones (Tsai *et al.*, 1990). **2)** Interaction of transcription factors with the hormone receptor (Review: Ptashne, 1988), synergistic in some cases (Schule *et al.*, 1988), may determine the rate of the transcription of a gene. Relative availability of these factors may determine tissue-specific hormonal response. **3)** Chromatin structural features may also be important. Some studies have suggested that nucleosomes, positioned critically, can prevent binding of various *trans* factors in the regulatory regions of the gene. After binding to hormone regulatory elements, the activated steroid receptor may help in moving up nucleosomes so that various specific factors could bind in those regions (Review: Beato, 1989).

MECHANISM OF ACTIVATION OF THE RECEPTOR

There are several interdependent and closely regulated steps which GR undergoes prior to the transcriptional regulation of the responsive genes. These steps are phosphorylation, binding of the hormone, dissociation of heat shock protein 90 (HSP 90), translocation to the nucleus, proper binding of the activated GR to the specific recognition sequences in the chromatin, receptor dimerization and interactions with other nuclear factors. However, the exact biochemistry of these steps is still being studied.

It is generally believed that a phosphorylated form of the GR, which binds steroids, is needed for optimal functioning (Schmidt and Litwack, 1982; Mendel *et al.*, 1990; Hoeck and Groner, 1990). However, this step of the GR activation pathway is not fully understood. In its non-activated form, the GR is found associated *in vivo* with a heat shock protein, HSP 90 (Housely *et al.*, 1985; Mendel *et al.*, 1986; Pratt *et al.*, 1989). Hormone dependent dissociation of HSP90 from the GR is required for the activation of the receptor (Sanchez *et al.*, 1987; Pratt *et al.*, 1989; Pratt, 1990). Binding of hormone is essential for the GR to be translocated to the nucleus, and withdrawal of hormone causes reverse translocation of the GR back to the cytosol (Hock *et al.*, 1989). Sanchez et al (1990) have identified a unique 56-59 kDa (p56-59). protein which complexes with inactivated GR-HSP 90 complex. The homodimer form of the receptor may be needed for optimal specific binding to DNA. Loss of the N-terminal domain of the receptor disrupts these contacts, which results in decreased specificity of DNA binding (Ericksson and Wrange, 1990). Thus the picture that is emerging is that the unactivated GR HSP90 complex (possibly + p56-59) binds steroid, releasing the holoreceptor, which translocates and cooperatively binds to GREs as a homodimer, possibly associating with other transcription factors.

MODELS FOR THE GLUCOCORTICOID-RECEPTOR ACTIONS IN HEMATOLOGIC DISEASES OF THE YOUNG AND OLD

As a model for the effects of glucocorticoids and their receptors in a typical childhood leukemia, we have worked extensively with clones from a cell line known as CEM (Foley *et al.*, 1965). These cells are primitive T lymphoblasts, CD-4 positive, and our standard "wild-type" clone is known as C7. CEM-C7 cells are quite sensitive to dexamethasone and contain receptors for that class of ligand. The biological and biochemical effects seen, following addition of glucocorticoid to these cells, depend on occupancy of receptor (Norman *et al.*, 1981; Harmon *et al.*, 1984). Figure 3 shows a simple time line of some of the major effects that we have described in these cells. In an hour or so after addition of dexamethasone, one sees the beginning of induction of glutamine synthetase and soon thereafter of the glucocorticoid receptor itself (Harmon *et al.*, 1982; Eisen *et al.*, 1988). Also, in this early time period, there is rapid down regulation of the messenger RNA for the c-*myc* protooncogene (Yuh and Thompson, 1989). These events reach their full effect

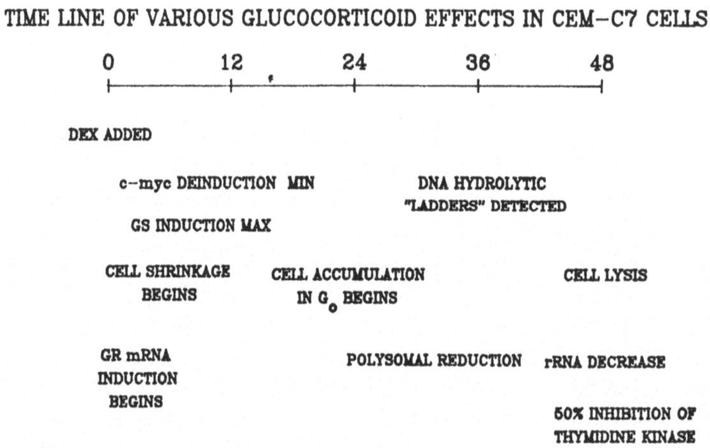

Approximate times of selected events in CEM-C7 cells following addition of glucocorticoid.

Figure 3. *Sequence of Several Events Known to Follow Addition of Glucocorticoid (DEX) to CEM-C7 Cells.*

at about 12 to 18 hours, depending on the specific response. Up to and including about 24 hours, if all steroid is washed from the cells, no effect is seen on cell viability as measured by the ability of the cells to clone (Norman *et al.*, 1978; Harmon *et al.*, 1979). Beginning at about 24 hour and increasingly thereafter, other events occur. These include sequestration of cells in a G1-like cell cycle phase, the beginning of cell death which occurs in a stochastic fashion, and a number of biochemical parallels such as deinduction of ornithine decarboxylase, thymidine kinase and rRNA synthesis (E.B. Thompson, unpublished results). Starting around 36 hours, one sees increasing degrees of DNA fragmentation. By 72 hours or so, there has been considerable cell kill, and few cells of the original population survive.

We have shown that spontaneous resistance to high dose of dexamethasone occurs in this clone of cells, at a rate of about 10-5 per cell per generation, and we have derived mutant subclones from C7 with or without mutagenesis, followed by selection in dexamethasone (Harmon and Thompson, 1981). In these clones growth continues unabated, even in the presence of up to $1O^{-5}$M dexamethasone. We have shown that all such clones contain one or another form of receptor defect (Harmon and Thompson, 1981; Harmon *et al.*, 1984, 1985, 1989; Schmidt *et al.*, 1980; Thompson *et al.*, 1988). In addition, we have isolated a clone from the original uncloned CEM stock without a selection in hormone. This clone has glucocorticoid receptors which appear to be normal, but is none the less resistant to cell lysis by dexamethasone (Zawydiwski *et al.*, 1983). These results combine to show the receptor dependence of cell kill, the need for continued steroid at receptor-saturating concentrations for a long period before death occurs, and the correlation of certain biochemical events with the kill process. The most striking of these correlation is the deinduction of the protooncogene c-*myc*. We recently found that this deinduction is tightly correlated with the ability of the hormone to elicit eventual cell lysis (Yuh and Thompson 1989). In this sense it is quite unlike certain other biochemical parameters, such as the induction of glutamine synthetase. Its induction occurs normally in CEM-C1 cells, the clone that has receptors but is not growth inhibited or lysed by glucocorticoids (Zawydiwski et al., 1983). Such inducible markers are a measure of the functionality of the receptor but are dissociable from growth inhibition. In clone C1, c-*myc* is not deinduced and the cells are not growth inhibited, showing that although the receptor functions, its ability to provoke cell lysis can be dissociated from that event by some blockage. Somatic cell hybrids between clone CEM-C1 and one of our receptor deficient clones, showed that this block is not dominant and that the receptor in C1 could complement the defect in the receptor mutant (Yuh and Thompson, 1987). We have confirmed that result in subsequent experiments by supplying the same mutant clone (ICR 27) with a transfected DNA coding for the entire human GR. This also restored the ability of this mutant to respond to dexamethasone with cell lysis (Harbour *et al.*, 1990). We have now begun to map the regions of the glucocorticoid receptor necessary for cell lysis by further transfections of various modified human glucocorticoid receptor genes to see whether they restore the lysis response of the receptor-defective mutant clone. Our initial gene transfection experiments pointed to the importance of the DNA binding region for this process. An insertion mutant in the first zinc finger of the hGR blocked the lytic effect in the transfected cells, and a chimeric gene containing the DNA binding region of the hGR, replacing that of the estrogen receptor, converted signal for the lytic response from glucocorticoid to estrogen (Harbour *et al.*, 1990). Pursuing these results, we have now carried out transfection experiments with a larger number of mutant glucocorticoid receptors (Figure 4). We are now preparing a full report of this work, but our preliminary results indicate that neither the steroid binding region of the receptor nor the amino terminal region preceding the DNA binding site, is essential for provoking the lytic response. Furthermore, they show that loss of the steroid binding region leaves a receptor form which in itself is lytic, even in the absence of ligand. The potency of this form is equal to that of holoreceptor + ligand, in contrast with the results for induction of genes from GRE sites. The role of the myc protooncogene product in control of normal and malignant lymphoid cell growth with age, and the function and behavior of the glucocorticoid receptor therefore obviously represent areas of relevance to the intentions of this workshop.

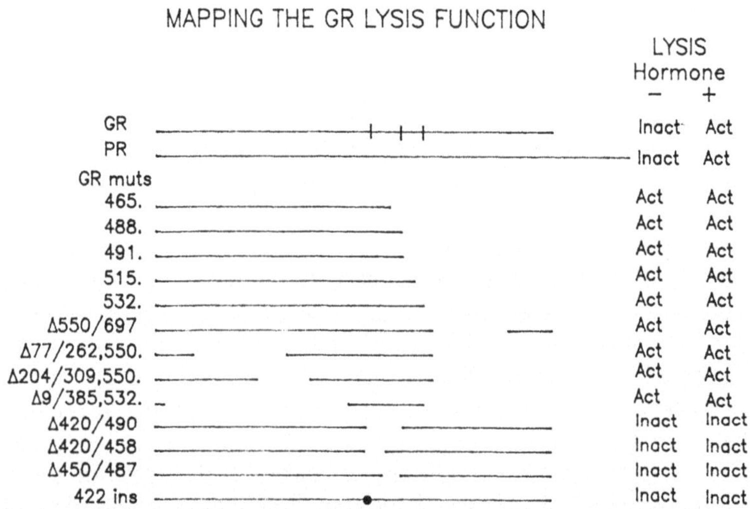

Figure 4. *Functional Mapping of The Regions of The Steroid Receptor Necessary for Lysis of Receptor-Deficient ICR-27 Leukemic Cells.* The diagram shows each receptor or receptor mutant as a horizontal line, to scale according to its amino acid sequence. GR, holo glucocorticoid receptor; PR holo progesterone receptor; GR muts, glucocorticoid receptor mutants. For the mutants, the numbers at the left signify the termini of truncated or deleted fragments; 422 ins. signifies an insertion mutant in the zinc finger. The columns at the right tell whether the receptor or receptor fragment was active (Act) or inactive (Inact) in causing lysis of the recipient cells in the absence (-) or presence (+) of hormone. For all the glucocorticoid receptor forms, Hormone was 10^{-5}M dexamethasone; for the PR, Hormone was 10^{-5}M progesterone.

As a second model system typical of one of the hematologic malignancies more often seen in the elderly, we have been studying several cell lines derived from multiple myeloma. With these we have been able to show that some are glucocorticoid sensitive and others are resistant, although all have glucocorticoid receptors. Thus we have shown formally that those myelomas which are responding to glucocorticoid therapy can be doing so as a result of the direct effects of the steroid on the myeloma cell itself, even though these are of B cell derivation, a class of lymphoid cell traditionally thought to be relatively resistant to glucocorticoids. In the clone of myeloma cells which are sensitive to growth inhibition by glucocorticoids, we have made a singular observation. As background to this data it is important to point out that many studies have shown in a variety of tissues,'that often the effect of administration of glucocorticoid is down regulation of its own receptor, which may occur by any of several mechanisms (Okret *et al.*, 1986; Kalinyak *et al.*, 1987; Dong *et al.*, 1988; Rosewicz *et al.*, 1988). Recently however, Harmon's laboratory found that dexamethasone induces rather than reduces the glucocorticoid receptor and its message in a clonal line of glucocorticoid-inhibited acute lymphoblastic leukemic cells (Eisen *et al.*, 1988). We carried out similar studies in the myeloma cell lines under study in our laboratory. The results (Figure 5) showed that OPM-II, the line sensitive to inhibition of growth by glucocorticoid, also showed induction of the GR message. The concentrations of hormone to carry out this induction were consistent with those for occupancy of receptor; so there was a rough proportionality between extent of GR mRNA induction and extent of occupancy of receptor, based on the affinity of ligand for receptor in those cells. Only at extremely high concentrations was there a very slight induction of receptor in OPM-I, the line of growth insensitive cells (Gomi et al., 1990).

These findings provoked our curiosity about the nature of the promoter of the glucocorticoid receptor gene. How could this gene in some cells respond to ligand by induction and in others by repression? Accordingly, we have cloned and sequenced the genomic gene for human GR (Zong *et al.*, 1990). We found that it contains no authentic GRE sites in the 3,000 bases prior to the transcription start sites. Instead, the promoter is rich in GC boxes, known as binding sites for the ubiquitous transcription factor SP1. As in other GC-rich promoters, the hGR promoter lacks other canonical promoter regulatory sites (i.e. TATA box and CAAT box). At approximately -2.5 kb, the hGR regulatory region shows two sequences consistent with the nGRE found in the POMC gene. Whether these function to convey down-regulation of hGR by its own ligand in those cells and tissues where that effect is seen, remains to be shown. Since there is no GRE in the promoter of the human GR, it seem likely that the ligand-dependent induction of the gene occurs as a result of indirect rather than direct actions of glucocorticoids. It is possible also that true GREs will be found even farther upstream. Since the content of GR in cells is related to their degree of response, the regulation of this gene in aging populations and in the cancers of old versus young patients, will be important to understand.

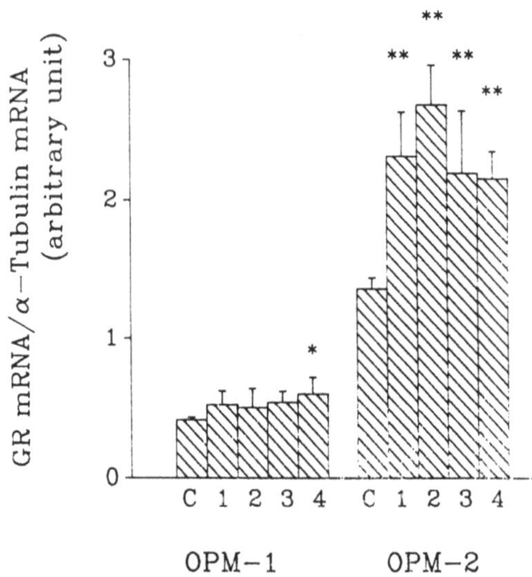

Figure 5. *Regulation of GR mRNA by DEX.*

Cells were treated with 10^{-9}M (1), 5 x 10^{-9}M (2), 10^{-8}M (3), or 10^{-7}M (4) DEX for 24 h. Total cellular RNA was extracted and slot blotted onto Gene Screen Plus filters. The filters were first probed for GR and reprobed for tubulin after stripping the GR probe. Autoradiograms were scanned densitometrically and the GR signal was normalized to the tubulin control, to adjust for slight variations in RNA applied. Data are mean ± SD, n = 4 or 5. Significant difference from control (C):*P<0.05; **P<O.Ol. Reprinted from Gomi, *et al.*, 1990, with permission of the publisher.

SUMMARY

In this paper we have briefly reviewed the nature of leukemias and lymphomas in the old and the young. We surveyed in general the ways in which lymphoid cells and other hematologic elements respond to glucocorticoids, mentioning that there may be direct or indirect effects on their growth by these ligands. We have reviewed the current general model for the action of glucocorticoids in all cells, namely the fact that the actions of these steroids are mediated to a large extent through binding with ligand-activated transcription factors, their receptors. The growing wealth of detail about the nature of the interaction of these receptors with regulatory sites in the genome is discussed. Finally, we have described our results with lines of tissue culture cells representing clones from a typical leukemia of the young, and of myeloma, a typical hematologic malignancy of the elderly. Several features of the effects of glucocorticoids on these cells point up areas that would be pertinent to explore in aging and in the relationship of hematologic diseases to survival and response to therapy in the older versus the younger patient.

REFERENCES

Akerblom, I. E., Slater, E. P., Beato, M., Baxter, J. D. and Mellon, P. L. Negative regulation by glucocorticoids through interference with a cAMP responsive enhancer. *Science* 241:350-353 (1988).

Altschmied, J., Muller, M., Baniahmad, A., Steiner, E. and Renkawitz, R. Cooperative interaction of chicken lysozyme enhancer sub-domains partially overlapping with a steroid receptor binding site. *Nucleic Acid Research* 17:4975-4991 (1989).

Antakly, T., Thompson, E. B. and O'Donnell, D. Demonstration of the intracellular localization and up-regulation of glucocorticoid receptor by *in situ* hybridization and immunocytochemistry. *Cancer Research* 49:2230s-2234s (1989).

Beato, M., Arnemann, J., Chalepakis, G., Slater, E. and Willmann, T. Gene regulation by steroid hormones. *J. Steroid Biochem.* 27:9-14 (1987).

Beato, M. Gene regulation by steroid hormones. *Cell* 56:335-344 (1989).

Beaulieu, S., Gagne, B. and Barden, N. Glucocorticoid regulation of proopiomelanocortin messenger ribonucleic acid control of rat hypothalamus. *Mol. Endocrinol.* 2:727-731 (1988).

Berczi, I. The influence of pituitary-adrenal axis on the immune system. In: Berczi, I. (ed.) **Pituitary Function and Immunity**. CRC Press Inc., Boca Raton, FL., pp. 54-134 (1986).

Bloomfield, C. D. Glucocorticoid receptors in leukemia and lymphoma. *J. Clin. Oncol.*, 2:323-328 (1984).

Bronnegard, M., Andersson, 0., Edwell, D., Lund, J., Norstedt, G. and Carlstedt-Duke, J. Human calpactin H (Lipocortin 1) messenger ribonucleic acid is not induced by glucocorticoid. *Mol. Endocrinol.* 2:732-739 (1988).

Buetti, E. and Diggelmann, H. Glucocorticoid regulation of mouse mammary tumor virus: identification of a short essential DNA region. *EMBO J.* 2:1423-1429 (1983).

Burnstein, K. L. and Cidlowski, J. S. Regulation of gene expression by glucocorticoids. *Ann. Rev. Physiol.* 51:683-699 (1989).

Camper, S.A., Yao, Y.A.S., and Rottman, F.M. Hormonal regulation of the bovine prolactin promoter in rat pituitary tumor cells. *J. Biol. Chemistry* 260:12246-12251 (1985).

Carlstedt-Duke, J., Okret, S., Wrange, 0. and Gustafsson, J-A. Immunochemical analysis of the glucocorticoid receptor: Identification of a third domain separate from the steroid-binding and DNA-binding domains. *Proc. Natl. Acad. Sci. (USA).* 79:4260-4264 (1988).

Carlstedt-Duke, J., Stromstedt, P. E., Wrange, 0., Bergamn, T., Gustafsson, J-A. and Jornvall, H. Domain structure of the glucocorticoid receptor protein. *Proc. Natl. Acad. Sci. (USA)* 84:4437-4440 (1987).

Carlstedt-Duke, J., Stomstedt, P. E., Persson, B., Cederlund, E., Gustafsson, J-A. and Jornvall, H. Identification of hormone interacting amino acids residues with the steroid binding domain of the glucocorticoid receptor in relation to other steroid hormone receptors. *J. Biol. Chem.* 263:6842-6846 (1982).

Carson-Jurica, M. A., Schrader, W. T. and O'Malley, B. W. Steroid receptor superfamily: Structure and functions. *Endocrin. Rev.* 11:201-220 (1990).

Cavanaugh, A. H., Gokal, P. K., Lawther, R. P. and Thompson E. A. Jr. Glucocorticoid inhibition of initiation of transcription of the DNA encoding rRNA (rDNA) in lymphosarcoma P1798 cells. *Proc. Natl. Acad. Sci. (USA).* 81:718-721 (1984).

Chalepakis, G., Arnemann, J., Slater, E., Bruller, H. J., Gross, B. and Beato, M. Differential genes activation by glucocorticoids and progestins through the hormone regulatory element of mouse mammary tumor virus, Cell. 53:371-382 (1988).

Charron, J. and Drouin, J. Glucocorticoid inhibition of transcription from episomal proopimelancortin gene promoter. *Proc. Natl. Acad. Sci. (USA).* 83:8903-8907 (1986).

Dalman, F. C., Bresnick, E. H., Patel, P. D., Perdew, G. H., Watson, J.J., Jr. and Pratt, W. B. Direct evidence that the glucocorticoid receptor binds to hsp 90 at or near the termination of receptor translation *in vitro. J. Biol. Chem.,* 264:19815-19821 (1989).

Danesch, U., Gloss, B., Schmid, W., Schutz, G., Schule R. and Renkawitz, R. Glucocorticoid induction of the rat tryptophan oxygenase gene is mediated by two widely separated glucocorticoid responsive elements. *EMBO J.* 6:625-630 (1987).

Danielsen, M., Northrop, J. P. and Ringold, G. M. The mouse glucocorticoid receptor: Mapping of functional domains by cloning, sequencing and expression of wild-type and mutant receptor proteins. *EMBO J.* 5:2513-2522 (1986).

Danielsen, M., Hinck, L. and Ringold, G. M. Two amino acids within the knuckle of the first zinc finger specify DNA response element activation by the glucocorticoid receptor. *Cell* 57:1131-1138 (1989).

Danison, S. H., Sands, A. and Tindall, D. J. A tyrosine aminotransferase glucocorticoid response element also mediates androgen enhancement of gene expression. *Endocrinol.* 124:1091-1093 (1989).

Denis, M., Gustafsson, J. A., Wikstrom, A.-C. Interaction of the Mr 90,000 heat shock protein with the steroid-binding domain of the glucocorticoid receptor. *J. Biol. Chem.* 263:18520-18523 (1988).

Distelhorst, C. W. and Benitto, B. M. Glucocorticoid receptor content of T-lymophocytes: Evidence for heterogeneity. *J. Immunol.* 126:1630-1634 (1981).

Dong, Y., Poellinger, L., Gustafsson, J-A. and Okret, S. Regulation of glucocorticoid receptor expression: evidence for transcriptional and postranslational mechanisms. *Mol. Endocrinol.* 2:1256-1264 (1988).

Drouin, J., Sun, Y. L. and Nemers, M. Glucocorticoid repression of pro-opiomelanocortin gene transcription. *J. Steroid Biochem.* 34:63-39 (1989).

Eberwine, J. H. and Roberts, J. L. Glucocorticoid regulation of pro-opiomelanocortin gene trnascription in the rat pituitary. *J. Biol. Chem.* 259:2166-2170 (1984).

Eisen, L. P., Elsasser, M. S. and Harmon, J. M. Positive regulation of the glucocorticoid receptor in human T-cells sensitive to the cytolytic effects of glucocorticoids. *J. Biol. Chem.* 263:12044-12048 (1988).

Eriksson, P. and Wrange, 0. Protein-protein contacts in the glucocorticoid receptor homodimer influence its DNA binding properties. *J. Biol. Chem* . 265:3535-3542 (1990).

Evans, R. M. The steroid and thyroid hormone receptor superfamily. *Science* 240:889-895 (1988).

Evans, R. M. Molecular characterization of the glucocorticoid receptor. *Rec. Prog. Hormone Res.* 45:1-22 (1989).

Fawell, S. E., Lees, J. A., White, R. and Parker, M. G. Characterization and colocalization of steroid binding and dimerization activities in the mouse estrogen receptor. *Cell* 60:953-962 (1990).

Foley, G. E., Lazarus, H., Farber, S., Uzman, B. G., Boone, B. A. and McCarthy, R. E. *Cancer* 18:522-529 (1965).

Foon, K. A., Gale, R. P. and Todd, R. F. III Recent advances in the immunologic classification of leukemia. *Semin. Hematol.* 23:257-283 (1986).

Francke, U. and Foellmer, B. E. The glucocorticoid receptor gene is in 5q-q32. *Genomics* 4:610-612 (1989).

Freedman, L. P., Luisi, B. F., Korszun, Z. R., Basavappa, R., Sigler, P. B. and Yamamoto, K. R. The function and structure of the metal coordination sites within the glucocorticoid receptor DNA binding domain. *Nature* 334:543-546 (1988).

Fuxe, K., Wikstrom, A. C., Okret, S., Agnati, L. F., Hartstrand, A., Yu, Z. Y., Grandholm, L., Zoli, M., Vale, W., Gustafsson, J. A. Mapping of glucocorticoid receptor immunoreactive neurons in the rat tel- and diencephalon using a monoclonal antibody against rat liver glucocorticoid receptor. *Endocrinol.* 117:1803-1812 (1985).

Gessani, S., McCandless, S. and Baglioni, C. The glucocorticoid dexamethasone inhibits synthesis of interferon by decreasing the level of its mRNA. *J. Biol. Chem.* 263:7454-7457 (1988).

Giguere, V., Hollenberg, S. M., Rosenfeld, M. G. and Evans, R. M. Functional domains of the human glucocorticoid receptor. *Cell* 46:645-652 (1986).

Giguere, V., Ong, E. S., Segui, P. and Evans, R. Identification of a receptor for the morphogen retinoic acid. *Nature* 330:624-629 (1987).

Glass, C. K., Holloway, J. M., Devary, 0. V. and Rosenfeld, M. G. The thyroid hormone receptor binds with opposite transcriptional effects to a common sequence motif in thyroid hormone and estrogen response elements. *Cell* 54:313-323 (1988).

Godowski, P. J., Rusconi, S., Miesfeld, R. and Yamamoto, K. R. Glucocorticoid receptor mutants that are constitutive activators of transcriptional enhancement. *Nature* 325:365-368 (1987).

Gomi, M., Moriwaki, K., Katagiri, S., Kurata, Y. and Thompson, E. B. Glucocorticoid effects on myeloma cells in culture: correlation of growth inhibition with induction of glucocorticoid receptor messenger RNA. *Cancer Research* 50:1873-1878 (1990).

Grange, T., Roux, J., Rigaud, G. and Pictet, R. Two remote glucocorticoid responsive units interact cooperatively to promote glucocorticoid induction of rat tyrosine aminotransferase. *Nucleic Acid Research* 17:8695-8709 (1989).

Graupner, G., Wills, K. N., Tzukerman, M., Zhang, X. K. and Pfahl, M. Dual regulatory role for thyroid-hormone receptors allows control of retinoic acid receptor activity. *Nature* 340:653-656 (1989).

Green, S. and Chambon, P Oestradiol induction of a glucocorticoid-responsive gene by a chimeric receptor. *Nature* 325:75-81 (1987).

Green, S., Kumar, V., Theulaz, 1., Wahli, W. and Chambon, P. The N-terminal DNA binding 'zinc finger' of the oestrogen and glucocorticoid receptors determines target genes specificity. *EMBO J.* 7:3037-3044 (1988).

Gustafsson, J-A., Carlstedt-Duke, J., Stromstedt, P. E., Wikstrom, A. C., Denis, M., Okret, S. and Dong, Y. Structure function and regulation of the glucocorticoid receptor. *Prog. in Clin. and Biol. Res.* 322:65-80 (1990).

Ham, J., Thompson, A., Neddham, M., Webb, P. and Parker, M. Characterization of response elements for androgens, glucocorticoids and progestins in mouse mammary tumor virus. *Nucleic Acid Research* 16:5263-5277 (1988).

Harbour, D. V., Chambon, P. and Thompson, E. B. Steroid mediated lysis of lymphoblasts requires the DNA binding region of the steroid hormone receptor. *J. Steroid Biochem.* 35:1-9 (1990).

Hard, T., Kellenbach, E., Boelens, R., Maleo, B. A., Dahlman, K., Freedman, L. P., Carlstedt-Duke, J., Yamamoto, K. R., Gustafsson, J.-A. and Kaptein, R. Solution structure of the glucocorticoid receptor DNA binding domain. *Science* 249:157-160 (1990).

Harmon, J. M., Norman, M. R., Fowlkes, B. J. and Thompson, E. B. Dexamethasone induces irreversible GI arrest and death of a human lymphoid cell line. *J. Cell Physiol.* 98:267-278 (1979).

Harmon, J. M. and Thompson, E. B. Isolation and characterization of dexamethasone-resistant mutants from human lymphoid cell line CEM-C7. *Mol. Cell. Bio.* 1:512-521 (1981).

Harmon, J. M., Schmidt, T. J. and Thompson, E. B. Deacylcortivazol acts through glucocorticoid receptors. *J. Steroid Biochem.* 14:273-279 (1981).

Harmon, J. M. and Thompson, E. B. Glutamine synthetase induction by glucocorticoids in the glucocorticoid-sensitive human leukemic cell line CEM-C7. *J. Cell Physiol.* 110:155-160 (1982).

Harmon, J. M., Schmidt, T. J. and Thompson, E. B. Molybdate-sensitive and molybdate-resistant activation-labile glucocorticoid receptor mutants of the human lymphoid cell line CEM-C7. *J. Steroid Biochem.* 21:227-236 (1984).

Harmon, J. M., Thompson, E. B. and Baione, K. A. Analysis of glucocorticoid-resistant human leukemic cells by somatic cell hybridization. *Cancer Research* 45:1587-1593 (1985).

Harmon, J. M., Elsasser, M. S., Eisen, L. P., Urda, L. A., Ashraf, J. and Thompson, E.B. Glucocorticoid receptor expression in 'receptorless' mutants isolated from the human leukemic cell line CEM-C7. *Mol. Endocrinol.* 3:734-743 (1989).

Hock, W., Martin, F., Jaggi, R. and Groner, B. Regulation of glucocorticoid receptor activity. *J. Steroid Biochem.* 34:71-78 (1989).

Hoeck, W. and Groner B. Hormone-dependent phosphorylation of the glucocorticoid receptor occurs mainly in the amino-terminal transactivation domain. *J. Biol. Chem.* 265:5403-5408 (1990).

Hollenberg, S. M., Weinberger, C., Ong, E. S., Cerelli, G., Oro, A., Lebo, R., Thompson, E. B., Rosenfeld, M. G. and Evans, R.M. Primary structure and expression of functional human glucocorticoid receptor cDNA. *Nature* 318:635-641 (1985).

Hollenberg, S. M., Giguere, V., Segui, P. and Evans, R. M. Colocalization of DNA-binding and transcriptional activation functions in the human glucocorticoid receptor. *Cell* 49:39-46 (1987).

Hollenberg, S. M. and Evans, R. M. Multiple and cooperative transactivation domains of the human glucocorticoid receptor. *Cell* 55:899-906 (1988).

Hollenberg, S.M., Giguere, B., Evans, R. Identification of two regions of the human glucocorticoid receptor hormone binding domain that block activation. *Cancer Research* 49:2292s-2294s (1989).

Homo-Delarche, F. Glucocorticoid receptors and steroid sensitivity in normal and neoplastic human lymphoid tissues: A review. *Cancer Research* 44:431-437 (1984).

Housley, P. R., Sanchez, E. R., Westphal, H. M., Beato, M. and Pratt, W. B. The molybdate-stabilized L-cell glucocorticoid receptor isolated by affinity chromatography or with a monoclonal antibody is associated with a 90-92 kDa non-steroid-binding phosphoprotein. *J. Biol. Chem.* 260:13810-13817 (1985).

Iacobelli, S., Marchetti, P., De-Rossi, G., Mandelli, F. and Gentiloni, N. Glucocorticoid receptors predict response to combination chemotherapy in patients with acute lymphoblastic leukemia. *Oncology* 44:13-16 (1987).

Jantzen, H. M., Strahle, U., Gloss, B., Stewart, F. B., Schmid, W. Cooperativity of glucocorticoid response elements located far upstream of the tyrosine amino transferase gene. *Cell* 49:29-38 (1987).

Kalinyak, J. E., Dorin, R. L., Hoffman, A. R. and Perlman, A. J. Tissue-specific regulation of glucocorticoid receptor mRNA by dexamethasone. *J. Biol. Chem.* 262:10441-10444 (1987).

King, W. J. and Greene, G. L. Monoclonal antibodies localize estrogen receptor in the nuclei of target cells. *Nature* 307:745-747 (1984).

Klock, G., Strahle, U. and Schutz, G. Oestrogen and glucocorticoid responsive elements are closely related but distinct. *Nature* 329:734-736 (1987).

Kumar, V., Green, S., Staub, A. and Chambon, P. Localization of the oestradiol-binding and putative DNA binding domains of the human oestrogen receptor. *EMBO J.* 5:2231-2236 (1986).

Lee, S. L., Stewart, K. and Goodman, R. H. Structure of the gene encoding rat thyrotripin releasing hormone. *J. Biol. Chem.* 263:16604-16609 (1988).

Makinodan, T. and Hirayama, R. Age related change in immunologic and hormonal activities. *IARC Sci. Publ.* 58:55-70 (1985).

McDonnell, D. P., Mangelsdorf, D. J., Pike, J. W., Haussler, M. R. and O'Malley, B. W. Molecular cloning of complementary DNA encoding the avian receptor for vitamin D. *Science* 235:1214 (1987).

Mendel, D. B., Bodwell, J. E., Gometchu, B., Harrison, R. W. and Munck, A. Molybdate-stabilized non-activated glucocorticoid receptor complexes contain a 90-kDa non-steroid-binding phosphoprotein that is lost on activation. *J. Biol. Chem.* 261:3758-3763 (1986).

Mendel, D. B., Orti, E., Smith, L. I., Bodwell, J. and Munck, A. Evidence for a glucocorticoid receptor cycle and nuclear dephosphorylation of the steroid-binding protein. *Prog. in Clin. and Biol. Res.* 322:65-80 (1990).

Miesfeld, R., Okret, S. Wikstrom, A.-C., Wrange, 0., Gustafsson, J.A., Yamamoto, K. R. Characterization of a steroid hormone receptor gene and mRNA in wild-type and mutant cells. *Nature* 312:779-781 (1984).

Miesfeld, R., Rusconi, S., Godowski, P. J., Maler, B. A., Okret, S., Wikstrom, A-C., Gustafsson, J-A. and Yamamoto, K. R. Genetic complementation of a glucocorticoid receptor deficiency by expression of cloned receptor cDNA. *Cell* 46:389-399 (1986).

Miesfeld, R., Godwski, P. J., Maler, B. A. and Yomamoto, K. A. Glucocorticoid receptor mutants that define a small region sufficient for enhancer activation. *Science* 236:423-427 (1987).

Miesfeld, R. L. The structure and function of steroid receptor proteins. In: Fasman, G.D. (ed.) **Critical Review in Biochemistry and Molecular Biology**. CRC Press, Baco Raton, FL, pp. 101-117 (1989).

Miller, J., McLachlan, A. D. and Klug, A. Repetitive zinc-binding domains in the protein transcription factor III A from xenopus oocytes. *EMBO J.* 4:1609-1614 (1985).

Munck, A., Guyre, P. M. and Holbrook, N. J. Physiological funcitons of glucocorticoid in stress and their relation to pharmacological actions. *Endocrine Reviews* 5:25-44 (1984).

Nordeen, S. K., Kuhnel, B., Lawler-Heavner, J., Baber, D. A. and Edwards, D. P. A quantitative comparison of dual control of a hormone response element by progestins and glucocorticoids in the same cell line. *Mol. Endocrinol.* 3:1270-1278 (1989).

Norman, M. R., Harmon, J. M. and Thompson, E. B. Use of a human lymphoid cell line to evaluate interactions between prednisolone and other chemotherapeutic agents. *Cancer Research* 38:4273-4278 (1978).

Norman, M. R., Harmon, J. M. and Thompson, E. B. The use of human cell culture systems for studying the action of glucocorticoids in human lymphoblastic leukemias. In: Foltherby, K. and Pal, S. B. (eds.), **Hormones in Normal And Abnormal Human Tissues**. deGruyter, New York, pp. 437-474 (1981).

Okret, S., Poellinger, L., Dong, Y. and Gustafsson, J-A. Down-regulation of glucocorticoid receptor mRNA by glucocorticoid hormones and recognition by the receptor of a specific binding sequence within a receptor cDNA clone. *Proc. Natl. Acad. Sci. (USA).* 83:5899-5903 (1986).

Payvar, F., DeFranco, D., Firestone, G. L., Edgar, B., Wrange, 0., Okret, S., Gustafsson, J-A. and Yamamoto, K. R. Sequence-specific binding of glucocorticoid receptor to MTV DNA at sites within and upstream of the transcribed region. *Cell* 35:381-392 (1983).

Perrot-Applanat, M., Logeat, F., Groyer-Picard, M. T., Milgrom, E. Immunocytochemical study with monoclonal antibodies to progesterone receptor in human breast tumors. *Cancer Research* 47:2652-2661 (1985).

Petkovich, M., Brand, N. J., Krust, A. and Chambon, P. A human retinoic acid receptor which belongs to the family of nuclear receptors. *Nature* 330:444-450 (1987).

Picard, D. and Yamamoto, K. R. Two signals mediate hormone-dependent nuclear localization of the glucocorticoid receptor. *EMBO J.* 6:3333-3340 (1987).

Picard, D., Salser, S. J. and Yamamoto, K. R. A movable and regulatable inactivation function within the steroid binding domain of the glucocorticoid receptor. *Cell* 54:1073-1080 (1987).

Pratt, W. B., Sanrhnz, F. R., Bresnick, F. H., Meshinchi, S., Scherrer, L. C., Dalman, F. C. and Welsh, M. J. Interaction of the glucocorticoid receptor with the Mr 90,000 heat shock protein: An evolving model of ligand-mediated receptor transformation and translocation. *Cancer Res.* 49:2220s-2221s (1989).

Pratt, W. B. Glucocorticoid receptor structure and the initial events in signal transduction. *Prog. in Clin. and Biol. Res.* 322:119-132 (1990).

Ptashne, M. How eukaryotic transcriptional activators work. *Nature* 335:683-689 (1988).

Raghow, R., Gossage, D. and Kang, A. H. Pretranslational regulation of type 1 collagen fibronectin and a 50-kilodalton noncollagenous extracellular protein by dexamethasone in rat fibroblasts. *J. Biol. Chem.* 261:4677-4677 (1986).

Riegel A. T., Aitken S. C., Martin, M. B. and Schoenberg, D. R. Posttranscriptional regulation of albumin gene expression in xenopus liver: evidence for an estrogen receptor-dependent mechanism. *Mol. Endocrinol.* 1:160-167 (1987).

Ringold, G. M. Steroid hormone regulation of gene expression. *Ann. Rev. Pharmacol. Toxico.* 25:529-566 (1985).

Rosewicz, S., McDonald, A. R., Maddox, B. A., Goldfine, 1. D., Miesfeld, R. L. and Longsdon, C. D. Mechanism of glucocorticoid receptor down-regulation by glucocorticoid. *J. Biol. Chem.* 263:2581-2584 (1988).

Rusconi, S. and Yamamoto, K. Functional dissection of glucocorticoid receptor. *EMBO J.* 6:1309-1315 (1987).

Ryseck, R. P., MacDonald-Bravo, H., Mattei, M. G., Ruppert, S., and Bravo, R. Structure, mapping and expression of a growth factor inducible gene encoding a putative nuclear hormonal binding receptor. *EMBO J.* 8:3327-3335 (1989).

Sakai, D. D., Helms, S., Carlstedt-Duke, J., Gustafsson, J-A., Rottman, F. and Yamamoto, K. R. Hormone-mediated repression: a negative glucocorticoid response element from the bovine prolactin gene. *Gene Dev.* 2:1144-1154 (1988).

Sanchez, E. R., Meshinchi, S., Tienrungroj, W., Schlesinger, M. J., Toft, D. 0. and Pratt, W. B. Relationship of the 90-kDa murine heat shock protein to the untransformed and transformed states of the L cell glucocorticoid receptor. *J. Biol. Chem.* 262:6986-6991 (1987).

Sanchez, E. R., Faber, L. E., Hanzel, W. J. and Pratt, W. B. The 56-59 kilodalton protein identified in untransformed steroid receptor complex is a unique protein that exists in cytosol in a complex with both the 70 and 90 kilodalton heat shock proteins. *Biochemistry* 29:5145-5152 (1990).

Sap, J. Munoz, A., Damm, K., Goldberg, Y., Ghysdael, J., Leutz, A., Beug, H. and Vennstrom, B. The c-*erb* A protein is a high affinity receptor for thyroid hormone, *Nature* 324:635-640 (1986).

Scheidereit, C., Geisse, S., Westphal, H. M. and Beato, M. The glucocorticoid receptor binds to defined nucleotide sequences near the promoter of mouse mammary tumor virus. *Nature* 304:749-752 (1983).

Schlecte, J. A., Simons, S. S., Jr., Lewis, D. A. and Thompson, E. B. [^{3}H]-cortivazol a unique high affinity ligand for the glucocorticoid receptor. *Endocrinol.* 117:1355-1362 (1985).

Schlecte, J. A. and Schmidt, T. J. Use of [^{3}H]-cortivazol to characterize glucocorticoid receptors in a dexamethasone-resistant human leukemic cell line. *J. Clin. Endocrinol. and Metabol.* 64:441-446 (1987).

Schmidt, T. J. and Litwack, G. Activation of the glucocorticoid receptor complex, *Physiol. Rev.* 62:1131-1192 (1982).

Schmid, W., Strahle, U., Schutz, G., Schmitt, J. and Stunnenberg, H. Glucocorticoid receptor binds cooperatively to adjacent recognition sites. *EMBO J.* 8:2257-2263 (1989).

Schmidt, T.J., Harmon, J.M. and Thompson, E.B. Activation-labile glucocorticoid-receptor complexes of a steroid-resistant variant of CEM-C7 human lymphoid cells. *Nature* 286:507-510 (1980).

Schule, R., Muller, M., Kaltschmidt, C. and Renkawitz, R. Many transcription factors interact synergistically with steroid receptors. *Science* 242:1418-1420 (1988).

Simons, S. S., Jr. and Thompson, E. B. Dexamethasone-21-mesylate: An affinity label of glucocorticoid receptors from rat hepatoma tissue culture cells. *Proc. Natl. Acad. Sci. (U.S.A.)* 78:3541-3545 (1981).

Simons, S. S., Jr., Pumphrey, J. G., Rudikoff, S. and Eisen, H. Identification of cysteine 656 as the amino acid of hepatoma tissue culture cell glucocorticoid receptors that is covalently labeled by dexamethasone-21-mesylate. *J. Biol. Chem.* 262:9676-9680 (1987).

Slater, E. P., Rabenau, 0., Karin, M., Baxter, J. D. and Beato, M. Glucocorticoid receptor binding and activation of a heterologous promoter by dexamethasone by the first intron of the human growth hormone gene. *Mol. Cell. Biol.* 5:2984-2992 (1985).

Smith, L. I., Bodwell, J. E., Mendel, D. B., Ciardelli, T., North, W. G. and Munch, A. Identification of cysteine 644 as the covalent site of attachment of dexamethasone 21-mesylate to murine glucocorticoid receptors in WEH 1-7 cells, *Biochemistry* 27:3747-3753 (1988).

Soler, J., Baiget, M., Rubiol, E., Guanabens, C., Nunes, V., Estivill, X. and Bosch, M. A. Genotype study of T-receptors in the diagnosis and classification of leukemias and lymphomas. *Med. Clin. (Barc.)* 91:135-138 (1988).

Strahle, U., Klock, G. and Schutz, G. A DNA sequence of 15 base pairs is sufficient to mediate both glucocorticoid and progesterone induction of gene expression. *Proc. Natl. Acad. Sci. (U.S.A.)* 84:7871-7875 (1987).

Thompson, E. B., Yuh, Y. S., Ashraf, J., Gametchu, B., Johnson, B. H. and Harmon, J. M. Mechanisms of glucocorticoid function in human leukemic cells: Analysis of receptor gene mutants of the activation-labile type using the covalent affinity ligand dexamethasone mesylate. *J. Steroid Biochem.* 30:63-70 (1988).

Thompson, E. B., Srivastava, D. and Johnson, B. H. Interactions of phenylpyrazolo steroid cortivazol with glucocorticoid receptors in steroid-sensitive and resistant human leukemic cells. *Cancer Research* 49:2253s-2258s (1989).

Tsai, S. Y., Tsai, M. J., O'Malley, B. W. Cooperative binding of steroid hormone receptors contributes to transcriptional synergism at target enhancer elements. *Cell* 57:443-448 (1989).

Tsai, S. Y., Srinivasan, G., Allan, G. F., Thompson, E. B., O'Malley, B. W., and Tsai, M. J. Recombinant human glucocorticoid receptor induces transcription of hormone response genes *in vitro*. *J. Biol. Chem.* 265:17055-17061 (1990).

Umesono, K. and Evans, R. M. Determinants of target gene specificity for steroid/thyroid hormone receptors. *Cell* 57:1139-1146 (1989).

Vacca, C., Martinotti, S., Screpanti, I., Maroder, M., Felli, M. P., Farina, A. R., Gismondi, A., Santoni, A., Frati, L. and Gulino, A. Transcriptional regulation of the interleukin 2 gene by glucocorticoid hormones. Role of steroid receptor and antigen-responsive 5' flanking sequences. *J. Biol. Chem.* 265:8075-8080 (1990).

von der Ahe, D., Janich, S., Scheidereit, C., Renkawitz, R., Schutz, G. and Beato, M. Glucocorticoid and progesterone receptors bind to the same sites in two hormonally regulated promoter. *Nature* 313:706709 (1985).

Walters, M. Steroid hormone receptors and the nucleus. *Endocr. Rev.* 6:512-543 (1985).

Walters, M. A. and Milbrandt, J. The NGFI-Bgene, a transcriptionally inducible member of the steroid receptor gene superfamily: genomic structure and expression in rat brain after seizure induction. *Mol. Cell. Biol.* 9:4213-4219 (1989).

Webster, N. J. G., Green, S., Jin, J. R. and Chambon, P. The hormone binding domains of the estrogen and glucocorticoid receptors contain an inducible transcription activation function. *Cell* 54:199-207 (1988).

Weinberger, C., Hollenberg, S. M., Rosenfeld, M. G. and Evans, R. M. Domain structure of human glucocorticoid receptor and its relationship to the v-*erb* A oncogene product. *Nature* 318:670-672 (1985).

Weinberger, C., Thompson, C. C., Ong, E. S., Lebo, R., Gruol, D. J. and Evans, R. M. The c-*erb* A gene encodes a thyroid hormone receptor. *Nature* 324:641-646 (1986).

Wu, K. C. and Phahl, M. Variable responsiveness of hormone-inducible hybrid genes in different cell lines. *Mol. Endocrinol.* 2:1294-1301 (1988).

Yamamoto, K. R. Steroid receptor transcription of specific gene and gene networks. *Ann. Rev. Genet.* 19:209-252 (1985).

Yuh, Y. S. and Thompson, E. B. Complementation between glucocorticoid receptor and lymphocytolyis in somatic cell hybrids of two glucocorticoid resistant human leukemic clonal cell lines. *Somatic Cell and Mol. Genet.* 13:33-45 (1987).

Yuh, Y. S. and Thompson, E. B. Glucocorticoid effect on oncogene/growth gene expression in human T-lymphoblastic leukemic cell line CCRF-CEM: Specific c-*myc* mRNA suppression by dexamethasone. *J. Biol. Chem.* 264:10904-10910 (1989).

Zawydiwski, R., Harmon, J. M. and Thompson, E. B. Glucocorticoid-resistant human acute lymphoblastic leukemic cell line with functional receptor. *Cancer Res.* 43:3865-3873 (1983).

Zong, J., Ashraf, J. and Thompson, E. B. The promoter and first, untranslated exon of the human glucocorticoid receptor gene are GC rich but lack concenus glucocorticoid response element sites. *Mol. Cell. Biol.* 10:5580-5585 (1990).

GENERAL ASPECTS OF CANCER CHEMOTHERAPY IN THE AGED

Ronald A. Fleming and
Robert L. Capizzi

Comprehensive Cancer Center
Wake Forest University
Bowman Gray School of Medicine
Department of Medicine
Section on Hematology/Oncology

INTRODUCTION

Age is one of the most important prognostic factors affecting outcome in the treatment of patients with neoplastic diseases. The negative impact of age is almost uniformly encountered with any solid tumor or hematologic malignancy. Detailed analysis of the negative implications of age on therapeutic outcome uncover tumor-related factors, host-related factors and some degree of the interaction between tumor and host-related factors. For example, it is generally accepted that histologic or cytologic subtype of Hodgkin's Disease or the acute leukemias have an important effect on outcome. The general observation is that the prognosis for Hodgkin's Disease is worse on older i.e. > 60 years of age compared to younger patients i.e. in the 20-30 year age group. However, it is not the diagnosis of Hodgkin's Disease per se that has a poorer prognosis in elderly patients but rather the impact of a more aggressive variant of Hodgkin's Disease (lymphocyte depleted) which has a higher frequency of occurrence in elderly patients compared to younger patients. Likewise, the frequency and duration of response as well as curability of ALL[1] in elderly patients is much lower than that possible in children. Reasons for this lesser effect

[1]ALL - Acute Lymphocytic Leukemia; AML - Acute Myelogenous Leukemia;

The Underlying Molecular, Cellular, and Immunological Factors in Cancer and Aging, Edited by S.S. Yang and H.R.Warner, Plenum Press, New York, 1993

include the fact that elderly patients with ALL have not only a higher frequency of biphenotypic ALL but also a higher frequency of Philadelphia chromosome positive ALL, both of which have negative prognostic implications in any age group. Older patients with AML[1] more commonly have a history of antecedent myelodysplasias or secondary leukemias, historical features that have a negative prognostic impact in any age group.

Host-related factors include features related to the impact of aging and co-morbid diseases on loss of organ reserve or function. These consequences of aging and co-morbid disease have profound effects on drug tolerance, physiologic pharmacology and various pharmacokinetic features as noted below. These host factors limit the possibility for treating the patient as aggressively as one might approach younger patients. This limitation is accentuated by the narrow therapeutic index of most anticancer drugs and declining organ reserve, both of which are manifested as poor drug tolerance.

The combined effects of co-morbid disease and neoplasias will have further negative implications on outcome of therapy. For example, the combined effects of chronic obstructive pulmonary disease inpatients with lung cancer; alcoholism and its consequent nutritional deficiencies in patients with head and neck cancer; cirrhosis in patients with hepatomas.

While age is a well recognized poor prognostic feature, its implications have greater impact when considered as physiological age rather than chronological age with due consideration for co-morbid diseases. This paper will summarize general aspects of cancer drug pharmacokinetics and the impact of changes in various physiologic parameters that are associated with increasing age on these pharmacokinetic parameters. To date very little work has been done in this important area of cancer medicine. Given that the median age and the incidence of cancer in the U.S. population is increasing, further attention to the clinical pharmacology of anticancer drugs in the aged is clearly warranted. The following will summarize the effects of age on various pharmacologic parameters along with conjecture as to how these changes might influence cancer drug clinical pharmacology.

PHARMACOKINETICS: BASIC DEFINITIONS

Pharmacokinetics, the measurement of blood concentration of a drug over time, encompasses the processes of absorption, distribution, metabolism, and elimination. Although absorption of a drug or drug formulation can occur at different sites (oral, sublingual, rectal, topical, etc.), the following discussion of absorption will only consider absorption after oral administration. Absorption of a drug is influenced by several host factors including gastrointestinal pH and gastrointestinal transit time. The physicochemical properties of a drug (solubility, pKa) will influence the extent of drug dissolution, membrane transport, and subsequent gastric absorption. ***Absorption*** can be defined as the transport of a drug across the gastrointestinal mucosa and into the systemic circulation. Because of portal blood flow, drugs absorbed into the systemic circulation enter directly into the liver. Once in the liver, certain drugs may be metabolized extensively with little drug reaching the systemic circulation and the targeted site of drug action. ***Bioavailability*** includes processes affecting drug absorption and the extraction of the drug by the liver during its "first-pass" through this organ. Thus, if hepatic disease is present, the bioavailability of a compound which is normally extracted extensively by the liver may increase without any change in absorption occurring.

The apparent volume of distribution of a drug reflects the diffusion of the drug into extravascular fluid, muscle tissue and the adipose tissue, as well as its binding to plasma proteins. The apparent volume in which the drug distributes is determined by dividing the amount of drug administered by the plasma/serum concentration of the drug. This volume is described as the apparent volume of distribution because it does not necessarily reflect a "true" volume but is indicative only of the distribution of a drug.

Although ***metabolism*** of most drugs can occur throughout the body, the organ responsible for the greatest degree of drug metabolism is the liver. There are two major categories of hepatic drug metabolism; phase I metabolism and phase II metabolism. Phase I processes are involved in the oxidative and reductive modification of drugs into either active or inactive compounds. The majority of drug metabolism occurs by phase I processes. Thus, diseases or concomitant drugs which alter or compete for this enzyme system may alter the pharmacokinetic disposition of several drugs. Phase II processes involve the conjugation of a drug into a water soluble compound by the attachment of a polar functional group (e.g. glucuronide). The metabolism of compounds in this system is generally altered only in the presence of very severe hepatic dysfunction.

The ***elimination*** of drugs can occur via a number of processes. Major routes of drug elimination include hepatic, biliary, and renal elimination. The kidney is an important route of elimination for several compounds. Depending on the physicochemical properties of the drug, a drug may be filtered at the glomerulus, secreted by renal tubules, or absorbed back into the systemic circulation after renal tubular absorption. These processes may all be involved in the elimination of certain renally eliminated compounds. Compounds which compete for renal elimination may cause elevations in plasma concentrations of other drugs eliminated through similar mechanisms. Additionally the presence of kidney disease may alter the disposition of certain drugs.

PHARMACOKINETIC CHANGES IN THE ELDERLY

With advancing age, a decline in several physiologic processes has been observed. A decline in respiratory, renal, and cardiac function is associated with advanced age (Figure 1). It is important to mention that the decline in certain physiologic functions depicted in Figure 1 represents trends for the entire aged population. As has been indicated by other authors, the elderly have a greater variability in biochemical and physiologic processes as compared to younger individuals (Williams, T. F., 1987). Thus, a decline in various physiologic or biochemical processes may be dramatic in some individuals but minimal in others. Depending on the magnitude of changes in various physiologic and biochemical processes that occur with aging, the disposition of may drugs may be altered.

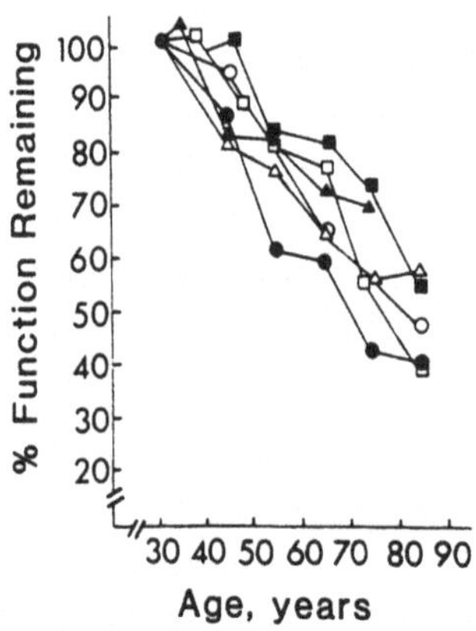

Figure 1. *Percentage of Function Remaining vs. Age*
The values shown are relative to those at age 30 years. Key: maximal breathing capacity (●); renal plasma flow by para-amino hippurate clearance (□); renal plasma flow by diodrast clearance (o); vital capacity (△); glomerular filtration rate by inulin clearance (■); cardiac index (▲). Adapted from Mayersohn M. "Special pharmacokinetic considerations in the elderly. In: Applied Pharmacokinetics. (Eds.) Evans W. E., Schentag, J. J., and Jusks, W. J. Applied Therapeutics Inc., Spokane, 1986.

Antineoplastic compounds have been traditionally regarded as having a narrow therapeutic index. Alterations in the pharmacokinetic profile (i.e. absorption, distribution, metabolism, elimination) of anticancer agents may result in increased host toxicity. A lack of knowledge concerning specific physiologic processes which may affect drug disposition in the aged and a poor understanding of the clinical pharmacology of individual antineoplastic agents may bias judgement on the choice of an inappropriate dose for potentially effective chemotherapeutic agents. Specific pharmacokinetic processes which may be altered in the elderly and examples of individual anticancer agents which may be affected by alterations of these processes are discussed below.

Alterations in Gastrointestinal Function

A number of anticancer agents are available as oral preparations (Table 1). Alterations in gastrointestinal absorption could significantly reduce the bioavailability of certain compounds. Gastrointestinal function is altered with advancing age. The gastric emptying time has been reported to be delayed in the elderly (Van Liere E. J. and Northup D. W., 1941). However this finding is complicated by other age-independent factors (drugs, stress, disease states) which may alter gastric emptying in the elderly patient. Recent studies have attempted to discern whether a difference exists in the gastric emptying rate in the elderly person (Evans M. A. et al., 1981; Moore J. G. et al., 1983). Moore et al. observed a significant delay in liquid emptying rates of elderly males as compared to young males. However, no significant difference was observed in solid food emptying rates between the two groups. Evans et al also observed a significant increase in the liquid emptying rates in the older as compared to young, healthy volunteers. Drugs which require a rapid onset of action or have a rapid clearance can potentially be altered in the presence of delayed gastric emptying. However, the effect of delayed gastric emptying on the bioavailability of oral anticancer agents is unknown.

Table 1. Oral Antineoplastic Agents

Busulfan	Hydroxyurea
Chlorambucil	Procarbazine
Cyclophosphamide	Prednisone
Melphalan	Aminogluthethimide
Lomustine	Tamoxifen
Semustine	Estrogens
Mercaptopurine	Progestins
Methotrexate	Etoposide
Thioguanine	

Studies have shown that the elderly have significant elevations in gastric pH as compared to younger individuals (Vanzant F. R. et al., 1932). Alterations in gastric pH could potentially affect the absorption, stability, and dissolution of several orally administered drugs, including chemotherapeutic agents. Studies assessing the influence of gastric pH have found absorption to be unaltered when comparing young normal subjects versus elderly patients with elevated gastric pH (Kramer, P.A. et al., 1978). Although potential alterations in gastric pH could affect drug dissolution, membrane transport and hence, drug bioavailability, there are no detailed studies of the effect of changes in gastric pH on the absorption of anticancer compounds.

Despite the potential for diminished absorption in the elderly due to alterations in gastrointestinal function, several studies have noted that the absolute bioavailability of medications in elderly individuals is not significantly different from that in younger individuals (Divoll, M. et al., 1983; Cusack, B. et al., 1979). Alterations in drug absorption in the elderly may be more influenced by concomitant drug therapy, concurrent disease states, and nutritional status rather than age per se.

Alterations in Body Composition

With advancing age, several changes have been noted in body composition. The elderly have decreased body water, decreased lean body mass, and increased body fat. Because of these alterations in body composition, the distribution of several drugs, including chemotherapeutic agents may be altered in elderly patients. Compounds which primarily distribute into water will have a smaller apparent volume of distribution, resulting in higher peak concentrations after intravenous bolus administration. Likewise, compounds which are lipid soluble will have a larger apparent volume of distribution. Because the elimination half-life is influenced by changes in either the systemic clearance or volume of distribution, such changes in observed in the elderly may increase or decrease the elimination half-life. In general terms, an increase in the volume of distribution (Vc) with no change in systemic clearance results in a prolongation of the elimination half-life. A decrease in the Vc (observed with hydrophilic compounds in the elderly) results in a shortening of the elimination half-life (the clearance remains unchanged).

Other factors influencing antineoplastic drug distribution in the elderly include changes in plasma protein and tissue binding due to decreases in both plasma proteins and decreased lean body mass. These changes may influence the apparent volume of distribution and steady-state concentrations of certain antineoplastic agents. Several anticancer drugs are extensively bound to plasma proteins (Table 2). Due to the narrow

Table 2. Serum/Plasma Protein Binding of Anticancer Drugs

Drug	Binding
Carboplatin	(parent <10%)
	(active species >90%)
Cisplatin	(parent <10%)
	(active species >90%)
Daunorubicin	(50%)
Doxorubicin	(50%)
Mitoxantrone	(75–95%)
Etoposide	(95%)
Teniposide	(99%)
Methotrexate	(50%)

therapeutic index of anticancer drugs, alterations in the binding of highly bound anticancer drugs may result in higher concentrations of unbound drug. Since the unbound drug is the pharmacologically active species, an increase in unbound concentrations of anticancer compounds may lead to excessive toxicity.

Numerous studies have demonstrated a difference in the plasma protein binding of drugs in young and elderly subjects (Shin, S. et al, 1988; Patterson, M. et al., 1982; Divoll, M. and Greenblatt, D.J., 1982). Of significance for drugs primarily bound to serum albumin, there is an age related decline in serum albumin concentrations (Greenblatt DJ, 1979). Several drugs, including anticancer drugs (e.g. etoposide, teniposide) are extensively bound to serum albumin (Stewart, C.F. et al., 1989). With the decline in lean body mass in advancing age, potential alterations in the tissue binding of drugs could be affected. Anticancer drugs with extensive tissue binding include doxorubicin and daunorubicin.

Alterations in hepatic function

In addition to alterations in hepatic function which may occur due to the involvement of tumor within the liver, there is a decline in hepatic function with increasing age. Given the large number of anticancer agents extensively metabolized by the liver (Table 3), reduction in liver function with advancing age could influence the therapeutic index of several anticancer agents. Unlike the use of creatinine clearance to quantitate renal function, hepatic function has no well accepted biological marker. Given the number of drugs which are metabolized by the liver, it is very difficult for clinicians to determine proper dosage adjustments necessary for patients with various degrees of hepatic function.

Table 3. Anticancer Drugs with Extensive Hepatic Metabolism

Cyclophosphamide
Daunorubicin
Doxorubicin
Etoposide
5-Fluorouracil
Ifosfamide
Nitrosureas
Teniposide
Vincristine
Vinblastine

Because of the lack of a suitable endogenous marker for liver function, researchers have attempted to quantitate hepatic function through the administration of model substrates. These substrates are administered to quantitate hepatic oxidative processes (antipyrine), conjugative processes (lorazepam), and liver blood flow (indocyanine green).

The clearance of antipyrine, a compound eliminated totally by hepatic oxidative processes, has been observed to be diminished with advanced age (Vestal, R. E. et al., 1975; Liddell, D. E. et al., 1975). The unbound clearances of both diazepam and theophylline (both extensively metabolized by hepatic oxidative processes) have been shown to be significantly diminished in the elderly, thus reflecting reduced hepatic enzymatic activity (Shin, S. et al, 1988; Greenblatt, D. J. et al., 1980). Several anticancer compounds e.g. cyclophosphamide and ifosfamide, are metabolized by hepatic oxidative processes. If hepatic oxidative function was reduced by age related or disease-related processes, less drug may be converted to the active phosphoramide mustard with a consequent reduction in therapeutic efficacy. Unlike hepatic oxidative function, hepatic conjugative processes (phase II) are generally not affected by age.

Alterations in Renal Function

Of all of the physiologic changes in the elderly which influence the disposition of drugs, none is more dramatic than the decline in renal function. Tubular absorption (Miller, J. H. et al., 1952), secretion, and glomerular filtration (Davies, D. F. and Shock, N.W., 1950) all decrease in elderly individuals. However, the degree of decline in renal function in elderly patients may vary substantially. This may require little or no dosagé adjustment in some patients or substantial dosage reductions for others. There are several anticancer agents whose disposition is altered in either moderate or severe renal impairment or should be used with caution due to risk of further renal impairment (Table 4).

Table 4. Anticancer Drugs Requiring Dosage Reduction in Renal Dysfunction

Bleomycin
Carboplatin
Cisplatin
Methotrexate
Streptozocin
Aminoglutethimide?
Cyclophosphamide?
Etoposide?

Because the availability of clinical assays for methotrexate[R] in serum, serum concentrations can be closely followed and leucovorin[R] administered as needed depending on the serum concentration of methotrexate and its degree of renal impairment. Nomograms for selecting doses of carboplatin based on creatinine clearance and desired decline in platelet count have been published (Egorin, M.J. et al., 1985). Additionally, other investigators have adjusted cyclophosphamide and methotrexate doses according to creatinine clearance in elderly patients with breast cancer (Gelman, R.S. and Taylor, S.G., 1984). Toxicity in the elderly was reduced in this study with apparently equivalent efficacy to patients requiring no dosage adjustment. Whether adjusting doses of cyclophosphamide in the presence of renal insufficiency reduces toxicity is unclear. The elimination of cyclophosphamide and its metabolites has been reported to be prolonged in patients with renal dysfunction (Bagley, C. M. et al., 1973; Mouridsen, H. T. and Jacobsen, E., 1975). Despite these alterations, other investigators have noted that no difference in toxicities occur when patients with renal insufficiency are administered full doses of cyclophosphamide (Humphrey, R. L. and Kvols, L.K., 1974).

DOSE AND DOSE INTENSITY VERSUS ANTICANCER RESPONSE

Several animal (Bruce, W. B. et al., 1966; Griswold, D. P. et al., 1963; Schabel, F. M. et al., 1984; Skipper, H. E. et al, 1964) and clinical studies (Bonnadonna, G. and Valagussa, P., 1981; Cohen, M. H. et al., 1977; Pinkel, D. et al., 1971) have demonstrated a positive correlation between anticancer drug dose and response or survival. In addition, other studies have determined the dose intensity of treatment (e.g. mg/m^2/week) to be an important determinant of response and/or survival (Carde, .P et al., 1983; Hyrniuk, W. and Bush, H., 1984; Hyrniuk, W. and Levine, M. N., 1986; Hyrniuk, W. M., 1987). The importance of dose and dose intensity have been the subject of recent editorials (DeVita, V. T., 1986; Hyrniuk, W. M., 1988).

AGE-RELATED DIFFERENCES IN CANCER TREATMENT

Elderly cancer patients have been reported to have less favorable outcomes (decreased response, shorter duration of response) as compared to disease-matched younger patients. Although several explanations have been proposed to account for these differences (i.e. increased incidence of advanced disease, comorbid disease, advanced disease at diagnosis), several studies have demonstrated that the elderly receive less intensive therapy (i.e. lower doses of first-line chemotherapeutic agents or selection of second-line agents associated with fewer toxicities) than younger cancer patients (Allen, C. et al., 1986; Greenfield, S. et al., 1987; Mor, V. et al., 1985; Samet, J., 1986). Even after accounting for concomitant diseases, elderly patients received less intensive therapy.

Although it is generally perceived that elderly cancer patients may have more complications from chemotherapy than younger patients, several studies have demonstrated that elderly cancer patients do not differ in toxicities or response to therapy as compared with younger patients (Begg, C. B. and Carbone, P. P., 1983; Cohen, H. J. et al., 1983; Cohen, H. J. and Bartolucci, A., 1985) although other studies have reported differences (Peterson, B. A. et al., 1982). The evidence suggests that anticancer drug dosage reductions should not be made on the basis of chronological age but in the presence of conditions which may alter the disposition of anticancer agents and predispose the patients to excessive toxicities. Thus, certain elderly patients with preexisting health problems (renal dysfunction, hepatic dysfunction, poor nutritional status) will require adjustment of anticancer drug dose but other elderly patients may be able to tolerate equivalent dose intensity as that given to younger individuals.

Many anticancer drugs demonstrate steep dose-response relationships. Although dose is a critical determinant of response for chemosensitive malignancies, failing to lower doses of anticancer doses in patients with altered drug disposition may also affect response. As noted above, several studies have demonstrated that dose intensity (dose per unit time, e.g. mg/m2/week) correlates with response. Patients who have excessive toxicities may have to have their treatment delayed or missed entirely and thus receive a lower dose intensity than what was originally prescribed. Therefore giving a elderly patient an excessive dose of an anticancer agent without adjustment for alterations in the pharmacokinetic disposition of that agent may result in excessive toxicity (myelosuppression, mucositis) which will delay further therapy, thus altering the overall dose intensity and perhaps influencing their treatment outcome. Clinicians treating elderly cancer patients with the goal of cure, must identify patients which may have alterations in the disposition of anticancer agents and make suitable dosage reductions while also identifying patients who will need only minimal or no changes in their therapy to ensure the maximum benefit of therapy for all elderly patients.

INDIVIDUALIZATION OF THERAPY IN THE ELDERLY CANCER PATIENTS - A SUMMARY

As has been discussed by others (Reidenburg, M. M., 1987), individualization of therapy is critical in the treatment of the elderly patient. Thus, dosage reductions should be made with evidence of compromised organ function or other factors affecting the disposition of anticancer drugs and not based on age alone.

The pharmacokinetics of many drugs, including anticancer drugs, are highly variable. In young patients with normal indices of hepatic and renal function, the clearance rate and systemic exposure (area under the curve or AUC) of various antineoplastic agents has been observed to vary by a factor greater than five (Smyth,

R. D. et al., 1985; Evans, W. E. and Relling, M. V., 1989). As discussed above, several physiologic processes affecting the disposition of drugs decline with advancing age. However, as pointed out, the degree in which these alterations occur in the elderly population are highly variable. Certain patients may have dramatic decreases in physiologic function while other patients may have only a slight decline. With these findings, one would anticipate the clearances and AUCs of antineoplastic drugs in the elderly to be highly variable. However there are very few studies which have evaluated the pharmacokinetic variability of antineoplastic agents in the elderly.

Given the lack of studies that address pharmacokinetic variability of anticancer agents in the elderly, it is possible that pharmacodynamic differences seen in certain elderly patients (excessive toxicity) may be linked to the variability in the systemic exposure (AUC) of antineoplastic agents. Several studies have correlated pharmacokinetic parameters of antineoplastic agents with indices of antitumor response or toxicity (Bennett, C. L. et al., 1987; Egorin, M. J. et al., 1985; Egorin, M. J. et al., 1986; Evans, W. E. et al., 1986; Rodman et al., 1987). Similar studies are needed for elderly cancer patients. Because of large interpatient pharmacokinetic variability in the elderly population, adaptive control of antineoplastic dosing based on pharmacokinetic and pharmacodynamic data may ensure the individualization of therapy in the elderly. Investigators have noted that adaptive control of antineoplastic drug administration is feasible (Forrest, A. et al., 1988; Ratain, M. J. et al., 1989).

Until studies that relate anticancer drug disposition to effect (response or toxicity) in the elderly become available, basic knowledge of altered physiologic processes in the elderly can allow individualization of drug dose for certain anticancer agents. With the knowledge that the most dramatic difference between the elderly and the young is renal function and the knowledge of specific chemotherapeutic agents requiring dosage reductions in renal dysfunction, appropriate dose intensity can be delivered to elderly cancer patients. As discussed previously, Gelman and Taylor (1984) were able to reduce the toxicity of anticancer agents in elderly patients (without compromising outcome) by adjusting anticancer dose based on creatinine clearance. Oncologic practice now routinely measures methotrexate serum concentrations with identification of patients at high risk for developing toxicities and individualization of leucovorin rescue'. Additionally, nomograms have been published which allow for individualization of carboplatin dose based on creatinine clearance (Egorin, M. J. et al., 1985).

Thus, clinical oncologists must maintain a thorough knowledge of the clinical pharmacology of anticancer compounds to ensure the rational use of anticancer compounds and prevent arbitrary dose reductions in the elderly cancer patient. Likewise, in the presence of organ dysfunction, knowledge of the metabolism and elimination of anticancer drugs and their active metabolites is essential in order to prevent severe toxicity and treatment delays. With an increasing number of elderly cancer patients, more research into the clinical pharmacology of cancer drugs in the aged is clearly needed.

REFERENCES

Allen, C., Cox, E.B., Manton, K.G., Cohen, H.J. Breast cancer in the elderly. Current patterns of care. *J. Amer. Geriatr. Soc.* 34:637-642 (1986).

Bagley, C.M. Jr., Bostick, F.W. and DeVita, V.T. Jr. Clinical pharmacology of cyclosphosphamide. *Cancer Res.* 33:226-233 (1973).

Begg, C.B. and Carbone, P.P. Clinical trials and drug toxicity in the elderly. The experience of the Eastern Cooperative Oncology Group. *Cancer* 52:1986-1992 (1983).

Bennett, C.L., Sinkule, J.A., Schilsky, R.L., Senekjian, E., Choi, K.E. Phase I clinical and pharmacological study of seventy-two hour continuous infusion of etoposide in patients with advanced cancer. *Cancer Res.* 47:1952-1956 (1987).

Bonnadonna, G. and Valagussa, P. Dose-response effect of adjuvant chemotherapy in breast cancer. *New Engl. J. Med.* 304:10-15 (1981).

Bruce, W. B., Meeker, B. E., Valeriote, F. A. Comparison of the sensitivity of normal hematopoietic and transplanted lymphoma colony forming cells to chemotherapeutic agents administered in vivo. *J. Natl. Cancer Inst.* 36:233-247 (1966).

Carde, P., MacKintosh, F. R. and Rosenberg, S. A. A dose and time response analysis of the treatment of Hodgkin's disease with MOPP chemotherapy. *J. Clin. Oncol.* 1:146-153 (1983).

Cohen, H. J., Silberman, H.R., Forman, R., Bartolucci, A. and Liu, C. Effects of age on responses to treatment and survival of patients with multiple myeloma. *J. Amer. Geriatr. Soc.* 31:272 (1983).

Cohen, H.J. and Bartolucci, A. Age and the treatment of multiple myeloma. Southeastern Cancer Study Group experience. *Amer. J. Med.* 79:316-324 (1985).

Cohen, M.H., Creaven, P.J., Fossiek, B.E. Jr., et al. Intensive chemotherapy of small cell bronchogenic carcinoma. *Cancer Treat Rep.* 61:349-354 (1977).

Cusack, B., Kelly, J., O'Malley, K. et al. Digoxin in the elderly: Pharmacokinetic consequences in old age. *Clin. Pharmacol Ther.* 25:772-776 (1979).

Davies, D.F., Shock, N.W. Age changes in glomerular filtration rate, effective renal plasma flow, and tubular excretory capacity in adult males. *J. Clin. Invest.* 29:496-507 (1950).

DeVita, V. T. Dose-response is alive and well. *J. Clin. Oncol.* 4:1157-1159 (1986).

Divoll, M. and Greenblatt, D. J. Effect of age and sex on lorazepam protein binding. *J. Pharmacol.* 34:122-123 (1982).

Divoll, M., Greenblatt, D. J., Ochs, H. R., Shader, R. I. Absolute bioavailability of oral and intramuscular diazepam: effects of age and sex. *Anesth. Analg.* 62:1-8 (1983).

Egorin, M. J., Van Echo, D.A., Olman, E. A., Whitacre, M. Y., Forrest, A., and Aisner, J. Prospective validation of a pharmacologically based dosing scheme for the cis-diammine dichloroplatimun(II) analogue diamminecyclobutane dicarboxylatoplatinum. *Cancer Res.* 45:6502 (1985).

Egorin, M. J., Van Echo, D. A., and Whitacre, M. Y. Human pharmacokinetics, excretion, and metabolism of the anthracycline menogaril (7-0MEN, NSC 269148) and their correlation with clinical toxicities. *Cancer Res.* 46:1513-1520 (1986).

Evans, M. A., Triggs, E. J., Cheung, M., Broe, G. A., Creasey, H. Gastric emptying rate in the elderly: implications for drug therapy. *J. Am. Geriatr. Soc.* 29:201-205 (1981).

Evans, W. E., Crom, W. R., Abromowitch, M., Dodge, R., Look A. T., Bowman, W.P., George, S. L. Clinical pharmacodynamics of high-dose methotrxate in acute lymphocytic leukemia. Identification of a relation between concentration and effect. *New Engl. J. Med.* 314:471-477 (1986).

Evans, W. E. and Relling, M. V. Clinical pharmacokinetics-pharmacodynamics of anticancer drugs. *Clin Pharmacokin.* 16:327-336 (1989).

Forrest, A., Conley, B.A., Egorin, M.J., Zuhowski, E., Jasman, N.M., Van Echo, D.A. Adaptive control of hexamethylene bisacetamide (HMBA) pharmacodynamics [Abstract]. *Proc. Am. Soc. Clin. Oncol.* 7:61 (1988).

Gelman, R. S., Taylor, S. G. Cyclophosphamide, methotrexate and 5-fluorouracil chemotherapy in women more than 65 years old with advanced breast cancer: The elimination of age trends in toxicity by using doses based on creatinine clearance. *J. Clin. Oncol.* 2:1404-1413 (1984).

Greenblatt, D. J. Reduced serum albumin concentrations in the elderly: a report from the Boston Collaborative Drug Surveillance Program. *J. Am. Geriatr. Soc.* 27:20=-22 (1979).

Greenblatt, D. J, Allen, M.D., Harmatz, J. S., Shader, R. I. Diazepam disposition determinants. *Clin. Pharmacol. Ther.* 27;301-312 (1980).

Greenfield, S., Blanco, D. M., Elashoff, R. M., Ganz, P. A. Patterns of care related to age of breast cancer patients. *J. Am. Med. Assoc.* 257:2766-2770 (1987).

Griswold, D. P., Laster, W. R., Snow, M. Y., Schabel, F. M., Jr. and Skipper, H. E. Experimental evaluation of potential anticancer agents. *Cancer Res.* 21(suppl 23):271-519 (1963).

Humphrey, R.L. and Kvols, L.K. The influence of renal insufficiency on cyclophosphamide-induced hematopoietic depression and recovery. *Proc. Am. Assoc. Cancer Res.* 15:84 (1974).

Hymiuk, W. and Bush, H. The importance of dose intensity in chemotherapy of metastatic breast cancer. *J. Clin. Oncol.* 2:1281-1288 (1984).

Hyrniuk, W. and Levine, M. N. Analysis of dose intensity for adjuvant chemotherapy trials in stage II breast cancer. *J. Clin. Oncol.* 4:1162-1170 (1986).

Hryniuk, W. M. Average dose intensity and the impact on design of clinical trials. *Semin. Oncol.* 14:65-74 (1987).

Hryniuk, W. M. More is better. *J. Clin. Oncol.* 6:1365-1367 (1988).

Kramer, P.A., Chapron, D.J., Benson, Mercik, S.A. Tetracycline absorption in elderly patients with achlorhydria. *Clin. Pharmacol. Ther.* 23:467-472 (1978).

Liddell, D. E., Williams, F. M., Briant, R. H. Phenazone (antipyrine) metabolism and distribution in young and elderly adults. *Clin. Exp. Pharmacol. Physiol.* 2:481-487 (1975).

Miller, J. H., McDonald, R. K., Schock, N. W. Age changes in the maximal rate of tubular reabsorption of glucose. *J. Gerontol.* 7:196-200 (1952).

Moore, J. G., Tweedy, E. J., Christian, P. E., Datz F.L. Effect of age on gastric emptying of liquid-solid meals in man. *Digestive Dis. Sci.* 28:340-344 (1983).

Mor, V., Masterson-Allen, S., Goldberg, R. J., Cummings, F. J., Glicksman, A. S., Fretwell, M. D. Relationship between age at diagnosis and treatments received by cancer patients. *J. Am. Geriatr. Soc.* 33:585-589 (1985).

Mouridsen, H. T. and Jacobsen, E. Pharmacokinetics of cyclophosphamide in renal failure. *Acta. Pharmacol. Toxicol.* 36:409-414 (1975).

Ozols, R. F. Cisplatin dose intensity. *Semin. Oncol.* 16(suppl 6):22-30 (1989).

Patterson, M., Heazelwood, R., Smithurst, B., Eadie, M.J. Plasma protein binding of phenytoin in the aged: *in vivo* studies. *Br. J. Clin. Pharmacol.* 13:423-425 (1982).

Peterson, B.A., Pajak, T.F., Cooper, M.R., Nissen, N.I., Glidewell, O.J., Holland, J.F., Bloomfield, C.D., Gottlieb, A.J. Effect of age on therapeutic response and survival in advanced Hodgkin's disease. *Cancer Treat. Rep.* 66:889-898 (1982).

Pinkel, D., Hernandez, K., Borella, L., Holton, C., Aur, R., Samoy, G., Pratt, C. Drug dosage and remission duration in childhood lymphocytic leukemia. *Cancer* 27:247-256 (1971).

Ratain, M.J., Schilsky, R.L., Choi, K.E., Guarnieri, C., Grimmer, D., Vogelzang, N.J., Sinckjian, E., Liebner, M.A. Adaptive control of etoposide administration: Impact of interpatient pharmacodynamic variability. *Clin. Pharmacol. Ther.* 45:226-233 (1989).

Reidenberg, M. M. Drug therapy in the elderly: the problem from the point of view of a clinical pharmacologist. *Clin. Pharmacol. Ther.* 42:677-680 (1987).

Rodman, J. H., Abromowitch, M., Sinkule, J. A., Hayes, F. A., Rivera, G. K., and Evans, W. E. Clinical pharmacodynamics of continuous infusion teniposide: Systemic exposure as a determinant of response in a phase I trial. *J. Clin. Oncol.* 5:1007-1014 (1987).

Samet, J., Hunt, W. C., Key, C., Humble, C. G., Goodwin, J. S. Choice of cancer therapy varies with age of patient. *J. Am. Med. Assoc.* 255:3385-3390 (1986).

Schabel, F. M., Griswold, D. P., Corbett, T. H., Laster, W. R., Jr. Increasing the therapeutic response rates to anticancer drugs by applying the basic principles of pharmacology. *Cancer* 54:1160-1167 (1984).

Shin, S., Juan, D. and Rammohan, M. Theophylline pharmacokinetics in normal elderly subjects. *Clin. Pharmacol. Ther.* 44:522-530 (1988).

Skipper, H. E., Schabel, F. M. Jr, Wilcox, W. S. Experimental evaluation of potential anticancer agents. XII. On the criteria and kinetics associated with "curability" of experimental leukemia. *Cancer Chemother Rep.* 51:125-165 (1967).

Smyth, R. D., Pfeffer, M., Sclazo, A. and Comis, R. L. Bioavailability and pharmacokinetics of etoposide (VP-16). *Semin. Oncol.* 12(suppl 2):48-51 (1985).

Stewart, C. F., Pieper, J. A., Arbuck, S. G., Evans, W. E. Altered protein binding of etoposide in patients with cancer. *Clin. Pharmacol. Ther.* 45:49 (1989).

Tannock, I. F., Boyd, N. F., DeBoer, G., Erlichman, C., Fine, S. Larocque, G., Mayers, C. Perrault, D. Sutherland, H. A. A randomized trial of two dose levels of cyclophosphamide, methotrexate, and fluorouracil chemotherapy for patients with metastatic breast cancer. *J. Clin. Oncol.* 6:1377 (1982).

Van Liere, E. J. and Northup, D. W. The emptying time of the stomach of old people. *Am. J. Physiol.* 134:719 (1941).

Vanzant, F. R., Alvarez, W. C., Eusterman, G. B. The normal range of gastric acidity from youth to old age. *Arch. Intern. Med.* 49:345 (1932).

Vestal, R. E., Norris, A. H., Tobin, Cohen, B. H., Shock, N. W., Andres, R. Antipyrine metabolism in man: influence of age, alcohol, caffeine, and smoking. *Clin. Pharmacol. Ther.* 18:425 (1975).

Williams, T. F. Aging or disease. *Clin. Pharmacol. Ther.* 42:663 (1987).

DRUG RESISTANCE AND CANCER

Charles S. Morrow and Kenneth Cowan

Medicine Branch, Division of Cancer Treatment
National Cancer Institute
Bethesda, Maryland 20892

INTRODUCTION

Systemic therapy with cytotoxic drugs is the basis of most effective treatments of disseminated cancers. Additionally, adjuvant chemotherapy can offer a significant survival advantage to selected patients following the treatment of localized disease with surgery or radiotherapy, presumably by eliminating undetected minimal or microscopic metastatic tumor. However, the responses of tumors to chemotherapeutic regimens vary and failures are frequent owing to the emergence of drug resistance. Patterns of treatment response and tumor sensitivity are conveniently divided into three groups. First, high complete response rates are common for some intrinsically drug-sensitive tumors such as childhood ALL, Hodgkin's disease, non-Hodgkin's lymphomas, and testicular cancer. A second group including tumors such as breast carcinomas, small cell lung cancers, and ovarian carcinomas are also usually highly responsive to initial treatments but more often become refractory to further therapy. Relapses in either group of tumors generally herald the emergence of tumor cells which are resistant to the antineoplastic agents used initially and often drugs to which the patient was never exposed. Therefore, success with salvage chemotherapies has been limited. Finally, a third common pattern of drug sensitivity is found in tumors which are intrinsically resistant to most chemotherapeutic agents. This group is represented by malignancies such as non-small cell lung cancers, malignant melanoma, and colon cancer. For these tumors, the number of active antineoplastic agents is few and significant chemotherapeutic responses are effected in a minority of cases.

The phenomenon of clinical drug resistance has prompted studies to clarify mechanisms of drug action and identify mechanisms of antineoplastic resistance. It

The Underlying Molecular, Cellular, and Immunological Factors in Cancer and Aging, Edited by S.S. Yang and H.R.Warner, Plenum Press, New York, 1993

is expected that through such information drug resistance may be circumvented by rational design of new non-cross-resistant agents, by novel delivery or combinations of known drugs, and by the development of other treatments which may augment the activity of or reverse resistance to known antineoplastics. Multiple mechanisms of antineoplastic failure have been identified using *in vitro* (tissue culture) and *in vivo* (animal and xenograft) models of antineoplastic failure. A list of these general mechanisms of cellular resistance to anti-cancer drugs are categorized in table I. Other factors including anatomic, pharmacologic, and various host-drug-tumor interactions

Table I. General Mechanisms of Drug Resistance

Cellular and Biochemical Mechanisms

- Decreased drug accumulation
  - Decreased drug influx
  - Increased drug efflux
  - Altered intracellular trafficking of drug
- Decreased drug activation
- Increased inactivation of drug or toxic intermediate
- Increased repair of drug induced damage to:
  - DNA
  - Protein
  - Membranes
- Drug targets altered (quantitatively or qualitatively)
- Altered cofactor or metabolite levels
- Altered gene expression
  - DNA mutation, amplification or deletion
  - Altered transcription, post-transcriptional processing or translation
  - Altered stability of macromolecules

do not involve specific cellular defenses (table II). The oral drug bioavailability and renal clearance of drug vary widely from patient to patient and may account for failure of drug therapy or result in excess toxicity. Furthermore, bone marrow stem cell reserve, especially in patients previously treated with chemotherapy or radiation therapy, can also severely limit the doses of chemotherapy tolerated by relapsed patients, thus compromising treatment effectiveness. These pharmacodynamic problems are particularly relevant in the elderly cancer patient.

Table II. Mechanisms Relevant to *In Vivo* Resistance

Host-tumor interactions
- Pharmacologic and anatomic drug barriers (tumor sanctuaries)

Host-drug interactions
- Increased drug inactivation by normal tissues
- Decreased drug activation by normal tissues
  - decreased bioavailability
- Pharmacogenetics or patient characteristics
  - relative increase of normal tissue drug sensitivity (toxicity)

The mechanisms of drug resistance have been largely determined in experimental systems. However, some have been implicated in clinical chemotherapeutic failure. Evidence which bears upon these mechanisms of resistance as well as strategies to circumvent them are discussed below. First, we discuss the general mechanisms of cellular drug resistance and then some specific examples in the sections that follow. Additionally, the important concept of resistance to multiple antineoplastic agents, resistance to specific classes of drugs, and resistance mechanisms unique to *in vivo* situations are discussed.

GENERAL MECHANISMS OF DRUG RESISTANCE

Experimental selection of drug resistance by repeated exposure to single antineoplastic agents will generally result in cross-resistance to some related agents of the same drug class. This phenomenon is explained on the basis of shared drug transport carriers, drug metabolizing pathways, and intracellular cytotoxic targets of these structurally and biochemically similar compounds. Generally, the resistant cells retain sensitivity to drugs of different classes with alternative mechanisms of cytotoxic action [36, 64]. Thus cells selected for resistance to alkylating agents or antifolates will usually remain sensitive to unrelated drugs such as anthracyclines. Exceptions include emergence of cross-resistance to multiple, apparently structurally and functionally unrelated drugs to which the patient or cancer cells were never exposed during the initial drug treatment. Despite apparent differences in the families of drugs associated with multiple drug resistance phenotypes, when the mechanisms underlying these phenotypes are identified, we frequently discover that the involved antineoplastic agents share common metabolic pathways, efflux transport systems, or sites of cytotoxic action. Conceptually then, the targets of multiple drug resistance mechanisms are similar to the targets of single agent resistance mechanisms.

Decreased drug accumulation

Decreased intracellular levels of cytotoxic agents is one of the most common mechanisms of drug resistance. This may result from decreased drug influx due to a defective carrier-mediated transport system. Decreased influx via a high affinity folate-transport system[2] is a well described cause of methotrexate resistance [34, 61]. A deficient membrane transport system has similarly been identified in cells resistant to nitrogen mustard [27]. Enhanced drug efflux may also lower intracellular steady state levels of drugs. Cells which are multiply resistant to antineoplastic drugs due to overexpression of the P-glycoprotein drug efflux pump (classical multidrug resistance or MDR) represent the most important example of this mechanism of resistance [20].

Altered drug metabolism

Decreased activation of pro-drugs and increased inactivation of active species can confer resistance to selected antineoplastic agents. For example, many antimetabolites and some alkylating agents (e.g. cyclophosphamide) are administered as pro-drugs which must be activated to their cytotoxic forms by the targeted tumor or by other tissues. Resistance to some nucleoside drugs such as cytosine arabinoside has been associated with decreased conversion to its cytotoxic species [7, 19]. Furthermore, enhanced inactivation of both pyrimidine and purine analogs by deaminases has been linked to resistance toward these agents [38, 63]. Finally, cofactor levels may modify drug toxicity. For example, optimal formation of inhibitory complexes between 5-fluorodeoxyuridine monophosphate (FdUMP) and its target enzyme, thymidylate synthetase require the cofactor 5,10-methylene tetrahydrofolate [37].

Increased repair

Cells contain multiple complex systems involved in the repair of membrane and DNA damage. Because such damage may occur as a direct or secondary consequence of cytotoxic drug action, altered intrinsic repair mechanisms can influence drug sensitivity. For example, resistance to cisplatin, a drug whose cytotoxic action is thought to involve intrastrand DNA cross-linkages, has been associated with altered activities presumed to reflect increased DNA repair.

Altered drug targets

The mechanisms of cell kill of several antineoplastic drugs involve interactions between the drug and an essential intracellular enzyme. These interactions result in alteration or inhibition of normal functions. Quantitative or qualitative changes in these enzyme targets of antineoplastic drugs can compromise drug efficacy. These changes have been demonstrated in several enzymes associated with drug resistance cells including dihydrofolate reductase [33], thymidylate synthetase [3], and topoisomerase II [54].

Altered gene expression

The cellular mechanisms of drug resistance outlined above depend upon altered levels or function of key gene products. One of the important findings observed in laboratory models of drug resistance has been the prevalence of somatic gene amplification as a common mechanism of drug resistance resulting in increased intracellular proteins.

RESISTANCE TO MULTIPLE DRUGS

De novo and acquired cross-resistance to multiple antineoplastic agents can result from several alternative factors and processes. Accordingly, we have grouped the major patterns of cross-resistance into three categories on the basis of their presumed underlying mechanisms: classical or P-glycoprotein-dependent multidrug resistance (MDR), multidrug resistance confined to drugs which are topoisomerase II poisons, and multidrug resistance in which the pattern of cross-resistance to particular agents may resemble the other two groups but apparently occurs independently of P-glycoprotein or topoisomerase II functions. Additionally, more speculative mechanisms of multidrug resistance mediated by non-specific xenobiotic metabolizing enzymes are discussed separately.

Classical (P-glycoprotein-dependent) MDR

An *in vitro* model of multidrug resistance (MDR) was described by Biedler and co-workers over two decades ago [6]. In these studies cultured cells selected for resistance by exposure to actinomycin D developed cross-resistance to a surprising array of structurally diverse compounds including Vinca alkaloids, puromycin, daunomycin, and mitomycin C. Subsequently, induction of this pattern of cross-resistance has been observed by numerous investigators who have selected cells in the presence of the same and other drugs. Generally, exposure of cells to any of the drugs (many of which are listed in table III) related to this MDR phenotype can result in cross-resistance to all other members of the phenotype [20]. Drug transport studies using parental and MDR cells have demonstrated that the reduced cytotoxicity of these drugs is the result of decreased drug accumulation secondary to enhanced drug efflux [39, 56]. Furthermore, the emergence of MDR has been associated with increased levels of a membrane bound glycoprotein, P-glycoprotein (P-170 or MDR-associated protein).

The view that P-glycoprotein is the energy-dependent drug efflux pump responsible for MDR is supported by pharmacologic, genetic, and biochemical data. First, the expression of P-glycoprotein is associated with concomitant increases in drug efflux and resistance. Furthermore, gene transfer experiments have shown that the expression of P-glycoprotein genes is sufficient to confer drug resistance [31, 67]. P-glycoproteins are encoded by members of a multigene family present in the mammalian genome. Analyses of these *mdr* genes have revealed a striking sequence homology between P-glycoproteins and several bacterial transport proteins [10, 32]. The deduced amino acid sequences of P-glycoproteins predict the presence of two pairs of six transmembrane domains and two ATP binding sites (Fig. 1). Photoaffinity labeling experiments have demonstrated direct binding of drugs to P-glycoprotein [58]. Finally, the distribution of P-glycoprotein on the luminal surfaces of normal tissues including renal tubules,

Table III. Cross-resistance Pattern of Classical MDR

Class	Drug
anthracyclines	doxorubicin daunorubicin mitoxantrone
antibiotics	actinomycin D plicamycin
anti-microtubule drugs	vincristine vinblastine colchicine
epipodphylotoxins	etoposide tenoposide

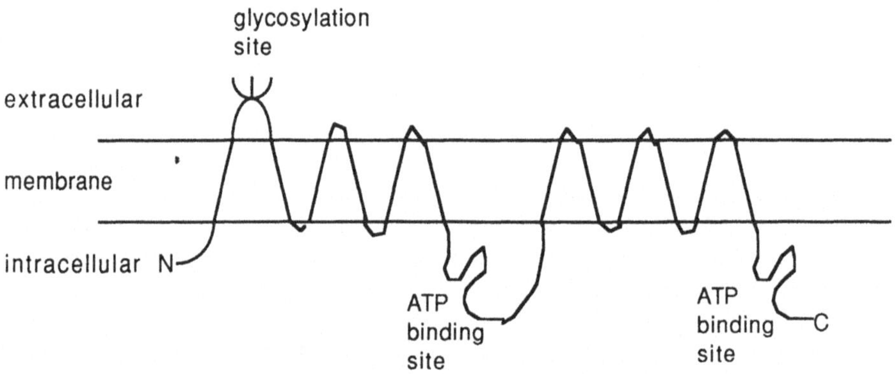

Figure 1. Model of P-glycoprotein

colon, small intestine, and bile canaliculi is consistent with its proposed role in excretory transport [30]. Thus, P–glycoprotein appears to fulfill the requirements predicted of a membrane–bound energy dependent drug carrier.

P–glycoprotein associated MDR is subject to significant phenotypic heterogeneity. The relative degree of cross–resistance to the drugs listed in table III will vary depending upon the cell line and the selecting drug. Moreover, the magnitude of the drug accumulation defect may appear insufficient to account for the degree of resistance. This phenotypic variability may result from the expression of alternative *mdr* alleles, by expression of different members of the *mdr* gene family, or through mutations in the *mdr* gene. While, the human genome contains two closely related *mdr* genes, only one of these genes, *mdr*1 has been shown to confer drug resistance in man [20]. Mutations in the coding region of the *mdr*1 gene have been reported to alter the relative resistance patterns of cells[14]. Post-translational modifications of P-glycoprotein may also alter its pump function. For example, P-glycoprotein can be phosphorylated by protein kinase C[8] and by a novel membrane associated protein kinase [62]. Activation of protein kinase C by a phorbol ester was associated with altered ^{3}H-vinblastine accumulation when cells were incubated in the presence of the MDR reversing agent, verapamil [8]. While the function of P-glycoprotein phosphorylation is poorly understood, these results suggest that altered kinase activities may influence drug resistance and MDR phenotypic diversity. Other cofactors involved in augmentation of P-glycoprotein function have been proposed but not yet identified [23]. Lastly, other mechanisms of drug resistance may co-exist with classical MDR.

A thorough understanding of the regulation of P-glycoprotein production and the means to suppress its expression might significantly influence future cancer treatment strategies. Studies addressing this issue have shown that high levels of P-glycoprotein expression *in vitro* are often associated with *mdr* gene amplification [20] and transcriptional activation. Increased expression of P-glycoprotein can be stimulated by heat shock [12], heavy metals [12], cytotoxic drugs [13, 22, 65], toxic and ablative liver insults [22, 65], differentiating agents [4, 48], and by repeated exposures to ionizing radiation [35]. However, the responses to these treatments appear to vary between species and are cell line specific. Thus, predictable modulation of *mdr* gene expression is not yet possible.

A considerable literature has been accumulated which concerns the importance of P-glycoprotein in human cancer. P-glycoprotein RNA or protein has been detected in tumor specimens derived from patients with acute and chronic leukemias [42, 57, 59], ovarian cancer [5], multiple myeloma [16], breast cancer [40, 60], neuroblastoma [28], soft tissue sarcomas [9], renal cell carcinoma [47], and others [29]. Although the numbers of patients with particular tumors in these studies were small, the results have tended to link P-glycoprotein expression with a history of prior therapy (usually with MDR-associated drugs) or toxin exposure, emergence of intrinsic or acquired drug resistance, and treatment outcome. Ma et al. [42] reported that in two patients with ANLL, disease progression with treatment (including an anthracycline), was associated with increasing P-glycoprotein levels in leukemic blasts. In a study of 15 additional patients with ANLL, Sato et al. [59] found that P-glycoprotein was commonly present in leukemic blasts but more prevalent in blasts derived from patients of poor prognostic groups including those with a history of prior toxin exposure. Although P-glycoprotein was frequently present in tumor specimens from both treated and untreated patients with neuroblastoma, P-glycoprotein RNA tended to be higher in patients treated with regimens including doxorubicin than in untreated patients [28]. In tumor specimens obtained from patients with childhood ALL [57] and soft tissue sarcomas [9], the presence of P-glycoprotein was associated with anthracycline pre-treatment, increased rate of remission induction failure, and increased frequency of relapse. Over 400 tumor specimens were tested for P-glycoprotein RNA levels in a recent large study [29]. Increased levels of P-glycoprotein RNA were more prevalent in tumors which tend to be intrinsically resistant to therapy (colon, renal, adrenal, hepatic, and pancreatic cancers) compared to intrinsically sensitive tumors. Furthermore, P-glycoprotein RNA was often increased in tumors at relapse (acute leukemias, breast cancer, neuroblastoma, pheochromacytoma, and nodular poorly differentiated lymphoma). Additional and prospective studies will be required to confirm the clinical significance of P-glycoprotein in human cancer. However, these preliminary results indicate that P-glycoprotein overexpression is associated with clinical evidence of drug resistance and treatment failure in a significant number of patients. Determinations of P-glycoprotein levels in patients at diagnosis or relapse may have a major role in the design of future treatment protocols.

Similar phenotypes of multiple resistance to antineoplastic agents have been described that are associated with the expression of other membrane proteins. In many of these examples resistance occurs independently of P-glycoprotein expression [11, 44, 45, 46, 52]. The mechanisms of multidrug resistance in these cell lines and whether these membrane proteins are directly involved in drug sensitivity or are merely markers of the resistant phenotype are subjects of current investigations.

Multidrug resistance associated with topoisomerase poisons

Topoisomerases are nuclear enzymes which catalyze the formation of transient single- or double-stranded DNA breaks, facilitate the passage of DNA strands through these breaks, and promote rejoining of the DNA stands [41, 68]. As a consequence of these activities, topoisomerases are thought to be critical for DNA replication, transcription, and recombination. The cytotoxicity of drugs which target topoisomerases (topoisomerase poisons) is thought to depend upon the DNA cleavage activities of topoisomerases. There are two classes of mammalian enzymes, topoisomerases I and II. Topoisomerase I catalyzes the formation of single stranded DNA breaks while topoisomerases II catalyze both single- and double-stranded breaks. During the cleavage reactions reversible DNA-topoisomerase complexes (cleavable complexes) can be stabilized by interactions with topoisomerase poisons. The formation of these stabilized DNA-topoisomerase-drug complexes is thought to initiate the production of lethal DNA strand breaks. Of the chemotherapeutic drugs that affect topoisomerase activities, the topoisomerase II poisons have been the most important clinically. A partial list of these agents, which include DNA intercalating and non-intercalating drugs appears in table IV.

The mechanism of resistance to topoisomerase II poisons is thought to involve altered topoisomerase II activity. Both qualitative and quantitative changes in enzyme activity have been demonstrated in resistant cell lines. Reduced levels of topoisomerase activity has been associated with decreased drug-induced DNA strand breaks as well as reduced drug cytotoxicity [18, 53]. Other studies have implicated intrinsic changes in drug-induced catalytic properties or associated cofactors as the basis of drug resistance in some cells [17, 26, 54, 69]. Indeed, the normal down regulation of topoisomerase II in non-dividing cells [41] may explain the relative insensitivity to topoisomerase II-poisons of some solid tumors containing a large proportion of quiescent cells.

Table IV. Topoisomerase II Poisons

	Class	Drugs
non-intercalators	epipodophyllotoxins	etoposide tenoposide
intercalators	anthracyclines	doxorubicin daunorubicin
	acridine	m-AMSA (amsacrine)
	anthracenedione	mitoxantrone
	antibiotic	actinomycin D
	ellipticine	9-hydroxy ellipticine

The cytotoxic agent, camptothecin has been shown to enhance topoisomerase I-mediated strand breaks. Until recently host toxicity has prohibited the clinical use of such topoisomerase I poisons. However, the prospect of less toxic analogs of this drug that maintain a high level of activity against topoisomerase I-rich human cancer cells, has renewed interest in the clinical application of this class of compounds [25]. Consequently, the emergence of resistance to these agents may become an increasingly important consideration. This problem is illustrated in a report by Andoh *et al.* [1] who have characterized a resistant leukemia cell line expressing defective topoisomerase I activity that mediates reduced camptothecin-induced DNA strand breaks.

Multidrug resistance associated with altered expression of drug metabolizing enzymes

The emergence of acquired drug resistance may be viewed as an acute or chronic adaptive response of tumor cells to environmental stress, primarily in the form of drug challenge. As discussed above rapid transient induction of P-glycoprotein may sometimes be mediated by an acute insult such as cytotoxic drug exposure, heavy metal exposure, or heat shock. Alternatively, chronic or repeated exposure to drugs may enhance P-glycoprotein levels by complex, stable genetic changes. In other models and tumor cells, challenges with cytotoxic agents result in alterations in the expression of several genes including those involved in drug metabolism. In the Solt-Farber model of chemical carcinogenesis [24], treatment of rats with various cytotoxins followed by partial hepatectomy results in the appearance of multiple pre-neoplastic nodules. A number of biochemical changes occur in these nodules including the overexpression of P-glycoprotein [22, 65], the induction of several phase II drug metabolizing (drug conjugating) enzymes, and the down-regulation of some phase I drug metabolizing (cytochrome P450-dependent mixed function oxidases) enzymes. These drug metabolizing enzymes are generally considered to be involved in the sequential oxidation of xenobiotics to more electrophilic, reactive intermediates followed by the formation of less toxic conjugated compounds which may be further metabolized or excreted (Fig. 2). A similar pattern of P-glycoprotein expression, phase I enzyme suppression, and phase II enzyme induction has been shown in a human breast cancer cell line made multidrug resistant by chronic doxorubicin exposure [15, 21]. The emergence of this phenotype appears to represent a programmed cellular stress response which might offer generalized protection from a variety of

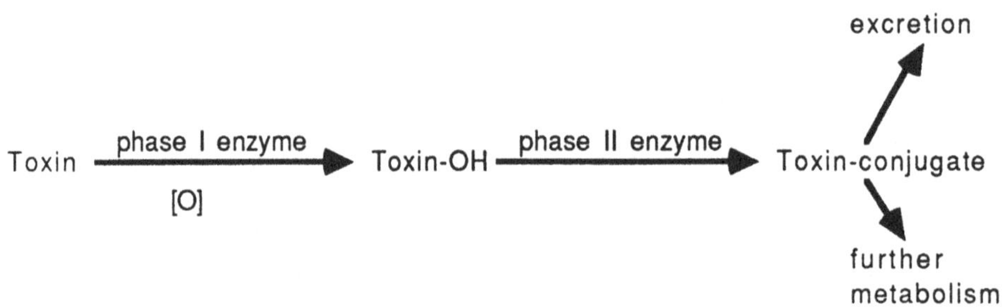

Figure 2. Phase I And II Drug Metabolizing Enzymes

exogenous toxins via increased drug efflux secondary to P-glycoprotein expression, decreased drug activation due to reduced phase I enzymes, and increased drug inactivation by phase II enzymes. Of the phase II enzymes, the glutathione *S*-transferases (GSTs) have been the most extensively studied.

GSTs [43, 49, 66] are comprised of multiple soluble and membrane-associated isozymes which catalyze the conjugation of electrophilic, hydrophobic compounds (R-X) with the thiol, glutathione (GSH). Circumstantial evidence has linked the increase in specific GST isozymes or bulk GST activity in cells with resistance to alkylating agents, doxorubicin, and other drugs [49, 66]. However direct evidence that GSTs are responsible for altering drug sensitivities is limited. Another catalytic activity, selenium-independent glutathione peroxidase activity has been attributed to some isozymes of GST. This and other GST-mediated reactions are of interest because of their potential to detoxify oxidative damage to membranes and DNA.

Table V. Some Important Substrates of GSTs Related to Drug Detoxification And Repair of Drug-mediated Damage

Antineoplastic drugs	Products of membrane and DNA oxidation
nitrogen mustards	fatty acid hydroperoxides
chlorambucil	4-hydroxy alkenals
melphalan	?DNA hydroperoxides
cyclophosphamide	
nitrosoureas	
1,3-bis(2-chloroethyl)-1-nitroso urea (BCNU)	
anthracenedione	
mitoxantrone	

Studies using cell–free preparations of GSTs have identified a limited number of antineoplastic drug substrates of these enzymes. These drugs and other substrates possibly associated with drug mediated–oxidative damage are listed in table V. Whether GST levels in tumor cells are sufficient to detoxify antineoplastic drugs to a clinically significant extent is a matter of considerable debate. Gene transfer experiments using recombinant *GST* genes and tissue culture cells have suggested that some GST isozymes may confer a very modest level of resistance to melphalan, chlorambucil, cisplatin [55], and doxorubicin [51]. Other experiments have failed to confirm any consistent resistance to doxorubicin, cisplatin, or melphalan in breast cancer cells transfected with the pi class isozyme of GST [50]. Clearly, additional studies are necessary to clarify the role of GSTs in drug resistance.

APPROACHES TO OVERCOMING RESISTANCE TO SPECIFIC GROUPS OF DRUGS

Approaches to overcome chemotherapeutic failures include efforts to prevent the emergence of drug resistance (table VI). An appreciation of factors which induce resistance mechanisms may lead to the choice of more efficacious treatment regimens. For example, drugs which may have only sporadic activity against a specific tumor yet are likely to select for cross–resistance to more active agents would be avoided. It is hoped that aggressive combination chemotherapy with non–cross reacting drugs will eliminate tumor rapidly enough to prevent the selection of multiple resistant tumor cell clones. Failures of the preventative approach require the incorporation of specific measures aimed at reversing or circumventing drug resistance.

Table VI. Approaches to Overcome or Circumvent Drug Resistance

prevention	* aggressive multiple agent therapy
	* appreciation of factors which induce resistance mechanisms
circumvention	* drug screening programs and rational drug design
	* circumvention of drug uptake defects dose escalation drugs which use alternative transport mechanisms
	* agents which reverse increased efflux
	* cofactors which augment drug activation or efficacy
	* inhibition of drug inactivation
	* novel treatment modalities immunotherapy and cytokines differentiating agents

CONCLUSIONS AND FUTURE DIRECTIONS

Through the kinds of studies done largely *in vitro* described in this chapter, many of the mechanisms of antineoplastic drug resistance have been identified. While several of these processes operate *in vivo*, their relative clinical importance must be better clarified in controlled, prospective examinations of patient tumor specimens and correlations with therapeutic responses to chemotherapy. Nevertheless, these mechanisms suggest potentially useful approaches to overcome clinical drug resistance. These approaches include the rational choice of conventional agents or design of novel drugs that are less likely to share resistance mechanisms. Additionally, many of the pathways of antineoplastic drug inactivation or transport are targets for pharmacologic manipulations that may reverse or circumvent the resistance of tumors to some drugs. Despite these efforts, many tumors will remain refractory to conventional chemotherapeutic drugs. Their successful treatment may require novel modalities such as biologic response modifiers. For example, the use of cytokines alone or in combination with adoptive immunotherapy, differentiating agents like retinoic acid, and pharmacologic agents capable of altering the responses of tumors to exogenous and autocrine growth factors may hold promise for the treatment of some cancers. Finally, dose escalation of conventional agents followed by hematologic rescue with cytokines or bone marrow transplantation is assuming a greater role in protocols designed to treat a variety of cancers.

REFERENCES

1. Andoh, T., Ishii, K., Suzuki, Y., Ikegami, Y., Kusunoki, Y. and Okada, K.: Characterization of a mammalian mutant with a camptothecin-resistant DNA topoisomerase I. *Proc. Natl. Acad. Sci.*, 84:5565, 1987.

2. Anthony, A. C., Kane, M. A., Portillo, R. M., Elwood, P. C. and Kolhouse, J.F.: Studies of the role of a particulate folate-binding protein in the uptake of 5-methyltetrahydrofolate by cultured human KB cells. *J. Biol. Chem.*, 260:14911, 1985.

3. Armstrong, R. A.: Fluoropyrimidine activity and resistance at the cellular level. In Resistance to antineoplastic drugs. Edited by D. Kessel, Boca Raton, Florida, CRC Press, 1989, p. 317.

4. Bates, S. E., Mickley, L. A., Chen, Y.-N., Richert, N., Rudick, J., Biedler, J. L. and Fojo, A. T.: Expression of a drug resistant gene in human neuroblastoma cell lines: modulation by retinoic acid-induced differention. *Mol. Cell Biol.*, 9:4337, 1989.

5. Bell, D. R., Gerlach, J. H., Kartner, N., Buick, R. N. and Ling, V.: Detection of P-glycoprotein in ovarian cancer: a molecular marker associated with multidrug resistance. *J. Clin. Onc.*, 3:311, 1985.

6. Biedler, J. L. and Riehm, H.: Cellular resistance to actinomycin D in Chinese Hamster ovary cells in vitro : cross resistance, radioautographic, and cytogenetic studies. *Cancer Res.*, 30:1174, 1970.

7. Brockmann, R. W.: Mechanisms of resistance to the anticancer agents. *Adv. Cancer Res.*, 7:129, 1963.

8. Chambers, T. C., McAvoy, E. M., Jacobs, J. W. and Eilon, G.: Protein kinase C phosphorylates P-glycoprotein in multidrug resistant human KB carcinoma cells. *J. Biol. Chem.*, 265:7679, 1990.

9. Chan, H. S. L., Thorner, P. S., Haddad, G. and Ling, V.: Immunohistochemical detection of P-glycoprotein: prognostic correlation in soft tissue sarcoma of childhood. *J. Clin. Oncol.*, 8:689, 1990.

10. Chen, C., Chin, J. E., Ueda, K., Clark, D. P., Pastan, I., Gottesman, M. M. and Roninson, I. B.: Internal depletion and homology with bacterial transport proteins in the *mdr*1 gene for multidrug-resistant human cells. *Cell*, 47:381, 1986.

11. Chen, Y.-N., Mickley, L. A., Schwartz, A. M., Acton, E. M., Hwang, J. and Fojo, A. T.: Characterization of Adriamycin resistant human breast cancer cells which display overexpression of a novel resistance-related membrane protein. *J. Biol. Chem.*, 265:10073, 1990.

12. Chin, K., Tanaka, S., Darlington, G., Pastan, I. and Gottesman, M. M.: Heat shock and arsenate increase expression of multidrug resistance (*MDR*1) gene in human renal carcinoma cells. *J. Biol. Chem.*, 265:221, 1990.

13. Chin, K.-V., Chauhan, S. S., Pastan, I. and Gottesman, M. M.: Regulation of *mdr* RNA levels in response to cytotoxic drugs in rodent cells. *Cell Growth Differentiation*, 1:361, 1990.

14. Choi, K., Chen, C., Kriegler, M. and Roninson, I. B.: An altered pattern of cross-resistance in multidrug-resistant human cells results from spontaneous mutations in the *mdr*1 (P-glycoprotein) gene. *Cell*, 53:519, 1988.

15. Cowan, K. H., Batist, G., Tulpule, A., Sinha, B. K. and Myers, C. E.: Similar biochemical changes associated with multidrug resistance in human breast cancer cells and carcinogen-induced resistance to xenobiotics in rats. *Proc. Natl. Acad. Sci.*, 83:9328, 1986.

16. Dalton, W. S., Grogan, T. M., Rybski, J. A., Scheper, R. J., Richter, L., Kailey, J., Broxterman, H. J., Pinedo, H. M. and Salmon, S. E.: Immunohistochemical detection and quantitation of P-glycoprotein in multiple drug-resistant human myeloma cells: association with level of drug resistance and drug accumulation. *Blood*, 73:747, 1989.

17. Danks, M. K., Schmidt, C. A., Cirtain, M. C., Suttle, D. P. and Beck, W. T.: Altered catalytic activity of and DNA cleavage by DNA topoisomerase II from human leukemia cells selected for resistance to VM-26. *Biochemistry*, 27:8861, 1988.

18. Deffie, A. M., Batra, J. K. and Goldenberg, G. J.: Direct correlation between DNA topoisomerase II activity and cytotoxicity in Adriamycin-sensitive and resistant P388 leukemia cell lines. *Cancer Res.*, 49:58, 1989.

19. Drahovsky, D. and Kreis, W.: Studies on drug resistance. II. Kinase patterns in P815 neoplasms sensitive and resistant to 1-ß-D-arabinofuranosyl cytosine. *Biochem. Pharmacol*, 19:940, 1970.

20. Endicott, J. A. and Ling, V.: The biochemistry of P-glycoprotein-mediated multidrug resistance. *Annu. Rev. Biochem.,* 58:137, 1989.

21. Fairchild, C. R., Ivy, S. P., Kao-Shaw, C.-S., Whang-Peng, J., Rosen, N., Israel, M. A., Melera, P. W., Cowan, K. H. and Goldsmith, M. E.: Isolation of amplified and overexpressed DNA sequences from adriamycin-resistant human breast cancer cells. *Cancer Res.*, 47:5141, 1987.

22. Fairchild, C. R., Ivy, S. P., Rushmore, T., Lee, G., Koo, P., Goldsmith, M.E., Myers, C. E., Farber, E. and Cowan, K. H. : Carcinogen-induced *mdr* overexpression is associated with xenobiotic resistance in rat preneoplastic liver nodules and hepatocellular carcinomas. *Proc. Natl. Acad. Sci.*, 84:7701, 1987.

23. Fairchild, C. R., Moscow, J. A., O'Brien, E. E. and Cowan, K. H.: Multidrug resistance in cells transfected with human genes encoding a variant P-glycoprotein and glutathione S-transferase-pi. *Mol. Pharmacol.*, 37:801, 1990.

24. Farber, E.: Cellular biochemistry of the stepwise development of cancer with chemicals. *Cancer Res.*, 44:5463, 1984.

25. Giovanella, B. C., Stehlin, J. S., Wall, M. E., Wani, M. C., Nicholas, A. W., Liu, L. F., Silber, R. and Potmesil, M.: DNA topoisomerase I-targeted chemotherapy of human colon cancer in xenografts. *Science*, 246:1046, 1989.

26. Glisson, B., Gupta, R., Smallwood-Kentro, S. and Ross, W.: Characterization of acquired epipodophylotoxin resistance in a Chinese hamster ovary cell line: loss of drug-stimulated DNA cleavage activity. *Cancer Res.*, 46:1934, 1986.

27. Goldenberg, G. J., Vanstone, C. L., Isreals, L. G., Isle, D. and Bihler, D.: Evidence for a transport carrier of nitrogen mustard in nitrogen mustard-sensitive and -resistant L5178Y lymphoblasts. *Cancer Res.*, 30:2285, 1970.

28. Goldstein, L. J., Fojo, A. T., Ueda, K., Crist, W., Green, A., Brodeur, G., Pastan, I. and Gottesman, M. M.: Expression of the multidrug resistant, *MDR*1, gene in neuroblastoma. *J. Clin. Oncol.*, 8:128, 1990.

29. Goldstein, L. J., Galski, H., Fojo, A., Willingham, M., Lai, S.-L., Gazdar, A., Pirker, R., Green, A., Crist, W., Brodeur, G. M., Lieber, M., Cossman, J., Gottesman, M. M. and Pastan, I.: Expression of a multidrug resistance gene in human cancers. *J. Natl. Cancer Inst.*, 81:116, 1989.

30. Gottesman, M. M. and Pastan, I.: Resistance to multiple chemotherapeutic agents in human cancer cells. *Trends Pharmacol. Sci.*, 9:54, 1988.

31. Gros, P., Ben Neriah, Y., Croop, J. M. and Houseman, D. E.: Isolation and expression of a complimentary DNA that confers multidrug resistance. *Nature*, 323:728, 1986.

32. Gros, P., Croop, J. and Houseman, D.: Mammalian multidrug resistant gene: complete cDNA sequence indicates strong homology to bacterial transport proteins. *Cell*, 47:371, 1986.

33. Haber, D. A., Beverly, S. M., Kiely, M. L. and Schimke, R. T.: Properties of altered dehydrofolate reductase encoded by amplified genes in cultured mouse fibroblasts. *J. Biol. Chem.*, 256:9501, 1981.

34. Hill, B. T., Bailey, B. D., White, J. C. and Goldman, I. D.: Characteristics of transport of 4-amino antifolates and folate compounds by two cell lines of LY5178Y lymphoblasts, one with impaired transport of methotraxate. *Cancer Res.*, 39:2440, 1979.

35. Hill, B. T., Deuchars, K., Hosking, L. K., Ling, V. and Whelan, R. D. H.: Over expression of P-glycoprotein in mammalian tumor cell lines after fractionated X irradiation *in vitro*. *J. Natl. Cancer Inst.*, 82:607, 1990.

36. Hill, B. T., Price, L. A. and Goldie, J. H.: The value of adriamycin in overcoming resistance to methotrexate in cell culture. *Eur. J. Cancer*, 12:541, 1976.

37. Houghton, J. A., Maroda, S. J., Phillips, J. O. and Houghton, P. J.: Biochemical determents of responsiveness to 5-fluorouracil and its derivatives in xenografts of human colorectal adenocarcinomas in mice. *Cancer Res.*, 41:144, 1981.

38. Hunt, S. W. and Hoffee, P. A.: Amplification of adenosine deaminase gene sequence in deoxycoformycin-resistant rat hepatoma cells. *J. Biol. Chem.*, 258:13185, 1983.

39. Juliano, R. L. and Ling, V.: A surface glycoprotein modulating drug permeability in Chinese hamster ovary cell mutants. *Biochem. Biophys. Acta*, 455:1252, 1976.

40. Keith, W. N., Stallard, S. and Brown, R.: Expression of *mdr*1 and GST π in human breast tumors: comparison to in vitro sensitivity. *Br. J. Cancer*, 61:712, 1990.

41. Liu, L.: DNA topoisomerase poisons as antitumor drugs. *Annu. Rev. Biochem.*, 58:351, 1989.

42. Ma, D. D., Scurr, R. D., Davey , R. A., Mackertich, S. M., Dowden, G. and Bell, D. R.: Detection of a multidrug resistant phenotype in acute non-lymphoblastic leukaemia. *Lancet*, 1(8525):135, 1987.

43. Mannervik, B. and Danielson, U. H.: Glutathione transferases-structure and catalytic activity. *Critical Reviews in Biochemistry,* 23:283, 1988.

44. Marquardt, D., McCrone, S. and Center, M. S.: Mechanisms of multidrug resistance in HL60 cells: detection of resistance-associated proteins with antibodies against synthetic peptides that correspond to the deduced sequences of P-glycoprotein. *Cancer Res.*, 50:1426, 1990.

45. Marsh, W. and Center, M.: Adriamycin resitance in HL60 cells and accompanying modification of a surface membrane protein contained in drug-sensitive cells. *Cancer Res.*, 47:5080, 1987.

46. McGrath, T., Latoud, C., Arnold, S. T., Safa, A. R., Felsted, R. L. and Center, M. S.: Mechanisms of multidrug resistance in HL60 cells. Analysis of resistance associated membrane proteins and levels of *mdr* gene expression. *Biochem. Pharmacol.,* 38:3611, 1989.

47. Mickisch, G., Bier, H., Bergler, W., Bak, M., Tschada, R. and Alken, P.: P-170 glycoprotein, glutathione and associated enzymes in relation to chemoresistance of primary human renal cell carcinomas. *Urol. Int.*, 45:170, 1990.

48. Mickley, L. A., Bates, S. E., Richert, N. D., Currier, S., Tanaka, S., Foss, F., Rosen, N. and Fojo, A. T.: Modulation of the expression of a multidrug resistance gene (mdr1/P-glycoprotein) by differentiating agents. *J. Biol. Chem.*, 264:18031, 1989.

49. Morrow, C. S. and Cowan, K. H.: Glutathione *S*-transferases and drug resistance. *Cancer Cells*, 2:15, 1990.

50. Moscow, J. A., Townsend, A. J. and Cowan, K.H.: Elevation of the π class glutathione *S*-transferase activity in human breast cancer cells by transfection of the GSTπ gene and its effect on sensitivity to toxins. *Mol. Pharmacol.*, 36:22, 1989.

51. Nakagawa, K., Saijo, N., Tsuchida, S., Sakai, M., Tsunokawa, Y., Yokota, J., Muramatsu, M., Sato, K., Tekada, M. and Tew, K. D.: Glutathione *S*-transferase π as a determinant of drug resistance in transfectant cell lines. *J. Biol. Chem.,* 265:4296, 1990.

52. Ohtsu, T., Ishida, Y., Tobinai, K., Minato, K., Hamada, H., Ohkodu, E., Tsuruo, T. and Shimoyama, M.: A novel multidrug resistance in cultured leukemia and lymphoma cells detected by a monoclonal antibody to 85kD protein, MRK20. *Japan. J. Cancer Res.*, 80:1133, 1989.

53. Per, S.-R., Mattern, M. R., Mirabelli, C. K., Drake, F. H., Johnson, R. K. and Crooke, S. T.: Characterization of a subline of P388 leukemia resistant to amsacrine: evidence of altered topoisomerase II function. *Mol. Pharmacol.*, 32:17, 1987.

54. Pommier, Y., Kerrigan, D., Schwartz, R. E., Swack, J. A. and A., M.: Altered DNA topoisomerase II activity in Chinese hamster cells resistant to topoisomerase II inhibitors. *Cancer Res.*, 46:3075, 1986.

55. Puchalski, R. B. and Fahl, W. E.: Expression of recombinant glutathione *S*-transferase π, Ya or Yb1 confers resistance to alkylating agents. *Proc. Natl. Acad. Sci.*, 87:1990.

56. Riordan, J. R. and Ling, V.: Genetic and biochemical characterization of multidrug resistance. *Pharmacol.Ther.*, 28:51, 1985.

57. Rothenberg, M. L., Mickley, L. A., Cole, D. E., Balis, F. M., Tsuruo, T., Poplack, D. and Fojo, A. T.: Expression of the *mdr*1 gene/P-170 gene in patients with acute lymphoblastic leukemia. *Blood,* 74:1388, 1989.

58. Safa, A. R., Glover, C. J., Meyers, M. B., Biedler, J. L. and Felsted, R. L.: Vinblastine photoaffinity labeling of a high molecular weight surface membrane glycoprotein specific for multidrug-resistant cells. *J. Biol. Chem.*, 261:6137, 1986.

59. Sato, H., Gottesman, M. M., Goldstein, L. J., Pastan, I., Block, A., Sandberg, A. A. and Preisler, H. D.: Expression of the multidrug reistance gene in myeloid leukemias. *Leukemia Res.*, 14:11, 1990.

60. Schneider, J., Bak, M., Efferth, T. H., Kaufmann, M., Mattren, J. and Volm, M.: P-glycoprotein expression in treated and untreated breast cancer. *Br. J. Cancer*, 60:815, 1989.

61. Sirotnak, F.M., Moccio, D.M., Kelleher, L.E. and Goutsas, L.J.: Relative frequency and kinetic properties of transport defective phenotypes among methotrexate-resistant L1210 clonal cell lines derived *in vivo*. *Cancer Res.*, 41:4447, 1981.

62. Staats, J., Marquardt, D. and Center, M. S.: Characteristics of a membrane-associated protein kinase of multidrug-resistant HL60 cells which phosphorylates P-glycoprotein. *J. Biol. Chem.*, 265:4084, 1990.

63. Steuart, C. D. and Burke, P. J.: Cytidine deaminase and the development of resistance to cytosine arabinoside. *Nature (London) New Biol.*, 233:109, 1971.

64. Teicher, B. A., Cucchi, C. A., Lee, J. B., Flatow, J. L., Rosowsky, A. and Frei, E., III: Alkylating agents : in vitro studies of cross-resistance patterns in human cell lines. *Cancer Res.*, 46:4379, 1986.

65. Thorgeirsson, S. S., Huber, B. E., Sorrel, S., Fojo, A., Pastan, I. and Gottesman, M. M.: Expression of the multidrug-resistant gene in hepatocarcinogenesis and regenerating liver. *Science*, 236:1120, 1987.

66. Townsend, A. J. and Cowan, K. H.: Glutathione *S*-transferases and antineoplastic drug resistance. *Cancer Bull.*, 41:31, 1989.

67. Ueda, K., Cardarelli, C., Gottesman, M. M. and Pastan, I.: Expression of a full-length cDNA from the human *mdr*1 gene confers resistance to colchicine, doxorubicin, and vinblastine. *Proc. Natl. Acad. Sci.*, 84:3004, 1987.

68. Zhang, H., D'Arpa, P. and Liu, L. F.: A model for tumor cell killing by topo-isomerase poisons. *Cancer Cells*, 2:23, 1990.

69. Zwelling, L. A., Hinds, M., Chan, D., Mayes, J., Sie, K. L., Parker, E., Silberman, L., Radcliffe, A., Beran, M. and Blick, M.: Characterization of an amsacrine-resistant line of human leukemia cells. Evidence for a drug-resistant form of topoisomerase II. *J. Biol. Chem.*, 264:16411, 1989.

SUMMATION AND SYNTHESIS:

FROM THE CANCER CELL BIOLOGY POINT OF VIEW[1]

Eric J. Stanbridge

Department of Microbiology and Molecular Genetics
University of California, Irvine
Irvine, CA 92717

I believe I speak for most people here in saying that I learned a lot about the interrelationship between aging and cancer the last couple of days, but I learned very little about the "why's". And I suppose that's why we are here. Very clearly, the phenomenon is out there; however, there is very little knowledge as to why it occurs.

Both Dr. Pereira-Smith and Dr. Cutler gave us a good start by posing some fundamental questions. Dr. Cutler put forward three theories for the age-dependent increase in cancer. These were: first, that aging and cancer are both time and multistage dependent, but they do not necessarily share a common mechanism. Second, the converse, that aging and cancer have common mechanisms, for example, differentiation. And, third, that there is no common mechanism. However, there is an increasing predisposition to cancer within age related disorders; for example, immune dysfunction.

Personally, I think that not a single one of these scenarios is a tenable hypothesis; however, we'll see a little bit of all three coming together as one goes through this extremely complex field.

---

[1]This is a direct transcript of Dr. Eric Stanbridge's wrap-up presentation in the Summation and Synthesis Session.

IMMUNE DYSFUNCTION, AN AGE RELATED DISORDER, AND ITS RELATIONSHIP TO INCREASING SENSITIVITY TO CELL TRANSFORMATION

With respect to immune dysfunction, we heard a couple of very interesting talks on immuno-senescence. It is clearly a definite phenomenon, but in my opinion, at least with respect to cancer, it will be somewhat limited when one thinks of it with respect to a lack of immune surveillance. There are some examples of where it might be important, such as some of the immunologic, malignancies. However, as a rule, I personally don't think that it will be a general mechanism. But one can think of ways - and we heard a bit about that from Bill Ershler - *vis à vis* so called immuno-enhancement. However, whether this or some other related physiological function provides the mechanism for immuno-senescence remains to be seen.

What, I think, can be said is that immuno-senescence is clearly an indication of a broader level of physiological dysfunction. And I think that's where we are going to find where some of the mechanistic inter-relationships occur, and I'll address that later.

THE INTERRELATIONSHIP BETWEEN CANCER AND AGING

I would like to turn to my own area of research, which is molecular genetics. And if I may qualify this further, it is primarily the genetics of cancer and senescence, and how they are inter-related. I would like to come back to Dr. Pereira-Smith's question of whether cellular senescence is related functionally to tumor suppression. And, echoing Dr. Cutler, I will say: Yes and No. I will give you some examples of this because, almost by definition, there has to be that kind of connection.

But first of all, let us start with what little we do know about the genetic basis of cancer. We know that there are oncogenes, but we do not know anything of the role they play in cancer. We have also heard a fair amount about tumor suppressor genes. The critical distinction with respect to function of these two classes of genes is that oncogenes are activated whereas there is loss of function of tumor suppressor genes. This is a very important concept to keep in mind. Many presentations (by Drs. J. Whang-Peng, Eric Fearon, and others) at this workshop discussed the multiple genetic alterations that occur in human malignancies, and that loss of genetic information is observed in many of these. I will use as an example a model of colorectal cancer (Figure 1), similar to the one that Eric presented, for the multiple step progression of a cell from a normal to a cancerous state. Let me emphasize that the high frequency of chromosome deletion is as important as the activation of oncogenes; e.g., 5q mutation or loss (APC gene) and 17p alterations, e.g. p53 loss or mutation, etc. However, there are a number of things to keep in mind. This is not a sequential order of events. There is a tendency to see these things

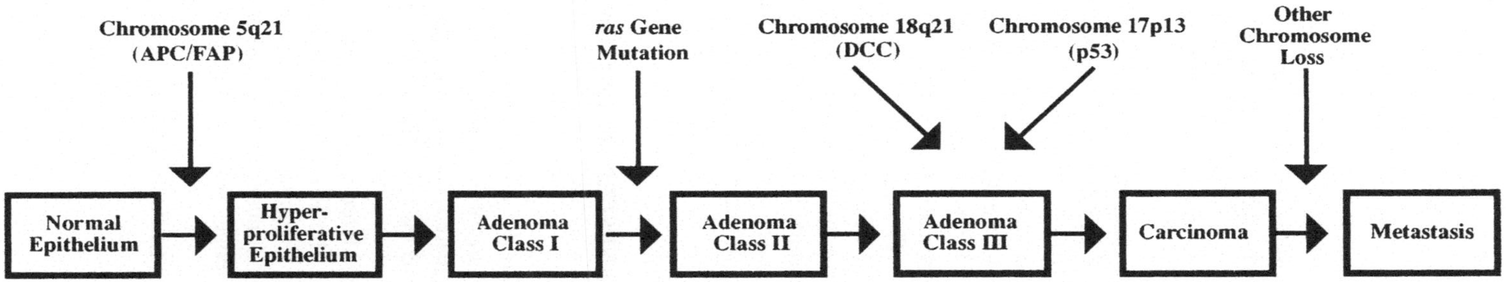
Chromosome 5q21
(APC/FAP)
ras Gene
Mutation
Chromosome 18q21
(DCC)
Chromosome 17p13
(p53)
Other
Chromosome
Loss
Normal
Epithelium
Hyper-
proliferative
Epithelium
Adenoma
Class I
Adenoma
Class II
Adenoma
Class III
Carcinoma
Metastasis

Figure 1.

in some sort of order, but there is no a priori reason for this to be. It is, rather, an accumulation of events.

The second thing to remember is the frequency with which one sees these sorts of phenomena. In sporadic colorectal cancer, one sees alterations in 5q in about 35 percent of cases. And if you listened to Jackie and others, you will find that this borders on the level of "significant gene alteration". It is important to keep in mind that there is a noise level of chromosome change. Further down the multi-step progression, you will see that about 50% of cases showed Ki-ras activation and that in the later stages of neoplastic progression, 70-80% showed 18q and 17p alterations.

Now, the way that this loss is measured is by RFLP (Restriction Fragment Length Polymorphism) analysis, using DNA probes mapping to the region of interest. It was, however, cytogenetic analysis that first convinced scientists of the changes in these regions of the chromosomes. Thus, they knew where to look for possible change and they did not just go blindly fishing. Leaving that aside, RFLP provides these percentages, which is impressive, because RFLP is an extremely crude measure of molecular alterations. And, unless one is fortunate enough that the alteration encompasses the RFLP site, you would not see it. Thus, RFLP analysis gives a minimal estimate of loss of genetic information. Clearly, what this also says is that not all colorectal cancers have all of these changes, and some may have none of them. This suggests that there are multiple, interconnecting or parallel independent pathways that go from the normal state to any particular (cancer) state. I think that it is very important to keep this in mind, because nothing is hard and fast, and these alterations do not appear to be 100 percent in most cases.

ESCAPE FROM CELLULAR SENESCENCE AND ONCOGENESIS: THE ROLE OF THE Rb GENE AND p53

Then we must ask what do these changes mean functionally with respect to aging. And I will ask, further, do any of these changes reflect an escape from cellular senescence? And, as I have indicated, the answer is both yes and no. I will give you two examples of that. Let us take the Rb gene and the p53 gene.

The Rb gene may be considered a cellular senescence gene. I think most of you are aware of the fact that the Rb protein has been implicated in cell cycle regulation, acting as a negative regulator. Let us introduce the Rb gene into retinoblastoma cells, which lack functional Rb, and ask what happens? Every retinoblastoma cell, to my knowledge, lacks the functional Rb protein. Following introduction of a wild-type Rb cDNA, the transformed cells express the Rb protein and are either stopped dead in their tracks - which is equivalent to cellular senescence-or proliferate extremely slowly.

On rare occasions the transfected cells continue to proliferate. These cells are found to have lost the transfected gene. Thus, the growth inhibitory effect is reversible and therefore presumably a dependent state of affairs, i.e., dependent on the expression of the Rb protein. Now, if one introduces the Rb gene into a prostate carcinoma cell line that is Rb negative, what we get is cells that are now Rb positive and nontumorigenic, but that continue to proliferate. Thus, here suppression of tumorigenicity need not necessarily involve senescence. And, a further caveat to this issue is the one that Eric gave us an example of; and now we are talking about the p53 gene. Accordingly, if one takes a colorectal carcinoma cell line that is p53-negative and again introduces into it the p53 gene, the cells undergo programmed cell death (apoptosis). The rare cell that grows out appears as though it has either now mutated the wild-type gene that was put in, or else the gene is no longer expressed. Thus, p53 has a very dramatic negative effect on the growth of these cells in culture; it is almost a return to senescence. If one takes an adenoma (which is wild-type for p53) and does the same experiment, there is no change. Even if one takes the adenoma from the same patient that has the colorectal cancer and does the same experiment, there is no change. So, there is something very strange going on here with respect to what p53 is doing. In this kind of scenario perhaps it has nothing to do with cellular senescence.

The final point to make is that Rb and p53 are expressed by virtually every tissue and every cell line in culture. To the best of my knowledge, and we have looked at a number of normal and tumor cell lines, in the human cell system, immortal, nontumorigenic cells tend to express wild-type Rb and p53 protein. So the escape from senescence in the experimental system appears not to involve these two genes. It is complicated, and I am sure in certain cell lineages p53 and Rb will be important, and how they play out in cell transformation and senescence in that regard remains to be seen. Arnie Levine made the comment that in rodent cell transformation, unlike human, one does see mutant p53 in immortalized cells. So there is a distinction, and an important distinction, between work with rodent cells and that with human cells.

So, this issue to my mind is one of the most important ones facing both cancer researchers and gerontologists and that is, if you like, the escape from cellular senescence. Cancer researchers are learning a great deal in one sense, as they are beginning to feel their way as to which genes may be playing a role in malignant progression. But all is not what it may seem to be. For example, activated cellular oncogenes: one can easily transform normal rodent cells with activated oncogenes, either singly or in combination. However, If you take normal human diploid fibroblasts that undergo normal cellular senescence and introduce one or more activated oncogenes via cDNA transfection the cells retain their normal phenotype. This suggests that there are intrinsically different mechanisms, I think, for the immortality of the human cell versus the rodent cell.

IMMORTALITY IN NATURE VERSUS IMMORTALIZATION *In Vitro*

What we do know is that there are less than a handful of what I would call *bona fide*, spontaneously immortalized human cell lines of either fibroblastic or epithelial origin. What we and others who have worked with these cells know is that if one takes these immortalized cell lines and adds activated oncogenes to them, one can get conversion to a malignant phenotype. And so that brings up the issue of genetic instability in an immortalized cell, i.e., genetically unstable, spontaneously immortalized ("normal") cell. This is a critical issue because when we talk abut progression, cancer researchers know nothing, in a sense, about this first step; and the only thing that reproducibly induces it experimentally, albeit at an extremely low frequency, are DNA tumor virus transforming genes. So to find out what is going on here is critical.

DOMINANCE OF CELLULAR SENESCENCE VERSUS DOMINANCE OF TUMOR SUPPRESSION

Somatic cell hybrids provided the initial experimental evidence for tumor suppression and indicated its dominance over the malignant phenotype. The dominance of cellular senescence has also been shown very nicely by such experiments. If you fuse a tumor cell with a normal cell you get a nontumorigenic hybrid cell. The cell is now immortal but not tumorigenic. Following prolonged culture genetic (chromosome) segregation occurs leading to reexpression of tumorigenicity. Where does one go from here? The answer to date has been to clone candidate tumor suppressor genes via positional cloning, assisted by RFLP "signposts". This approach was used by Fearon and colleagues to clone the DCC gene, which is considered a candidate colorectal carcinoma tumor suppressor gene, on chromosome 18q21. (DCC stands for Deleted in Colorectal Carcinoma.) But another thing, as you heard from Carl Barrett, that has been useful for both tumor suppression and cellular senescence is marked chromosome transfer. So rather than using a single gene, one can use a single chromosome. In this case one can transfer a neo-tagged chromosome #17 via microcell fusion into colon carcinoma cells that are mutant for p53, if one does not have a wt p53 cDNA, and ask what happens? What happens is that one gets cells that do not proliferate. But say that you also have neo-tagged chromosomes 5 and 18? Transfer of these chromosomes into the same cells does not result in altered growth in vitro but does cause tumor suppression in vivo.

With respect to cellular senescence genes, as Carl Barrett has indicated, there may be multiple chromosomes (genes) involved, since we know that there are four complementation groups. One can then regionalize this effect in obvious ways and eventually clone the gene or genes that convey this negative regulation of growth upon the cells. Then one can go back and ask "are these senescence genes involved in neoplastic progression?" If any thing brings the gerontologists and the cancer researchers together experimentally, in the short term, this is one of the areas where collaboration can occur in a very significant way.

THE MICRO ENVIRONMENT *In Vivo*

Even though we may learn which genes we should be investigating at the molecular level, biologically I think that one of the most neglected areas is the in vivo micro environment. (Although I was most pleased to hear people talking about it over the past few days.) The interaction between normal and malignant tissue, either assists or inhibits the growth of the tumor. And we have some very nice examples of that in breast and prostate cancer from a number of presentations here.

I want to come back to the point I just mentioned with regard to genetics. In the original experiments, a malignant cell was fused to a normal human cell to generate a hybrid cell that remains transformed in culture, since it has evaded cellular senescence, but is completely nontumorigenic. From this hybrid one can isolate rare tumorigenic segregants. I will give you an example. We fused HeLa cells to either fibroblasts or keratinocytes. In both cases nontumorigenic hybrids were generated. In the case of the HeLa/fibroblast hybrids, rare segregants arose in which there had been a loss of a very discrete amount of genetic information at the chromosome level. So these cells contain a great deal of genetic information of the normal parent, but are now tumorigenic. The HeLa/keratinocyte hybrids were also nontumorigenic, but formed very small, non-progressive nodules that histologically had the appearance of terminally differentiated keratinizing cysts. Tumorigenic segregants of these cells formed undifferentiated carcinomas, identical to HeLa tumors. In culture, both nontumorigenic and tumorigenic HeLA/fibroblast hybrids behave as transformed hybrid cells and appear almost identical. They both grow well in culture, are anchorage independent, and show the same growth factor dependence. It turns out that the cells that fail to form tumors are now induced to differentiate in vivo. In short, very interestingly, they take on the program of differentiation from the normal parent, i.e. forming mesenchymal tissue. So, while the HeLa/keratinocyte hybrids form keratinizing tissue in the host, the HeLa/fibroblast hybrids form mesenchymal tissue. Tumorigenic segregants form undifferentiated carcinomas. What that says is that the event of signalling which does not occur in tissue culture, occurs in a very dramatic way in the micro environment of the host. One may need that in vivo interaction in order for gene switching to occur. That is something that has been lost in the shuffle, particularly among molecular geneticists. It would seem then that one would have a requirement for this tumor-host interaction, both for tumor growth, because of enhancement, and also for inhibition. I would not mind betting that once we know a little more about the signals of this in vivo micro environment that we will find the differences between the young and the aged.

I draw you back to the "histological" cancer that we heard of yesterday, which made me think of the microscopic foci that you can see at autopsy. They also show features of malignant cells but they are not proceeding toward a full-blown malignant tumor. They can be held in abeyance in some way by the type of signalling that I'm talking about. If that signalling is relaxed in some way, I think that it does not take much to get a cell going. We have evidence from experiments with immortalized human keratinocytes where we have introduced an activated oncogene, that we get a series of clones, some of which are completely nontumorigenic, others of which form benign papillomas, and yet others that form invasive squamous cell carcinomas. All of them express the activated oncogene. And, what this suggests to us is that expression allows some limited proliferative advantage in vivo so that the cells can undergo some limited number of doublings that allows for further genetic alterations to occur. If the genetic changes don't occur, the cells remain controlled by the micro environment to some degree or other. Now it may be the same in real life. It is quite possible that a slight relaxation of the in vivo micro environmental signals may allow these "preneoplastic cells" enough of a chance for limited cell cycling, allowing for important genetic changes that eventually lead to the malignant condition. In this discussion I have used the term malignant synonymously with tumorigenic. Yet, we have hardly touched on malignancy. People have begun to look at this a little bit, but there has been very little done on the molecular genetics of malignancy. So without going into that in any more detail, I believe at least in these two areas there is room for very fruitful collaboration in a meaningful way between the gerontologists and the cancer researchers. All is left is to thank Sue Yang for putting together a stimulating workshop.

SUMMATION AND SYNTHESIS:

FROM THE IMMUNOLOGY POINT OF VIEW[1]

Gloria H. Heppner

Michigan Cancer Foundation
Detroit, Michigan 48201

The Rate-Limiting Change That Leads to Cancer Development

As Eric has said from the cancer point of view, cancer is a series of genetic changes, which from my, the immunology, point of view, only become meaningful under particular environmental conditions, and that is the environment of the host. I would certainly agree that the order in which the molecular genetic events appear to occur is probably a part of that. But, I do not know if the order is not an important part of that. I think that they can occur in any order, but what cannot be overlooked is that the recognized changes are found in *lesions*. The reasons that molecular genetic studies can be done is because the lesions are there; so that even though the order in which the particular molecular events occurred is somewhat irrelevant in the overall process, it may be highly relevant from the clinical point of view. In a sense this is a hierarchy of events that we are witnessing. And the reason that you have a lesion at any particular time is that *some* event has occurred. So, I think that it is important to do the map and try to see if there is a sequence of events that is being imposed on the whole process because I think, in fact, that might tell us something about what the *rate-limiting* processes are from the clinical point of view. Changes can occur in any order, but when you have a lesion, that is simple. And if those changes actually manifest themselves at some point along the line, then a clinically detectable entity can be teased out from among the others. They are then the rate-limiting changes.

[1] This is a direct transcript of Dr. Gloria Heppner's wrap-up presentation in the Summation and Synthesis Session.

They are the ones that will really matter from the point of view of ultimate prevention. I think this is important, practically.

Cancer as a "Cellular Society" or a Tissue

Now this kind of scheme[2] does not begin to show the "richness" of what is really going on here. When one looks at a scheme like this, you think that "there is a cell and there is a change". And then, there is another cell and another change, and so on. But that is **not** at all what is really going on here. What's really happening is that each of these stages are in fact tissues and they consist of multiple cells: that is, multiple abnormal cells, multiple cancer cells, as well as multiple host cells. This whole process is a process of cellular changes. Ken DeOme used to say there is no such thing as **a** cancer cell. It makes no sense to talk about a cancer cell. There are cancers. There are pre-neoplastic lesions. But there are no cancer cells. Cancer cells, *per se*, do not exist. What you are really dealing with when you go through this series of events is **population biology**, the unit of which happens to be cellular. What gives flavor to the whole process, the richness of the whole process, is the **interaction** among these different cells. When you get to the end here, at what we call cancer, the process has not stopped. Even when one has a fully malignant cell type, new cell populations continue to emerge and grow out a whole new cancer. You wind up with a very heterogenous population. It does not matter if you are looking for oncogenic changes, suppressor changes, or drug resistant changes. As cancer cells metastasize, in fact, you are dealing with a population of cells, some of which can and some of which cannot. Now these cells, by themselves, do not exist in a vacuum. There are tremendous interactions among the different cells that make up a cancer. So just as you can fuse together a normal and a malignant cell and wind up with a hybrid cell that behaves differently than the partners, in fact, you can put individual cells together and they will behave differently without having to fuse them at all. So, in a sense, a *cancer is a tissue*; it is a *cellular society*. Learning how to manipulate these societies and learning what the significance of the particular genetic changes are in these societies requires seeing both sides of the picture, and requires analyzing genetic changes within the context of the environment.

Genetic and the Environment

It seems to me that, from the point of view of trying to develop a program of cancer and aging, that the place to look for fruitful collaboration is in the environment because, in fact cancer and aging appear to be occurring during the same period. So what are the kinds of things that the environment can be doing? Knowing how

---

[2]This refers to the scheme presented by Dr. Eric Stanbridge in the Summation and Synthesis Section.

the environment in the host influences cancer development might give us a clue as to which direction we should approach. We have heard at this conference that there are at least three levels of regulation or control of the environment altering tumorigenic phenotypes.

First of all, the environment can actually influence and cause genetic change. We have heard from Dr. Cutler about oxy-radicals and the mutagenic activities of oxy-radicals and the possibility that they are involved in aging. There is a whole group of carcinogenesis investigators who are studying the role of oxy-radicals in the initiation and the early promotion phases. And some of us have looked at the role of oxy-radicals in later phases. Oxy-radicals come from outside the cancer cells. The inflammatory cells often have them. The dietary source is also a place to look. So, one area, it seems to me, that would encourage fruitful interaction between aging researchers and cancer biologists is in this whole area of oxy-radical and oxygen metabolism in the process of tumor tissue development. Other areas in which the environment can influence, at least, the gene expression is post transformation. Again, there is a dietary side of that.

Growth Factors, Cell-Cell Interaction and Other Three-Dimensional Structuralization

The second area in which the host influences the manifestation of this "tissue" is in the area of regulation. Now you have heard about regulation at the growth factor level and at the hormone level. But we have not heard much here about the effect of the extracellular matrix on the regulation of gene expression. This is a very hot area of research and investigators, like Mina Bissel, have shown that you can actually turn on and off genes depending on the kind of extracellular matrix that the cells are in.

Other types of cells that are found in a tumor are the inflammatory immune cells and the stromal cells. And, another important thing is the three-dimensional structure of the epithelium. What are the tumor cells adjacent to? Where is the lesion physically housing the cancer cells located? How are they related structurally to the blood supply? What does the three-dimension architecture of the tumor do to the shape of the tumor cells? It turns out the cell shape is very important in gene expression. So again, it is not what is happening between cells, it is the circumstances in which they find themselves and how that changes that impacts the development as they mature into a cancer.

Changes in Host Micro Environment and Its Impact on Cancer Development

Then, to me, there is a third area in which the environment - the host - can be said to regulate the expression, manifestation of the cancer phenotype. That is the area of selection the host provides. Because there is a series of genetic events and because we have heterogenous cell types, ample opportunity for particular cell populations to emerge, similar to an evolution, or progression, i.e. a shift in the population over the course of tumor development. The host's place obviously is to act to select against tumor variant cells.

I would like to say something about selection. Variant phenotypes are never selected for. Something is *selected against*. The agents of selection work to remove cell populations. It may be that, in fact, one cell population can live under circumstances which another one cannot. It may be that one cell population requires a different level of nutrition, or whatever, than another cell population. That cell population is therefore selected against. If everything is equal and there are enough resources, food, etc. for everybody, nobody is selected against. In fact, I have carried out experiments in which you mix cell populations together and one will double in culture twice as fast as the other one; but, if both populations have what they need, there is no selection. Only when the environment changes and things become limited in the environment, can you see selection. So, again, this is the environment within the host.

Now, this whole process of tumorigenicity, development of cancer, malignancy is played out against the back-drop of constant changes in aging. To try to bring these two things together, it seems to me, a fruitful place to start looking is at what happens during aging at the cellular level. We have heard about two types of changes that go on with aging. One is the quantitative one and that we all know about. Basically, with aging, all sorts of biological functions gradually deteriorate. We are going to find that in every system. Now, it seems to me that where this type of aging can have a profound catastrophic effect is in drug metabolism. It is certainly an area that we should investigate.

From the point of view of tumorigenicity, development and expression, the probability that *heterogeneity* may play a role has to be considered. Because one thing that is true about this process is that it is not only very variable from patient to patient, but is also variable within an individual tumor. It is a subtle process. This is not something that happens all the time, in the same way in everybody. So the kinds of changes that one has to look for over time, during aging, are not these catastrophic events of old age, but, in fact, changes that are much more subtle.

One of the things that I became interested in was the subtle qualitative changes that were mentioned in a number of presentations here. Dr. Thompson talked about a shift in hormone production and how that might regulate the time course of ovarian cancer manifestation. I thought that was a very interesting case. It was not that endocrine production was undergoing dramatic reduction, it was that it shifted and when it shifted it changed the kind of cancer one might see.

Another example was that of Dr. Thoman who looked at shifts in T-cells during aging. And what she found was that in aging mice, the predominant T-cells shifted from those that could produce IL-2 to those that could produce IL-4. It is not that all the T-cells decreased, it is that the type of T-cells and, particularly what kind of cytokines and growth factors they were capable of producing, changed. Again, one can imagine how that could very much influence the manifestation of the particular kind of cancer. If, in fact, you had a cancer that was IL-4 dependent, now it might become manifested where it would not have before. So it is not immunosuppression, it is an ***immunochange*** that will make the difference. It seems to me that if we want to find out where aging can impact on this kind of process, we are going to have to look, not at the catastrophic events, but at the **details**. That's where the "richness" is and, I think, that's where the money is. It is also where we know the least. It is easy to **say** that is where we have to look. Because it is precisely those kinds of subtle changes in physiology that occur during aging that we do not know much about.

Immunity in Aging and Cancer: Immunosenescence, Immunodeficiency and Immune Surveillance

That gets me to the discussion on the role of immunity in aging and in cancer. I also have never heard the term *immunosenescence* before and I also must say that it probably should not be heard again. I think that is a loaded word. Senescence suggests that there is a real loss of function. We do not go into immunosenescence. We may undergo change. We may not be as good as we once were, in some ways. But, in fact, senescence is not what we are looking at, and to imply that is what we are doing is to really load the deck. It makes that phenomenon seem more important than all the common sense and observation put together would tell us it can possibly be.

What do you mean when you say immunodeficient? If you measure the number of circulating T-cells or the ability to respond to mitogen, whatever, what does that really tell you? What is real deficiency? What is the "norm"? Does it really matter if one has half the number of T-cells? What does this mean in terms of function? I grew up in cancer immunology during the days when research support was abundant for immunology, measuring all immunological cells: T-cell subsets and T-cell functions, measuring T- to B- cells ratios: circulating lymphocytes in massive number of patients, on a day-by-day basis. All these efforts told very little about how patients respond in certain circumstances. It was just really a lot of hot air. So I, myself, I must say, would always advise very strongly against launching those kind of massive studies, massive epidemiological studies where you periodically measure a number of people in regard to their "immune profile".

That also brings us to the theory of surveillance. This is an old theory that is being revisited, and what is interesting to me is that there is not a thread of evidence to support the idea of immune surveillance. There is a great deal written on it. But let's not go around that again in the context of cancer and aging.

To begin with, immune surveillance suggests that there is such thing as cancer antigen. So what would be the target of the immune surveillance? Many proposals have been presented with models of immunized mice and repressed mice, etc. etc. giving one the idea that immunization can keep cancer from occurring. But there is the other idea that Bill Ershler brought up which dates back to 1967, and that is the idea that the *immune response somehow can stimulate the growth of the tumor.* This idea has lots of merit.

The Contribution of Immunology to the Understanding of Cancer and Aging

Before it was recognized that lymphocytes had anything to do with immunity, these cells were known as trevocytes. Many papers and books were written on these cells, the trevocytes, that ran around the body and delivered nutrition and so forth to organs and helped the organs grow and achieve homeostasis. Nobody knew that they were lymphocytes. I think we need to get back to this trevocyte, because it is not the role of *immunity*, it is the lymphocyte's role in growth factor production that makes lymphocytes important.

To me the most exciting thing about immunology right now is the recognition that the immune system, the neurological system, the endocrine systems are talking to each other by using a common language. The more people are involved in cloning, sequencing, and understanding what lymphokines, cytokines, peptide hormones, and neural peptides are, the more we are convinced that many of them turn out to be the same thing. This is an area where research should concentrate. I have an example in a mammary gland model, where a pre-neoplastic lesion progresses to a tumor, and NK cells aid in that progression, apparently by making prolactin. These are research areas, obviously, that are going to occupy us for a long period of time. But these are the kind of research areas again, where you are going to find subtlety; you are going to find differences that matter in the approach. And insofar as one is looking for the role of "immune system" in this, I would submit that rather than worrying about whether it stimulates, whether it inhibits, or whatever, you have to worry about what is it that the cells are making and how are they physically interacting with tumor cells. I would submit that this is the area of research where aging and cancer researchers really should get together and make some useful inquiries because these are the systems that control the switches.

SUMMATION AND SYNTHESIS:

FROM THE AGING POINT OF VIEW[1]

George H. Martin

Department of Pathology
School of Medicine
University of Washington
Seattle, Washington 98195

INTRODUCTION

I am pleased to represent the gerontological community in making these summary remarks. Given the enormous scope of this meeting, however, I can cover only a few topics. We can regard this general, introductory conference as a precursor to a series of more focused workshops on cancer and aging. The National Cancer Institute and the National Institute on Aging have much to learn from each other. I congratulate Drs. Huber Warner and Stringner Sue Yang for bringing their perspective constituencies together.

In planning any future workshops on the subject, it is important to keep in mind that we have been dealing with two distinct issues. The first issue, to which we have been devoting most of our time, has to do with basic mechanisms of aging and how these might set the stage for carcinogenesis. The second issue is to immediate practical interest to practicing oncologists and geriatricians, who are concerned with the special vulnerabilities of their cancer patients to chemotherapeutic agents, other pharmaceuticals, and complicating infectious and non-infectious illnesses that may complicate management. Older subjects with

---

[1] This is a direct transcript of Dr. George Martin's wrap-up presentation in the Summation and Synthesis Session.

cancer also may have special psychosocial and financial difficulties, subjects that are certainly worthy of research. Let us consider a few points under each of these headings.

BASIC MECHANISMS OF AGING AS THEY RELATE TO CARCINOGENESIS

What is Aging?

Botanists sharply differentiate between the terms aging and senescence. The former is used to refer to all changes in structure and function from the birth of an organism until its death. They reserve the term senescence for those alterations in structure and function that immediately precede tissue, organ and organismal death. Mammalian gerontologists, however, typically use these two terms interchangeably. While they are aware that development can have major effects on the subsequent patterns of senescence, they generally consider, as aging, only those changes in structure and function that unfold after the organism achieves it adult phenotype, including maturation. While many of these alterations are appropriate compensations for declines in the efficiency of physiological homeostasis, the overall picture is one of increasing vulnerability to the forces of mortality. At the population level, one eventually observes an exponential increase in age-specific death rate, generally considered to the hallmark of intrinsic biological aging. This is the famous Gompertz relationship. It must be emphasized, however, that such kinetics, which were derived from the study of populations of organisms, cannot be applied as a litmus test for what is aging at a molecular, cellular, tissue, organ and organismal levels. it is equally illogical to demand that, even given a phase of exponential kinetics, one must insist that such kinetics continue throughout the life span of the individual in order to be considered a manifestation of aging. Thus some tumor biologists have concluded that cancer cannot be related to intrinsic biological aging because the age-specific (80 years and older) incidence with certain cancers (e.g. nasal cavity, lung and bronchus, corpus uteri, kidney and renal pelvis, brain and nervous system[2]) is observed to decline during the latter decades of the life span. Tissues and organs do not all age synchronously, however, Consider the examples of the human female breast and ovary. Major involutional changes have already occurred in these organs by the time of menopause.

Why Do We Age?

Evolutionary biologists believe that there is straightforward answer to the question of ***why*** we age, as opposed to the question of ***how*** we age. In all age-

---

[2] Ries, L.A.G., Hankey, B.F. and Edwards, B.K. Cancer Statistics Review, 1973-1988. NIH Publication No. 90-2789. U.S. DHHS, National Cancer Institute, Bethesda, MD (1991).

structured populations, such as mammals, there is a decline in the force of natural selection in older members of the population. Thus, any gene action that might have deleterious effects in older animals cannot be readily selected against. In short, nature does not care about aging. She is only concerned with gene action that involves reproductive fitness at the level of the individual organism. There is very little evidence in support of adaptive theories of aging such as group selection.

There are two major nonadaptive evolutionary theories of aging. One theory invokes the accumulation of constitutional mutations that have neutral effects on reproductive fitness but that have deleterious expressions in postreproductive individuals. This could include a variety of gene actions which never reach any significant phenotypic threshold for expression until relatively late in the life course, when selection is ineffective. Perhaps more interestingly is the idea of antagonistic pleiotropy (also known as negative pleiotropy). Certain alleles at a variety of genetic loci, selected because of their enhancement of reproductive fitness, might, paradoxically, have deleterious effects postreproductively. An example cited by George C. Williams involved alleles which enhanced incorporation of calcium into bone. Over time, such gene action could have the undesirable effect of increasing the incorporation of calcium into arterial walls, thus contributing to a form of calcific arteriosclerosis. Are there such examples that might relates to the coupling of aging and cancer? Let me give you a speculative example relevant to our consideration below of the question of the loss of proliferative homeostasis in aging organisms. It involves the famous Hayflick model of cellular aging, the gradual decline of replicative potential of many different cell type. I prefer to use the term "clonal attenuation" to refer to this phenomenon, since I believe that this mechanism of regulating the proliferative behavior of populations of cells is a reflection of cell physiology rather than of cell injury, and that the mechanism was selected in order to more finely regulate growth and differentiation during organogenesis. Some of my colleagues believe that the mechanisms was selected in order to decrease the probability of neoplastic growth. If either of these speculations is correct, according the evolutionary definition of aging, clonal attenuation is not aging. There may, however, be very important ***consequences*** of clonal attenuation for the biology and pathobiology of aging. One can imagine that the price one may pay for this mechanism includes multifocal atrophies and hyperplasias. I would propose that the latter may develop because of asynchronous clonal attenuations among families of cells that regulate each other's proliferative states. Such multifocal hyperplasias could, of course, set the stage for subsequent steps in tumor progression.

ABERRATIONS IN PROLIFERATIVE HOMEOSTASIS IN MAMMALIAN AGING

A striking feature of the senescent phenotype of all mammalian species if the deregulation of proliferative homeostasis. Table 1 summarizes a number of such examples. It is often the case that inappropriate proliferations occur side-by-side with atrophic changes. This is the case in a variety of skin cancers of older human subjects, for example. Returning to our example of menopause, it is also the case that in the ovary, where, in the face of almost complete loss of primary ovarian follicles, one sees hyperplasia of stromal cells. The same basic theme of atrophy with hyperplasia plays out in such major age-related disorders as atherosclerosis and osteoarthritis (or better, osteoarthrosis). We see it in such diverse situations as brown atrophy of the pancreas (which is often associated with increases in

Table 1. Examples of Multifocal Hyperplasias Which Accompany in Humans and Other Mammals[3]

Cell Type Which Proliferates	Associated Age-Related Disorder
Adipocyte	regional obesity
Arterial myointimal cell	atherosclerosis
Cartilage osteocyte and synovial cells	osteoarthrosis (osteoarthritis)
Central nervous system astrocyte	gliosis
Epidermal basal cell	verruca senilis (seborrheic keratosis) (basal cell papilloma)
Epidermal melanocyte	senile lentigo ("liver spots")
Epidermal squamous cell	senile keratosis
Fibroblast	interstitial fibrosis (multiple tissues; e.g. thyroid)
Fibromuscular stromal cell and glandular epithelium of prostate	nodular hyperplasia (benign prostatic hypertrophy)
Lymphocyte	ectopic lymphoid tissue
Lymphocyte (suppressor T cell)	immunologic deficiency
Oral mucosal squamous cell	leukoplakia
Ovarian cortical stromal cell	cortical stromal hyperplasia
Endometrial glandular epithelium	postmenopausal hyperplasia
Pancreatic ductal epithelial cell	ductal epithelial hyperplasia and metaplasia
Sebaceous glandular epithelium	senile sebaceous hyperplasia (skin) Sordyce disease (oral mucosa)

[3]Adapted from Martin, G. M. *Ann. N.Y. Acad. Sci.* 621:401-417 (1991).

adipocytes ("fatty infiltration"), follicular atrophy of the thyroid (which is associated with interstitial fibrosis), and in the "senile" endometrium (which is often associated with hyperplasia).

Table 2. A Sample of Mutations in Man That Have the Potential to Elucidate Mechanisms Underlying the Loss of Proliferative Homeostasis in Somatic Tissues.

- Neurofibromatosis
- Tuberous Sclerosis
- Familial Polyposis of Colon
- Familial Breast Cancer
- Multiple Endocrine Neoplasms
- Chromosomal Instability Syndromes
    - Ataxia Telangiectasia
    - Werner's Syndrome
    - Fanconi's Anemia
    - Bloom's Syndrome
- Psoriasis
- Beckwith-Weidemann Syndrome
- Cervical Lipomatosis
- Familial Pancreatic Carcinoma
- Various Trisomies and Partial Trisomies
- Monosomies and Partial Monosomies

THE GENETIC APPROACH TO THE INVESTIGATION OF AGE-RELATED ABERRATIONS IN PROLIFERATIVE HOMEOSTASIS

As with so many other biomedical problems, an analysis of gene action in mutant individuals should help elucidate mechanisms of altered proliferative homeostasis in development, cancer and aging. A partial list of such constitutional mutations of man is given in Table 2.

ENVIRONMENTAL CARCINOGENS AND 'GERONTOGENS'

Mutagens, Clastogens and Aneugens: Are They "Gerontogenic" As Well As Carcinogenic?

The role of various types of somatic mutations in the pathogenesis of neoplasia is well established, although there are certainly grounds for also invoking an important role for epigenetic alterations. The role of somatic mutations in the genesis of various aspects of the senescent phenotype is more controversial. This is clearly an area deserving of more research and provides a logical bridge between the two disciplines. Given the popularity of the free radical theory of aging, we can expect to learn a great deal about the precise types of lesions in DNA that may result from active oxygen species. While the free radical theory postulates an intrinsic origin for the damaging radicals, as a byproduct of normal metabolism, we must consider the possibility that there are important positive and negative environmental modulations of these processes, including nutritional variables.

THE GERIATRIC CANCER PATIENT

Let us now turn to the second major issue of this conference, the special vulnerability of the geriatric cancer patient. Bob Capizzi and Charles Schiffer gave us an excellent example of the kind of research needed in this field. The high dose protocol of ARA-C for the treatment of hematological malignancy may cause central nervous system damage. While this analog acts primarily to inhibit DNA synthesis, there is evidence that it can also inhibit transcription in differentiated neural cells. There is very good evidence that, as normal human subjects age, they exhibit ***selective, regional*** neuronal loss. For example, there is about a 30% loss of Purkinje's cells over the life span of human subjects who have been free of such disorders as hypertensive cardiovascular disease and diabetes. There is also a roughly linear rate of loss of dopaminergic cells within the substantia nigra. While one could have to lose about 80% of such cells before reaching a phenotypic threshold of Parkinson's disease, it is apparent that certain classes of cytotoxic drugs could accelerate the process.

The extent to which the various measures of immunological decline in aging human subjects have functional significance is controversial. Apart from the problem of immunosenescence, however, virtually all systems are relatively more vulnerable to injury, so that, in considering the special vulnerability of the elderly cancer patient to intercurrent infections, one has to be aware of the more dangerous course of the influenza virus, for example, in subjects with impaired pulmonary function.

A striking feature of physiological decline in aging human subjects is the variability, from system to system, and from patient to patient, when one carries out longitudinal studies among groups of age-matched individuals. Thus, the clinician will have to assess the special strengths and weaknesses of any given patient when contemplating a course of management.

The goal of this initial workshop will have been achieved if by the presentations and interactions here, clinicians, oncologists, and gerontologists are brought to the awareness of the state-of-the-art in cancer and aging and of the need for rational designs for diagnosis and treatment of geriatric cancer patients in reducing cancer mortality among the underserved elderly (over 65) population.

PARTICIPANTS AND CONTRIBUTORS

Anderson, Elizabeth P., Ph.D.
Organ Systems Coordinating Branch
Centers, Training and Resources Program
Division of Cancer Biology
and Diagnosis
National Cancer Institute
Bethesda, MD 20892

Barrett, Carl J., Ph.D.*§
National Institute
of Environmental Health Sciences
P.O. Box 12233
Research Triangle Park, NC 27709

Campisi, Judith, Ph.D.
Department of Biochemistry
Boston University School of Medicine
Boston, MA 02215

Capizzi, Robert L., M.D. *§
Comprehensive Cancer Center of
Wake Forest University
Bowman Gray School of Medicine
Department of Medicine
Winston-Salem, NC 27292

Chiarodo, Andrew, Ph.D.
Organ Systems Coordinating Branch
Centers, Training and Resources Program
Division of Cancer Biology
and Diagnosis
National Cancer Institute
Bethesda, MD 20892

Cowan, Kenneth H., M.D. *§
Medicine Branch
Division of Cancer Treatment
National Cancer Institute
Bethesda, Maryland 20892

Cutler, Richard, Ph.D.*
Research Chemist
Gerontology Research Center
National Institute on Ageing
Baltimore, MD 21224

Dickson, Robert B., Ph.D. *§
Vincent T. Lombardi Cancer Center
Georgetown University Hospital
3900 Reservoir Road N.W.
Washington, D.C. 20007

Djakiew, Daniel, Ph.D.*§
Department of Anatomy and Cell Biology
Georgetown University Medical School
3900 Reservoir Rd. N.W.
Washington D.C. 20007

Emerson, Julia C., Ph.D. *§
Arizona Cancer Center
University of Arizona
Tucson, Arizona 85724

Ershler, William B., M.D.*§
Department of Medicine
University of Wisconsin
Madison, Wisconsin 53706

Fearon, Eric R., M.D., Ph.D.*
Oncology Research Laboratories
Johns Hopkins University
Baltimore, MD 21218

Freeman, Colette, Ph.D.
Cancer Biology Branch
Extramural Research Program
Division of Cancer Biology and Diagnosis
National Cancer Institute
Bethesda, MD 20892

Glenn, Gladys M., M.D., Ph.D.
Cancer Diagnosis Branch
Extramural Research Program
Division of Cancer Biology
and Diagnosis
National Cancer Institute
Bethesda, MD 20892

Gorelic, Lester S., Ph.D.
Cancer Prevention Branch
Division of Cancer Prevention
and Control
National Cancer Institute
Bethesda, MD 20892

Harris, Randall E., M.D., Ph.D.
Department of Preventive Medicine
Ohio State University
Columbus, OH 43210–1240

Heppner, Gloria H., Ph.D.*§
Michigan Cancer Foundation
Detroit, MI 48201

Isaacs, John T., Ph.D.*§
Johns Hopkins Oncology Center and
the Department of Urology
The Johns Hopkins School of Medicine
Baltimore, Maryland 21231

Jazwinski, S. Michal, Ph.D.*§
Department of Biochemistry and
Molecular Biology
Louisiana State University
Medical Center
New Orleans, LA 70112

Kimes, Brian W., Ph.D.*
Centers, Training and Resources
Program
Division of Cancer Biology
and Diagnosis
National Cancer Institute
Bethesda, MD 20892

Lane, Mary–Ann
Michigan Cancer Foundation
Detroit, MI 48201

Lavrin, David, Ph.D.
Immunology Program
National Institute on Ageing
Bethesda, MD 20892

Levine, Arnold J., Ph.D.*§
Department of Molecular Biology
Princeton University
Princeton, NJ 08544–1014

Longfellow, David D., Ph.D.
Chemical and Physical Carcinogenesis
Branch
Division of Cancer Etiology
National Cancer Institute
Bethesda, MD 20892

Mandelblatt, Jeanne S., M.D.*§
Memorial Sloan–Kettering
Cancer Center
Division of Cancer Control
New York, New York 10021

Martin, George M., M.D., Ph.D.*§
University of Washington
Department of Pathology
Seattle, Washington 98195

Martin, Mary Beth, Ph.D.*§
Lombardi Cancer Research Center
Georgetown University
Washington, DC 20007

McCormick, Anna, Ph.D.
Molecular and Cellular Biology
Branch
National Institute on Ageing
Bethesda, MD 20892

McIntyre, O. Ross, M.D.§
Norris Cotton Cancer Center
2 Maynard Street
Hanover, NH 03756

McKeehan, Wallace L., Ph.D.*§
W. Alton Jones Cell Science
Center, Inc.
10 Old Barn Road
Lake Placid, NY 12946

Nakamura, Masahiro, Ph.D.
Gerontology Research Center
National Institute on Ageing
Baltimore, MD 21224

Pereira–Smith, Olivia M., Ph.D.*
Division of Molecular Virology
Baylor College of Medicine
Baylor Plaza
Houston, TX 77030

Pipas, James M., Ph.D.*§
Department of Biological Sciences
University of Pittsburgh
Pittsburgh, PA 15260

Pollard, Morris, Ph.D.
Lobund Laboratory
University of Notre Dame
Notre Dame, IN 46556

Rabson, Alan S., M.D.
Division of Cancer Biology
and Diagnosis
National Cancer Institute
Bethesda, MD 20892

Satariano, William A., Ph.D.*§
School of Public Health
University of California at Berkeley
Berkeley, CA 94720

Schiffer, Charles A., M.D.*§
Division of Hematologic
Malignancies
University of Maryland
Cancer Center
School of Medicine
Baltimore, MD 21201

Slater, Stanley L., Ph.D.
Geriatric Research and Training Branch
National Institute on Ageing
Baltimore, MD 21224

Smith, Helene S., Ph.D.
Geraldine Brush Cancer Research Institute
San Francisco, CA 94115

Smith, James R., Ph.D.
Division of Molecular Virology
Baylor College of Medicine
Baylor Plaza
Houston, TX 77030

Sogn, John A., Ph.D.
Cancer Immunology Branch
Extramural Research Program
Division of Cancer Biology and
Diagnosis
National Cancer Institute
Bethesda, MD 20892

Stanbridge, Eric J., Ph.D.*§
Department of Microbiology and
Molecular Genetics
University of California, Irvine
Irvine, CA 92717

Straile, William, Ph.D.
Organ Systems Coordinating Branch
Centers, Training and Resources
Program
Division of Cancer Biology
and Diagnosis
National Cancer Institute
Bethesda, MD 20892

Thoman, Marilyn L., Ph.D.*§
Department of Immunology
Research Institute of Scripps Clinic
La Jolla, CA 92037

Thompson, E. Brad, M.D.*§
Department of Human Biological
Chemistry and Genetics
University of Texas
Medical Branch
Galveston, Texas 77550

Thompson, Margaret A., Ph.D.*§
Department of Obstetrics and
Gynecology
S.U.N.Y. Health Science Center
Syracuse, NY 13210

Trent, Jeffrey M., M.D.§
University of Michigan
Cancer Center
Ann Arbor, Michigan 48109

Warner, Huber R., Ph.D.§
Molecular and Cellular Biology
Branch
National Institute on Ageing
Bethesda, MD 20892

Whang-Peng, Jacqueline, M.D.*§
Cytogenetic Oncology Section
Medicine Branch
Division of Cancer Treatment
National Cancer Institute
Bethesda, MD 20892

Williams, T. Franklin, M.D.*
National Institute on Aging
Bethesda, MD 20892

Yamagami, Keiji, Ph.D.
Gerontology Research Center
National Institute on Ageing
Baltimore, MD 21224

Yang, Stringner Sue, Ph.D.§
Centers, Training and Resources
Program
Division of Cancer Biology
and Diagnosis
National Cancer Institute
Bethesda, MD 20892

*Speaker
§Contributor to the book

INDEX

The manufacturer's authorised representative in the EU is Springer
Nature Customer Service Centre GmbH, Europaplatz 3, 69115 Heidelberg,
Germany. If you have any concerns regarding our products, please
contact ProductSafety@springernature.com

Printed and bound by CPI Group (UK) Ltd, Croydon, CR0 4YY
12/08/2026
02194533-0001